T0213803

Lecture Notes in Computer Science   9352

Commenced Publication in 1973
Founding and Former Series Editors:
Gerhard Goos, Juris Hartmanis, and Jan van Leeuwen

Editorial Board

More information about this series at http://www.springer.com/series/7412

Luping Zhou · Li Wang
Qian Wang · Yinghuan Shi (Eds.)

Machine Learning in Medical Imaging

6th International Workshop, MLMI 2015
Held in Conjunction with MICCAI 2015
Munich, Germany, October 5, 2015
Proceedings

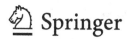

Editors
Luping Zhou
University of Wollongong
Wollongong, NSW
Australia

Qian Wang
Shanghai Jiaotong University
Shanghai
China

Li Wang
Radiology and BRIC
University of North Carolina
Chapel Hill, NC
USA

Yinghuan Shi
Department of Computer Science
Nanjing University
Nanjing
China

ISSN 0302-9743   ISSN 1611-3349   (electronic)
Lecture Notes in Computer Science
ISBN 978-3-319-24887-5   ISBN 978-3-319-24888-2   (eBook)
DOI 10.1007/978-3-319-24888-2

Library of Congress Control Number: 2015950024

LNCS Sublibrary: SL6 – Image Processing, Computer Vision, Pattern Recognition, and Graphics

Springer Cham Heidelberg New York Dordrecht London

Printed on acid-free paper

Springer International Publishing AG Switzerland is part of Springer Science+Business Media
(www.springer.com)

Preface

The 6th International Workshop on Machine Learning in Medical Imaging (MLMI 2015) was held in the Holiday Inn Hotel, Munich City Centre, and the Klinikum rechts der Isar, University Hospital of Technische Universität München at Max-Weber-Platz, Munich, Germany, on October 5, 2015, in conjunction with the 18th International Conference on Medical Image Computing and Computer Assisted Intervention (MICCAI).

Machine learning plays an essential role in the medical imaging field, including computer-assisted diagnosis, image segmentation, image registration, image fusion, image-guided therapy, image annotation, and image database retrieval. With advances in medical imaging, new imaging modalities and methodologies are developed, such as cone-beam computed tomography, tomosynthesis, electrical impedance tomography, and new machine learning algorithms/applications. Owing to large inter-subject variations and complexities, it is generally difficult to derive analytic formulations or simple equations to represent objects such as lesions and anatomy in medical images. Therefore, tasks in medical imaging require learning from patient data for heuristics and from prior knowledge, in order to facilitate the detection/diagnosis of abnormalities in medical images.

The main aim of the MLMI 2015 workshop was to help advance scientific research within the broad field of machine learning in medical imaging. This workshop focuses on major trends and challenges in this area, and presents works aimed at identifying new cutting-edge techniques and their use in medical imaging. We hope that the MLMI workshop becomes an important platform for translating research from the bench to the bedside.

The range and level of submissions for this year's meeting were of very high quality. Authors were asked to submit full-length papers for review. A total of 69 papers were submitted to the workshop in response to the call for papers. Each of the 69 papers underwent a rigorous double-blind peer-review process, with each paper being reviewed by at least two (typically three) reviewers from the Program Committee, composed of 51 well-known experts in the field. Based on the reviewing scores and critiques, the 40 best papers (58%) were accepted for presentation at the workshop and chosen to be included in this LNCS volume published by Springer. The large variety of machine-learning techniques applied to medical imaging were well represented at the workshop.

We are grateful to the Program Committee for reviewing the submitted papers and giving constructive comments and critiques, to the authors for submitting high-quality papers, to the presenters for their excellent presentations, and to all the MLMI 2015 attendees coming to Munich from all around the world.

August 2015

Luping Zhou
Li Wang
Qian Wang
Yinghuan Shi

Organization

Steering Committee

Dinggang Shen	University of North Carolina at Chapel Hill, USA
Kenji Suzuki	Illinois Institute of Technology, USA
Pingkun Yan	Philips Research North America, USA
Fei Wang	AliveCor Inc., USA

Program Committee

Shu Liao	Siemens Medical Solutions, USA
Shuiwang Ji	Old Dominion University, USA
Wei Liu	University of Utah, USA
Wenlu Zhang	Old Dominion University, USA
Gustavo Carneiro	University of Adelaide, Australia
Chong-Yaw Wee	National University of Singapore, Singapore
Yang Li	Allen Institute for Brain Science, USA
Clarisa Sanchez	Radboud University Nijmegen Medical Center, The Netherlands
Heung-Il Suk	Korea University, Korea
Jurgen Fripp	CSIRO, Australia
Feng Shi	University of North Carolina, Chapel Hill, USA
Jinah Park	KAIST, Korea
Kazunori Okada	San Francisco State University, USA
Adrienne Mendrik	University Medical Center Utrecht, The Netherlands
Marleen de Bruijne	University of Copenhagen, Denmark
Li Shen	Indiana University School of Medicine, USA
Lei Wang	University of Wollongong, Australia
Mert Sabuncu	MGH, Harvard Medical School, USA
Ghassan Hamarneh	Simon Fraser University, Canada
Siamak Ardekan	Johns Hopkins University, USA
Heang-Ping Chan	University of Michigan Medical Center, USA
Pierrick Bourgeat	CSIRO, Australia
Guorong Wu	University of North Carolina, Chapel Hill, USA
Brent C. Munsell	College of Charleston, USA
Gozde Unal	Sabanci University, Turkey
Yanrong Guo	University of North Carolina, Chapel Hill, USA
Ivana Isgum	University Medical Center Utrecht, The Netherlands
Gang Li	University of North Carolina, Chapel Hill, USA
Guoyan Zheng	University of Bern, Switzerland

Yaozong Gao	University of North Carolina, Chapel Hill, USA
Minjeong Kim	University of North Carolina, Chapel Hill, USA
Jian Cheng	NIH, USA
Yuanjie Zheng	University of Pennsylvania, USA
Bram van Ginneken	Radboud University Nijmegen Medical Center, The Netherlands
Pim Moeskops	University Medical Center Utrecht, The Netherlands
Ismail Ben Ayed	GE Healthcare, Canada
Emanuele Olivetti	Fondazione Bruno Kessler, Italy
Antonios Makropoulos	Imperial College London, UK
Hotaka Takizawa	University of Tsukuba, Japan
Rong Chen	The University of Maryland, Baltimore County, USA
Byung-Uk Lee	Ewha W. University, Korea
Daniel Rueckert	Imperial College London, UK
Yiqiang Zhan	Siemens Medical Solutions, USA
Gerard Sanroma	Universitat Pompeu Fabra, Spain
Hidetaka Arimura	Kyusyu University, Japan
Nathan Lay	NIH, USA
Shaoting Zhang	UNC Charlotte, USA
Kevin Zhou	Siemens Corporate Research, USA
Elizabeth Krupinski	University of Arizona, USA
Yan Jin	University of North Carolina, Chapel Hill, USA
Mitko Veta	Technische Universiteit Eindhoven, The Netherlands

Contents

Segmentation of Right Ventricle in Cardiac MR Images Using Shape Regression

Suman Sedai[✉], Pallab Roy, and Rahil Garnavi

IBM Research Australia, Level 5, 204 Lygon Street, Carlton, VIC 3053, Australia
{ssedai,pallroy,rahilg}@au1.ibm.com

Abstract. Accurate and automatic segmentation of the right ventricle is challenging due to its complex anatomy and large shape variation observed between patients. In this paper the ability of shape regression is explored to segment right ventricle in presence of large shape variation among the patients. We propose a robust and efficient cascaded shape regression method which iteratively learns the final shape from a given initial shape. We use gradient boosted regression trees to learn each regressor in the cascade to take the advantage of supervised feature selection mechanism. A novel data augmentation method is proposed to generate synthetic training samples to improve regressors performance. In addition to that, a robust fusion method is proposed to reduce the the variance in the predictions given by different initial shapes, which is a major drawback of cascade regression based methods. The proposed method is evaluated on an image set of 45 patients and shows high segmentation accuracy with dice metric of 0.87 ± 0.06. Comparative study shows that our proposed method performs better than state-of-the-art multi-atlas label fusion based segmentation methods.

1 Introduction

Segmentation of right ventricle (RV) structure in cardiac MRI images is an important task, required in management of most cardiac disorders, e.g. pulmonary hypertension, coronary heart diseases, dysplasia and cardiomypathies [1]. However, automatic segmentation of RV is challenging due to its complex anatomy - caused by highly variable and crescent structure - and adverse shape variation among patients. Moreover, thin and indistinguishable myocardial walls, along with inhomogeneous and ill-defined boundaries makes segmentation more difficult. Thus, while ample amount of research has been done on segmentation of the left ventricle (LV), fewer attempts have been made on RV segmentation. Existing methods mainly falls into three categories: pixels classification-based, statistical shape-based, and atlas-based methods.

In pixel classification-based methods, a classifier is generally trained using annotated RV labels, then segmentation is done by grouping the classified pixels. For example,[2] used motion information to detect the region of interest and segmentation was performed using Expectation Maximization based classifier and a Markov Random Field. In another approach [3], a graph cut based

© Springer International Publishing Switzerland 2015
L. Zhou et al. (Eds.): MLMI 2015, LNCS 9352, pp. 1–8, 2015.
DOI: 10.1007/978-3-319-24888-2_1

method was used to perform joint segmentation of cardiac RV and LV, using mutual context information. However, in these approaches shape's prior information has not been utilized, although it can improve the segmentation accuracy particularly in the presence of ill-defined and inhomogeneous RV boundary. Statistical shape based methods incorporate shape prior information by encoding expected shape variation using variants of Principal Component Analysis (PCA). For example, [4] modeled both ventricles using Point Distribution Model (PDM) followed by active shape and appearance based optimization [5]. However, such learned shape and appearance models have limited capability to capture the complex RV shape. Moreover, they are sensitive to the initialization due to gradient descent optimization. A number of methods based on multi-atlas label fusion is proposed to segment RV [6]. However, multi-atlas segmentation methods are computationally expensive, also highly dependent on the result of the registration step, therefore any inaccurate alignment in registration adversely affects the ultimate segmentation result.

In this paper, we propose a novel segmentation method of right ventricle in MR images, based on shape regression. In our method, RV shape is represented as a collection of landmark points, and a regression function that maps the image appearance to the target shape, is learned from the training data. Previous works such as [7] used boosting regression for predicting the shape of the left ventricle in echo-cardiogram images. Yet, their method would learn regressors for individual landmarks, and does not takes into account the appearance correlation between landmarks. We, however, propose to use the cascade regression framework based on layer-wise training of regressors to directly regress multidimensional RV shape landmarks from image appearance. Our method takes into account correlations between RV landmarks and uses shape invariant feature selection during regression. Cascade regression framework have been previously used for non-rigid pose estimation [8] and facial landmark points alignments [9] using random fern as a shape regressor. In this paper, we use gradient boosted regression trees to train each regressor at the cascade for supervised feature selection. Moreover, we have proposed a novel data augmentation method to generate synthetic data and demonstrate the positive effect of increasing the training data on segmentation performance. Cascade regression suffers from dependency of prediction to initializations. To make the final segmentation robust towards the initializations, we present a fusion method to combine predictions based on their confidence. Once the regression model is trained, our method does not need optimization in testing phase, hence provides faster segmentation.

2   Methodology

We represent the right ventricle shape as a collection of p landmark points $S = \{x_1, y_1, \cdots x_p, y_p\}$. In the cascade regression framework [8,9], a strong shape regressor is built by cascading T weak shape regressors $F_1, \cdots F_T$. Given an image I and an initial RV shape S_0, each regressor in the cascade is trained to predict a shape increment vector ΔS to update the previous shape:

$$S^t = S^{t-1} + F^t(I, S^{t-1}) \tag{1}$$

In this framework, each regressor F^t computes the feature relative to the previous shape S^{t-1}. Such relative indexing of features introduces weak geometric invariances into the cascade regression and have been shown to improve the performance when compared with the fixed feature indexing [8,9]. Moreover, final prediction always lies in the linear subspace of the training data as long as the initial shape S^0 is a valid right ventricle shape. Therefore, this approach automatically incorporates shape constraints in the learning stage.

Given a training examples $\left\{I_i, \hat{S}_i\right\}_{i=1}^N$ where I_i is a short-axis MRI image and $\hat{S}_i$ is a ground truth shape vector, the goal is to learn the cascade of regressors $\left\{F^1 ... F^T\right\}$. In landmark-based shape model, it is important that landmarks on all training samples are located at corresponding locations. To ensure each landmark (x_j, y_j) of all the training shapes represents approximately same location in the right ventricle boundary, the first landmark x_1, y_1 is taken to be the left insert point of the RV and q^{th} landmark point is taken to be the second insert point of the RV. Each training example needs an initial shape to train the regression framework. Next step of our proposed method involves data augmentation process to automatically generate initial shapes, which is explained in the following section.

2.1 Data Augmentation

In the cascade regression framework, the cascade needs to learn to predict from different initial shapes, therefore using multiple initial shapes for each training samples have been shown to improve the performance of the regression [8]. In previous approaches [8,9], initial shapes have been sampled from the training set. However, existing shapes in the training set may be limited and less diverse. In this paper, we propose a method to generate a collection of initial shapes, based on PDM [5]. First, all training shapes are normalized in common coordinate system using the two RV insert points as references. Then, the normalized training shapes are averaged to obtain a mean shape $\bar{S}$. Next, PCA is performed on the covariance matrix of the normalized training shapes to obtain the B unit eigenvectors $\mathbf{v}_1, \cdots \mathbf{v}_B$ corresponding to the B largest eigenvalues. A new RV shape, can then be generated by adding the mean shape to the weighted combination of the unit eigenvectors:

$$S^0 = \bar{S} + \sum_{j=1}^{B} \mathbf{v}_j b_j \tag{2}$$

where $\mathbf{b} = b_1, ... b_j$ are the weights of each eigenvectors. We learned the bound of $\mathbf{b}$ from the normalized training shapes. Hence, by varying the weights within the bound, we can generate large number of initial shapes that lies in the space of the training shapes. For each training example i, we randomly sample the K values of $\mathbf{b}$ within the bound and use Equation 2 to obtain K initial shapes. The sampled shapes are then transformed to absolute image coordinates by attaching them to the RV insert points in I_i. Therefore, the effective number of training samples in the augmented training set becomes $N_{ag}=N*K$. Ultimately, the augmented training set to train the first regressor F^1 in the cascade consist of $\left\{I_i, \hat{S}_i, S_i^0\right\}_{i=1}^{N_{ag}}$. Note that, in order to train the tth regressor in the cascade F^t, the augmented set is updated to form $\left\{I_i, \hat{S}_i, S_i^{t-1}\right\}_{i=1}^{N_{ag}}$ where S_i^{t-1} is computed using Equation 1.

2.2   Feature Extraction

In this section, we describe how to extract the feature vector $\mathbf{x}^t$ to train the regressor F^t in the cascade. Pixels around the RV boundary are likely to contain most discriminative features. In order to select such features, we index the pixels relative to the previously estimated shape S^{t-1}, rather than the original image coordinates. This leads to better geometric invariance against the shape variation, and in turn helps the regressors to converge more quickly [8]. First, we randomly sample Q pixels locations $u_1, \cdots u_Q$ in the space of the mean RV shape where each pixel u_j is indexed by its nearest RV shape landmark point l_j using an offset vector $\boldsymbol{\delta}^j = (\delta_x, \delta_y)$. Next, the pixels are transformed to the absolute image coordinate for each image I_i in the training set as $v_j^i = I_i(S_i^{t-1}(l_j) + \boldsymbol{\delta}^j)$ where $S_i^{t-1}(l_j)$ denotes the image location of the l_j^{th} landmark position with respect to the previous shape estimate S_i^{t-1}.

The features are then computed as intensity difference between any two pixels. The pixel difference features are not only cheap to compute but also they are insensitive to illumination variation in images. We compute the difference between intensity values for any two pixel v_j^i and v_k^i for $j = 1, \cdots Q; k = j, \cdots Q$ and $j \neq k$. The dimension of the pixel difference feature vector $\mathbf{x}_i^t$ is therefore $Q(Q-1)/2$.

2.3   Training the Regressors

Given the augmented training data $\left\{I_i, \hat{S}_i, S_i^{t-1}\right\}_{i=1}^{N_{ag}}$, our goal is to train each regressor F^t in the cascade. In doing so, we first compute the shape index feature vector $\mathbf{x}_i^t$ from I_i using the previous shape estimate S_i^t for all $i = 1, \cdots N_{ag}$. Then, the regressor F^t is trained to map from the shape indexed feature space $\mathbf{x}^t$ to the target shape increment vector $\Delta S_i^t = \hat{S}_i - S_i^{t-1}$. The regressor F^t is thus trained using $\{\mathbf{x}_i^t, \Delta S_i^t\}_{i=1}^{N_{ag}}$ as follows.

We approximate the regressor F^t using gradient boosting regression (GBR) [10] with sum of square loss. GBR is an iterative process to build a strong regressor from several weak regressors, which can be expressed in the following additive form:

$$F_m^t(\mathbf{x}^t) = F_{m-1}^t(\mathbf{x}^t) + \gamma \, f_m^t(\mathbf{x}^t), \tag{3}$$

where F_m^t is a regressor obtained at m^{th} iteration and f_m^t is an incremental weak regressor by which F_{m-1}^t should advance in order to minimize the expected value of the given loss function and γ is a shrinkage parameter that determines contribution of weak regressor on the ensemble. The shrinkage parameter $0 < \gamma \leq 1$ controls the learning rate and selecting $\gamma < 1$ helps to prevent overfitting [10]. The gradient boosting regression approximates f_m^t in the path of the steepest decent, which is given by the residuals of the training samples [10]. For the sum of square loss, residuals of the ith training sample is computed as $g_m(\mathbf{x}_t^t) = \Delta \mathbf{S}_i^t - F_{m-1}(\mathbf{x}_i^t)$. Next, the weak regressor f_m^t is trained using $\{\mathbf{x}_i^t, g_m(\mathbf{x}_i^t)\}_{i=1}^{N_{ag}}$.

We model the weak regressor $f_m(x)$ as the multi-dimensional version of the regression tree which recursively partitions the feature space into L disjoint regions $R_{l,m}, l = 1 \cdots L$. In normal regression tree, each partition is assigned a scalar constant. However, our output shape increment vector $\Delta S \in \mathbb{R}^{\mathbb{P}}$ is multidimensional, each of the partition $R_{l,m}$ in the terminal nodes of the tree is represented by a P-dimensional constant response vector. To train the regression tree, we select the best feature dimension and the split at each node by minimizing the sum of the squared deviations about the mean of $g_m(\mathbf{x}_i^t)$ for all i that belongs to the partition denoted by the node. The split can be found very efficiently as the response vector for the candidate partitions resulting from the splits is just a mean of the residuals in the partitions i.e, $\gamma_l^m = \sum_{x^i \in R_{l,m}} g_m(\mathbf{x}_i^t)/N_{lm}$, where N_{lm} is the number of training samples that falls in the partition $R_{l,m}$.

2.4   Prediction

Given a test image, we first generate J initial shapes using the method described in Section 2.1. These multiple initializations are fed to the trained cascade regressor in Equation 1 to obtain J predictions $\left\{\tilde{S}_j\right\}_{j=1}^{J}$. Previous approaches use median of these output without validating the prediction. We, however, compute the confidence score of a prediction using Gaussian distance transform. In doing so, we first detect edges in the test image by thresholding the gradient image to obtain a binary edge map. We then construct a Gaussian distance map E_g by convolving the binary edge image with a Gaussian kernel and rescaling the pixel values between 0 and 1. The Gaussian distance map gives the proximity of a pixel to the edge and hence can be used to determine the edge probability of the pixel.

The cost of prediction S is then obtained by computing the mean square error (MSE) of the edge probability values at the points in shape S as $Cost(S) = \frac{\sum_{p \in S}(1 - E_g(p))^2}{P}$, where P is the number of landmarks in shape S. The cost measures how well the predicted shape S is aligned with the right ventricular edges in the given image. The confidence of prediction of $\tilde{S}_j$ is computed as $w(\tilde{S}_j) = \exp(-Cost(\tilde{S}_j))/\sum_{i=1}^{J} \exp(-Cost(\tilde{S}_i))$. The final prediction is then obtained using weighted combination of all the predictions, $S_{final} = \sum_{j=1}^{J} w(\tilde{S}_j)\tilde{S}_j$.

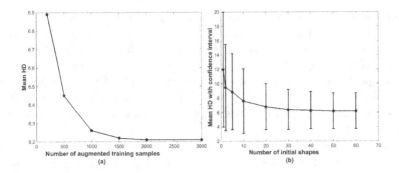

Fig. 1. (a) The effect of increasing the augmented training samples on the segmentation error (b) The effect of number of initial shapes used in our weighted fusion-based prediction.

3   Experiments

Our proposed method is evaluated on the Sunnybrook Cardiac Dataset (SCD)[11] which contains MRI volume of 45 subjects. Since SCD does not include any ground truth segmentation of right ventricle therefore boundaries and left/right insert points of the right ventricle has been manually annotated by our collaborator radiologist. SCD dataset is divided into three groups : training , validation and test set, each on them consists of 15 subjects. Training and parameter selection of our proposed method is done on the training and validation set respectively and evaluation is done on the test set.

Table 1. Comparative study between our proposed method and multi-atlas label fusion methods.

Method	Dice Metric (DM)	Hausdorff distance (HD)
WVLF[12]	0.80($\pm$0.11)	9.66($\pm$5.96)
JLF[13]	0.85($\pm$0.1)	10.45($\pm$6.67)
Proposed method	**0.87($\pm$0.06)**	**6.20 $\pm$ 2.50**

Our method has three main parameters: number of training samples , number of initial shapes and number of cascade regressor. Fig. 1 (a) shows that increasing the number of training samples using proposed data augmentation method (described in section 2.1) significantly reduces the segmentation error. In the proposed method optimal training sample number is set to 2000. To obtain the optimal number of initial shapes we evaluate the impact of increment in the number of initial shapes on the segmentation accuracy. Fig.1 (b) shows that increasing the number of initial shapes used in our weighted fusion-based prediction reduces the segmentation error. The optimal number of initial shape is set to 50. We set the number of cascade regressors $T = 10$ as we found that setting $T > 10$ did not improve the performance.

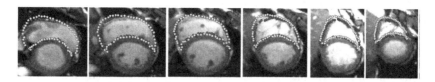

Fig. 2. Example outputs of our proposed segmentation method for a same volume at different slice location in a test set. The manual segmentation is outlined in red color and automatic segmentation is outlined in yellow color.

We compare our proposed method with joint label fusion (JLF) [13] and weighted voting label fusion (WVLF) [12] which are multi-atlas segmentation methods. Both method has two steps: registration and label fusion. In the registration step, we use two RV insert points and LV center point to perform affine registration followed by deformable registration [14] to align the atlas subject slices with the corresponding slices of the target subject. In the label fusion step, we evaluate both JLF and WVLF for final segmentation of RV. As shown in Table 1, mean dice metric (DM) and hausdorff distance (HD) of our proposed method is 0.87 and 6.20 which is significantly better than the results obtained by multi-atlas segmentation methods. Our proposed method shows lower standard deviation for both evaluation metrics compared to multi-atlas label fusion methods, which reflects the stability of our approach. Figure 2 shows the segmentation output of our proposed method and corresponding manual segmentations. The method proposed in this paper has been implemented in Java, and experiments have been performed on an Intel Core i5 CPU @ 3.10 GHz with 8 Gb of memory. Our proposed method took 3 seconds to segment RV in a single volume with 10 slices, which is remarkably faster compared to multi-atlas segmentation methods which took 20 minutes for segmenting the volume.

4 Conclusions

In this paper, we presented a method which uses cascades of non-linear regressor to accurately segment right ventricle, by minimizing the shape alignment error over the training data. The proposed approach involves a novel data augmentation method to generate synthetic data, which has shown to improve the performance. To overcome the drawback of the cascade shape regression (i.e. dependency of the predicted shape to variations in the initial shape), a fusion method was proposed to combine such predictions based on their confidence. Our method has been trained, validated and evaluated on a dataset of 45 patients [11] resulting in a high segmentation accuracy (DM 0.87 and HD 6.20) and shown to outperform two multi-altas label fusion based segmentation methods. For future work, we intend to automate the RV insert point selection and will investigate its effect on the segmentation accuracy.

References

1. Petitjean, C., Zuluaga, M.A., Bai, W., Dacher, J.-N., Grosgeorge, D., Jérôme Caudron, S., Ruan, I.B., Ayed, M.J., Cardoso, H.-C.C., et al.: Right ventricle segmentation from cardiac MRI: A collation study. Medical image analysis **19**(1), 187–202 (2015)
2. Gering, D.T.: Automatic segmentation of cardiac MRI. In: Ellis, R.E., Peters, T.M. (eds.) MICCAI 2003. LNCS, vol. 2878, pp. 524–532. Springer, Heidelberg (2003)
3. Mahapatra, D., Buhmann, J.M.: Cardiac LV and RV segmentation using mutual context information. In: Wang, F., Shen, D., Yan, P., Suzuki, K. (eds.) MLMI 2012. LNCS, vol. 7588, pp. 201–209. Springer, Heidelberg (2012)
4. Mitchell, S.C., Lelieveldt, B.P.F., van der Geest, R.J., Bosch, H.G., Reiver, J.H.C., Sonka, M.: Multistage hybrid active appearance model matching: segmentation of left and right ventricles in cardiac mr images. IEEE Transactions on Medical Imaging **20**(5), 415–423 (2001)
5. Cootes, T.F., Taylor, C.J., Cooper, D.H., Graham, J.: Active shape models-their training and application. Comput. Vis. Image Underst. **61**(1), 38–59 (1995)
6. Ou, Y., Doshi, J., Erus, G., Davatzikos, C.: Multi-atlas segmentation of the cardiac MR right ventricle. In: RV Segmentation Challenge at MICCAI (2012)
7. Zhou, S.K.: Shape regression machine and efficient segmentation of left ventricle endocardium from 2D B-mode echocardiogram. Medical Image Analysis **14**(4), 563–581 (2010)
8. Dollár, P., Welinder, P., Perona, P.: Cascaded pose regression. In: CVPR, pp. 1078–1085. IEEE (2010)
9. Cao, X., Wei, Y., Wen, F., Sun, J.: Face alignment by explicit shape regression. IJCV **107**(2), 177–190 (2014)
10. Friedman, J.H.: Greedy function approximation: A gradient boosting machine. Annals of Statistics **29**, 1189–1232 (2000)
11. Radau, P., Lu, Y., Connelly, K., Paul, G., Dick, A., Wright, G.: Evaluation framework for algorithms segmenting short axis cardiac MRI. The MIDAS Journal **49** (2009)
12. Sabuncu, M.R., Yeo, B.T., Van Leemput, K., Fischl, B., Golland, P.: A generative model for image segmentation based on label fusion. IEEE Trans. Med. Imaging **29**(10), 1714–1729 (2010)
13. Wang, H., Suh, J.W., Das, S.R., Pluta, J.B., Craige, C., Yushkevich, P.A.: Multi-atlas segmentation with joint label fusion. IEEE Transactions on PAMI **35**(3), 611–623 (2013)
14. Klein, S., Staring, M., Murphy, K., Viergever, M.A., Pluim, J.P.W.: Elastix: a toolbox for intensity-based medical image registration. IEEE Transactions on Medical Imaging **29**(1), 196–205 (2010)

Visual Saliency Based Active Learning for Prostate MRI Segmentation

Dwarikanath Mahapatra$^{(\boxtimes)}$ and Joachim M. Buhmann

Department of Computer Science, ETH Zurich, Zürich, Switzerland
`mahapatd@vision.ee.ethz.ch`

Abstract. We propose an active learning (AL) approach for prostate segmentation from magnetic resonance (MR) images. Our label query strategy is inspired from the principles of visual saliency that has similar considerations for choosing the most salient region. These similarities are encoded in a graph using classification maps and low level features. Random walks identify the most informative node which is equivalent to the label query sample in AL. Experimental results on the MICCAI 2012 Prostate segmentation challenge show the superior performance of our approach to conventional methods using fully supervised learning.

1 Introduction

According to the American Cancer society, prostate cancer is the second leading cause of cancer death in American men, and early diagnosis can potentially increase the survival rate amongst patients [1]. Accurate quantification of prostate volume (PV), and location relative to adjacent organs is also an essential part of image guided radiation therapy (IGRT). Magnetic resonance imaging's (MRI) popularity in treatment planning has increased due to high spatial resolution, soft-tissue contrast and absence of ionising radiations.

Manual segmentation of the prostate in MRI is time consuming, and prone to inter- and intra-expert variability. This necessitates the design of (semi-) automated segmentation algorithms that can overcome challenges like: 1) variability of prostate size and shape between subjects; 2) variable image appearance and intensity ranges from different MR scanning protocols; and 3) lack of clear prostate boundaries due to similar intensity profiles of surrounding tissues. Hence, machine learning (ML) methods have focused on learning discriminative image features from manual annotations. However, manual annotations are very expensive, time consuming and requires personnel with high expertise.

The growing importance of prostate MRI segmentation led to the prostate segmentation challenge in MICCAI 2012. Different approaches in the challenge include marginal space learning [2], multi-atlas segmentation [7] and ML [8]. Success of ML methods depends on the discriminative power of hand crafted features. To overcome this shortcoming Liao et al. in [11] propose a deep learning framework using independent subspace analysis (ISA) to automatically learn the most discriminative features. A detailed overview of the different methods and their performance is found in [12].

© Springer International Publishing Switzerland 2015
L. Zhou et al. (Eds.): MLMI 2015, LNCS 9352, pp. 9–16, 2015.
DOI: 10.1007/978-3-319-24888-2_2

In this paper we propose an active learning based segmentation method that requires significantly fewer labeled samples, yet achieves higher segmentation accuracy than conventional ML methods. The important contribution of this paper is a visual saliency based approach to select the most informative samples for active learning (AL). We show that many of the principles of salient image region detection are applicable to query selection in active learning. Hence selecting the most informative region in MRI becomes a problem of salient region detection by defining an appropriate measure of a region's importance.

2   Image Features

We calculate the mean, variance, skewness and kurtosis of intensity, texture and mean 3D curvature values from a 31×31 patch around every voxel. The texture maps are calculated for each slice of the supervoxel using $2D$ Gabor filters oriented at $0°, 45°, 90°, 135°$ at the original scale. Thus each voxel gives a 24 dimensional feature vector.

3   Semi Supervised Learning With Random Forests

Random forests (RF) [3] have become increasingly popular in classification tasks because of their computational efficiency for large training data and ability to handle multiclass classification. Semi supervised learning techniques train classifiers with a few labeled samples [4] and many unlabeled samples. This is a typical scenario in many medical applications where it is difficult to find qualified experts to label the large number of medical images. A 'single shot' RF method for SSL without the need for iterative retraining was introduced in [6]. We use this method for SSL as it is shown to outperform other approaches.

For labeled samples the information gain over data splits at each node is maximised and encourages separation of the labeled data [3,6]. However for SSL the objective function encourages separation of the labeled training data and simultaneously separates different high density regions. It is achieved via the following mixed information gain:

$$I_j = I_j^U + \beta I_j^S \tag{1}$$

where $I_j^S = H(S_j) - \sum_{i \in \{L,R\}} \frac{|S_j^i|}{|S_j|} H(S_j^i)$ is the information gain from the labeled data; H is the entropy of training points, S_j^L and S_j^R the subsets going to the left and right children of node j, and β is a user defined weight. I_j^U depends on both labeled and unlabeled data, and is defined using differential entropies over continuous parameters as

$$I_j^U = \log |\Lambda(S_j)| - \sum_{i \in \{L,R\}} \frac{|S_j^i|}{|S_j|} \log |\Lambda(S_j)| \tag{2}$$

Λ is the covariance matrix of the assumed multivariate distributions at each node. Further details are given in [6].

4   SSL-AL Based Segmentation From MR Images

Initial Preprocessing. The given images are first bias-corrected using the method in [5] and the intensities are then to $[0, 1]$. Learning starts with randomly chosen labeled samples (voxels) of the first training dataset (set L). The features of L and unlabeled voxels (set U from the remaining training datasets) are used as inputs to an RF based SSL classifier (denoted as $RF - SSL$) which predicts the class labels and probabilities of the unlabeled patches. The most informative sample is added to set L and the classifier is updated using online learning [15]. In online learning there is no need for retraining of classifiers. The RF classifier is updated based on the newly labeled samples only. The query strategy of AL is discussed in Section 4.1.

4.1   AL Query Strategy

Conventional query strategies like density weighting [16] use classification uncertainty and weigh samples according to their similarity with other neighbors. However conventional approaches do not exploit the contextual information over neighborhoods. Our query strategy selects a sample: 1) with high classification uncertainty to obtain novel information from each labeling instance; 2) situated in a dense region such that it is representative of many other samples; and 3) minimal overlap of influence with previously labeled samples to minimize redundancy in labeling effort. Salient image regions have the following characteristics: 1) feature values are significantly different from surroundings (high local contrast); and 2) contrast magnitude is higher than other regions. High contrast regions have maximum information and hence higher entropy [10]. High classification uncertainty also corresponds to high entropy, indicating a correspondence between information content of salient regions and classification uncertainty. Salient regions are located on regular objects (or dense regions of the sample space) and different salient regions are far away from each other, i.e. their influence areas have minimum overlap. Thus we see that the properties of salient regions have similarities with the desired characteristics of query samples. Hence saliency models can be adapted for active learning tasks using appropriate similarity metrics.

Image patches are represented as nodes V of a graph G, and connected by set of edges E. Based on the similarity between any two nodes i and j a weight w_{ij} is given by

$$w_{ij} = \exp\left(\frac{-\|F_i - F_j\|^2}{\sigma^2}\right), \tag{3}$$

where F_i is the feature vector of node i or the informativeness $Inf(i)$; $\sigma = 1$, and $\|.\|$ denotes L_2 norm. Informativeness of node i (or voxel x) is given by

$$Inf(i) = \{\phi(i),\ \gamma, \alpha\}. \tag{4}$$

ϕ is the classification uncertainty of i given by the entropy as

$$\phi(i) = - \sum_{\widehat{y}} P((\widehat{y}|i) \log P((\widehat{y}|i), \tag{5}$$

where $\widehat{y}$ indicates all possible labels (in this case two) for i, and $P((\widehat{y}|i)$ is calculated by RF-SSL. High entropy indicates greater uncertainty. α incorporates contextual information, and a is the collection of intensity, texture and curvature differences defined as

$$\gamma = [Int_{ij} \ Tex_{ij} \ Curv_{ij}]. \tag{6}$$

where $Int_{ij} = \sum_{j \in N} e^{-|Int_i - Int_j|/\sigma^2}$ is the sum of exponential of intensity differences between node i and all unlabeled nodes j in N (a 48×48 neighborhood of x), and $\sigma = 1$. For similar nodes, Int_{ij} takes higher values. Tex_{ij} and $Curv_{ij}$ are the corresponding texture (from the oriented map at $90°$) and curvature differences. Note that we do not average the feature differences over the neighborhood. In a high density region γ is calculated by summing over more voxels than in a sparsely populated region. Since γ is not divided by a normalization constant its value is higher in a high density region.

Context Information for Informativeness: An unlabeled sample close to a labeled sample is assigned lower importance because it has a higher probability of having the same label than a sample far away. If the radiologist were to annotate samples close to an already labeled sample it *does not* generally lead to significant information gain. Thus α incorporates context information and is equal to i's distance from the nearest labeled sample

$$\alpha = \min \left(\|i - i^L\| \right). \tag{7}$$

where i^L denotes all the labeled samples (or nodes), and $\|.\|$ denotes the Euclidean distance based on voxel co-ordinates.

4.2   Random Walks and Most Salient Node

The weights w_{ij} (Eqn.3) are used to define the affinity matrix A as

$$A_{ij} = \begin{cases} w_{ij}, i \neq j \\ 0, i = j. \end{cases} \tag{8}$$

The most salient node is identified by the random walks algorithm on the graph. Let us denote as $E_i(T_j)$ the expected number of steps to reach state j if a Markov chain is started in state i at time $t = 0$. It is also known as the hitting time, and can be derived from the fundamental matrix ($\mathbf{Z}$) of an ergodic Markov chain and its equilibrium probability distribution π. The global saliency of node i is given by the sum of hitting times from all other nodes to node i on a complete graph,

$$H_i = \sum_j E_j(T_i), \tag{9}$$

and the most salient node is given by the maximum H_i as $N_s = \arg\max_i H_i$. For details the reader is referred to [9]. Labels are queried for N_s.

Stopping Criteria: Irrespective of the number of labeled samples, there will always be one unlabeled sample with maximum informativeness. In order to ensure that the label query does not continue indefinitely, we determine the probability values of the two classes for the most informative sample. If the probability value for any one class is less than 0.45 (or greater than 0.55 for the other class) we do not query the label for that sample. If we encounter such samples for 5 consecutive iterations then we stop the label query because this indicates that the classifier has obtained sufficient samples to have high confidence on its classification output.

4.3 Graph Cut Segmentation

A spatially smooth solution is obtained by formulating the segmentation as a labeling problem within a second order Markov random field (MRF) cost function. The labels are obtained for each voxel and not the individual patches by optimizing the cost function using graph cuts. A second order MRF energy function is given by

$$E(L) = \sum_{s \in P} D(L_s) + \lambda \sum_{(s,t) \in N} V(L_s, L_t), \qquad (10)$$

where P denotes the set of pixels and N is the set of neighboring pixels for pixel s. λ is a weight that determines the relative contribution of penalty cost (D) and smoothness cost (V). $D(L_s)$ is given by

$$D(L_s) = -\log\left(Pr(L_s) + \epsilon\right), \qquad (11)$$

where Pr is the likelihood (from probability maps) previously obtained using RF classifiers and $\epsilon = 0.00001$ is a very small value to ensure that the cost is a real number. The penalty cost encourages high label probability. V ensures a spatially smooth solution by penalizing discontinuities and is defined as

$$V(L_s, L_t) = e^{-\frac{(I_s - I_t)^2}{2\sigma^2}} \cdot \frac{1}{\|s - t\|}, \qquad (12)$$

I denotes the intensity. Smoothness cost is determined over a 8 neighborhood system.

5 Experiments and Results

We apply our method on the MICCAI 2012 PROMISE prostate segmentation challenge (http://promise12.grand-challenge.org/). The training set consisting of 50 patients is used to train our classifier, which is then applied on the 30 test datasets of transversal T2-weighted MR images. We submit our results to the online evaluation system and get feedback on our performance as well as a ranking. The datasets are acquired under different clinical settings.

They are multi-center and multi-vendor, and have different acquisition protocols (e.g. differences in slice thickness, with/without endorectal coil). The volume dimensions and voxel resolutions are different for different images. Each slice of the different volumes is of size 512×512 (voxel resolution of $0.4 \times 0.4 \times 3.3$) or 320×320 (resolution $0.6 \times 0.6 \times 3.6$). Our whole pipeline was implemented in MATLAB on a 2.66 GHz quad core CPU running Windows 7. The quality of our segmentation results was evaluated by the organizers using: 1) Dice Metric (DM) and 2) 95% Hausdorff Distance (HD). λ (Eqn. 10) was set to 0.02. Our RF-SSL classifier had 50 trees with tree depth of 20. Due to space constraints we provide results only on the test set which is used to rank each algorithm.

5.1   Results on MICCAI PROMISE12 Online Challenge Dataset

We train our $SSL - AL$ classifier on all 50 volumes of the training data and submit our results for 30 challenge datasets for which the manual segmentations are not available to the participants. The ranking methodology is explained in [12]. Our proposed $SSL - AL$ method is ranked **third** among all the methods while a competing fully supervised learning (FSL) based method [13] is ranked 14.

$SSL - AL$'s quantitative values are $DM = 86.7 \pm 4.9$, $95\%HD = 5.9 \pm 1.9$ mm, and boundary distance $= 2.25 \pm 0.77$ mm. The corresponding values for FSL are $DM = 80.6 \pm 6.5$, $95\%HD = 7.6 \pm 1.7$ mm, and boundary distance $= 3.38 \pm 0.84$ mm. A plot of DM and HD values for our method on individual datasets is shown in Fig. 1.

[17]'s method is ranked first followed by [2] with the following scores: 1) [17] - $DM = 88.0 \pm 4.0$, $95\%HD = 5.94 \pm 2.14$ mm, and boundary distance $= 2.1 \pm 0.68$ mm; and 2) [2] - $DM = 87.0 \pm 4.0$, $95\%HD = 5.58 \pm 1.49$ mm, and boundary distance $= 2.13 \pm 0.48$ mm. For DM, $SSL - AL$ ranked fourth with [14] having $DM = 87.0 \pm 4.0$, ranked third. For all other metrics our method was ranked third. Importantly, our method's DM and HD values are very close to the two methods ranked higher than us. The significant improvement in performance of $SSL - AL$ over FSL clearly indicates the advantage of using SSL and AL in training a classifier. The difference in their performance is also significant ($p < 0.0001$). Fig. 2 shows segmentation results on Patient 15 from the training data using different methods. Since we do not have access to the manual segmentations of the online challenge dataset, we are unable to show the comparative performance of the difference methods.

5.2   Savings in Labeling Effort and Time

By querying labels of most informative patches we reduce the redundancy of labels such that new labels provide truly novel information to the classifier. In $5-$fold cross validation FSL uses approximately 80% of manual labels for training while $SSL - AL$ requires 42% of manual annotations and still achieves higher segmentation accuracy. Although FSL has access to more training samples it performs poorly. More training samples does not necessarily translate to better performance since they could introduce noise, particularly if the annotations are

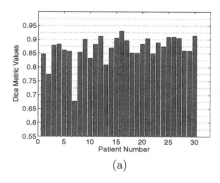
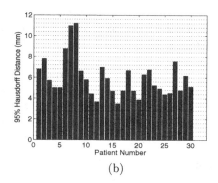

(a)   (b)

Fig. 1. Individual values for $SSL - AL$ on 30 patients of the MICCAI 2012 online challenge dataset: (a) DM; (b) 95% HD

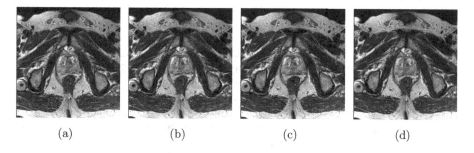

(a)   (b)   (c)   (d)

Fig. 2. Segmentation results for Patient 15. The manual annotations are shown in red with the algorithm segmentations in green: (a) $SSL - AL$ (b) FSL (c) $SSL - AL_{n\alpha}$ and (d) $FSL - AL$.

not accurate enough. In such a scenario it is beneficial to ask experts to label only the most informative samples. This leads to savings in time, effort and also improves algorithm's performance.

Online learning leads to significant time savings. Updating the classifiers with every new label requires about $0.03 - 0.1$ seconds. On the other hand, lots of time is required to retrain the entire classifier using the entire training set.The total *training time* for the 50 training patients is 38 minutes using FSL (as reported in [13]) and 20 minutes using $SSL - AL$. The lower training time for $SSL - AL$ is due to fewer training samples, leading to time savings of $(1 - 20/38 =)47\%$. However, $FSL - AL$ takes a longer training time (32 minutes) than $SSL - AL$ since it does not make use of unlabeled samples. However it is still less than FSL since many of the manually labeled samples are redundant.

6   Discussion and Conclusion

We have developed a novel query strategy for active learning based prostate segmentation. The problem of query sample selection is similar to detecting visually salient regions on a graph. Our method combines semi supervised classification and active learning to achieve higher segmentation accuracy than fully supervised methods, but with fewer labeled samples. Experimental results on real patient prostate MR volumes from the public MICCAI 2012 Prostate segmentation challenge dataset show our method is ranked third amongst 16 methods. Our performance is quite close to the two methods ranked above us. This clearly demonstrates the improvement in segmentation accuracy obtained using SSL and AL even without knowledge of labels of the test image.

References

1. Cancer facts and figures (2014). amer. cancer soc. http://www.cancer.org
2. Birkbeck, N., et. al.: Region-specific hierarchical segmentation of MR prostate using discriminative learning. In: Proc. MICCAI PROMISE 2012, pp. 4–11 (2012)
3. Breiman, L.: Random forests. Machine Learning 45(1), 5–32 (2001)
4. Chapelle, O., Scholkopf, B., Zien, A.: Semi-Supervised Learning. MIT Press, Cambridge (2006)
5. Cohen, M., et al.: Rapid and effective correction of RF inhomogeneity for high field magnetic resonance imaging. Human Brain Map 10(4), 204–211 (2000)
6. Criminisi, A., Shotton., J.: Decision Forests for Computer Vision and Medical Image Analysis. Springer
7. Gao, Q., et. al.: An automatic multi-atlas based prostate segmentation using local appearance-specific atlases and patch-based voxel weighting. In: Proc. MICCAI PROMISE 2012, pp. 12–19 (2012)
8. Ghose, S., et. al.: A random forest based classification approach to prostate segmentation in MRI. In: Proc. MICCAI PROMISE 2012, pp. 20–27 (2012)
9. Harel, J., Koch, C., Perona, P.: Graph based visual saliency. In: NIPS, pp. 545–552 (2006)
10. Kadir, T., Brady, M.: Saliency, scale and image description. International Journal of Computer Vision 45(2), 85–105 (2001)
11. Liao, S., Gao, Y., Oto, A., Shen, D.: Representation learning: a unified deep learning framework for automatic prostate MR segmentation. In: Mori, K., Sakuma, I., Sato, Y., Barillot, C., Navab, N. (eds.) MICCAI 2013, Part II. LNCS, vol. 8150, pp. 254–261. Springer, Heidelberg (2013)
12. Litjens, G., et al.: Evaluation of prostate segmentation algorithms for MRI: The PROMISE12 challenge. Med. Imag. Anal. 18(2), 359–373 (2014)
13. Mahapatra, D., Buhmann, J.: Prostate mri segmentation using learned semantic knowledge and graph cuts. IEEE Trans. Biomed. Engg. 61(3), 756–764 (2014)
14. Malmberg, F., et. al.: Smart paint a new interactive segmentation method applied to MR prostate segmentation. In: Proc. MICCAI PROMISE 2012, pp. 4–11 (2012)
15. Saffari, A., Leistner, C., Santner, J., Godec, M., Bischof., H.: On-line random forests. In: IEEE ICCV Workshops, pp. 1393–1400 (2009)
16. Settles, B., Craven, M.: An analysis of active learning strategies for sequence labeling tasks. In: Empirical Methods in Natural Language Processing, pp. 1070–1079 (2008)
17. Vincent, G., et. al.: Fully automatic segmentation of the prostate using active appearance models. In: Proc. MICCAI PROMISE 2012, pp. 75–81 (2012)

Soft-Split Random Forest for Anatomy Labeling

Guangkai Ma[1,2], Yaozong Gao[2], Li Wang[2], Ligang Wu[1(✉)], and Dinggang Shen[2]

[1] Space Control and Inertial Technology Research Center,
Harbin Institute of Technology, Harbin, China
ligangwu@hit.edu.cn
[2] Department of Radiology and BRIC, University of North Carolina at Chapel Hill,
Chapel Hill, NC, USA

Abstract. Random Forest (RF) has been widely used in the learning-based labeling. In RF, each sample is directed from the root to each leaf based on the decisions made in the interior nodes, also called splitting nodes. The splitting nodes assign a testing sample to *either* left *or* right child based on the learned splitting function. The final prediction is determined as the average of label probability distributions stored in all arrived leaf nodes. For ambiguous testing samples, which often lie near the splitting boundaries, the conventional splitting function, also referred to as *hard split* function, tends to make wrong assignments, hence leading to wrong predictions. To overcome this limitation, we propose a novel *soft-split* random forest (SSRF) framework to improve the reliability of node splitting and finally the accuracy of classification. Specifically, a *soft split* function is employed to assign a testing sample into *both* left *and* right child nodes with their certain probabilities, which can effectively reduce influence of the wrong node assignment on the prediction accuracy. As a result, each testing sample can arrive at multiple leaf nodes, and their respective results can be fused to obtain the final prediction according to the weights accumulated along the path from the root node to each leaf node. Besides, considering the importance of context information, we also adopt a Haar-features based context model to iteratively refine the classification map. We have comprehensively evaluated our method on two public datasets, respectively, for labeling hippocampus in MR images and also labeling three organs in Head & Neck CT images. Compared with the *hard-split* RF (HSRF), our method achieved a notable improvement in labeling accuracy.

1   Introduction

Many anatomy labeling methods have been proposed recently. These methods can be roughly categorized into two classes: 1) multi-atlas based and 2) learning-based methods. In the multi-atlas based methods, a set of already-labeled images, namely atlases, are used to guide the labeling of new target image [1]. Specifically, given a new target image, multiple atlas images are first registered onto this target image, and then the estimated deformation fields are applied to transform the corresponding label maps of atlases to the target image. Finally, all warped atlas label maps are fused for labeling the target image. Specially, in the label fusion step, patch-based similarity is often used as weight to propagate the neighboring atlas labels to the target image, for

© Springer International Publishing Switzerland 2015
L. Zhou et al. (Eds.): MLMI 2015, LNCS 9352, pp. 17–25, 2015.
DOI: 10.1007/978-3-319-24888-2_3

potentially overcoming errors from the registration. The limitation of multi-atlas based methods is that 1) the labeling accuracy highly depends on registration between atlas and target images; 2) the patch similarity is often handcrafted based on the pre-defined features (e.g., image intensity), which might not be effective for labeling all types of anatomical structures, thus potentially limiting the labeling accuracy.

On the other hand, learning-based labeling methods have attracted much attention recently. In the learning-based methods, a strong classifier, such as Adaboost [2], random forests [3] and artificial neural networks [4], is often used to classifying whether a voxel belongs to the interested anatomical structure, based on the local appearance features. In the testing stage, the learned classifiers are applied to voxel-wisely classify the whole target image. These learning-based labeling methods can identify the discriminative features specific to each anatomical structure and make full use of appearance information for anatomy labeling. For example, Zikic et al. [5] developed so-called atlas forest to learn a classification forest for each atlas. Tu et al. [6] adopted the probabilistic boosting tree (PBT) for labeling the MR brain images with Haar features and texture features. Also, Kim et al. [7] utilized Adaboost algo-rithm to train classifiers in multiple atlas image spaces. Then, the final segmentation of a target image is achieved by averaging the labeling results from all classifiers. In addition to just using local appearance information, many researches have shown that the context information is also very useful in identifying an object from a complex scene. In the field of anatomy labeling, many learning-based methods combined ap-pearance with context features to improve the labeling accuracy. For example, Zikic et al. [5] constructed a population mean atlas to provide the rough context information for the target image. Tu et al. [6] proposed an auto-context model (ACM) to extract the context information embedded in the tentative labeling map of the target image for iterative refinement of labeling results. Kim et al. [7] extracted the context informa-tion from an initial labeling probability map of the target image, obtained by using the multi-atlas based method. Compared to the multi-atlas based methods, the learning-based methods can easily learn discriminative features and further utilize context information to improve the labeling performance.

Our method belongs to the learning-based labeling methods. Specifically, we use random forest as classifier for voxel-wise labeling. *The major contribution of our paper is proposing a novel variant of random forest, namely* soft-split *random forest (SSRF), which improves the performance of the conventional RF in anatomical labe-ling.* In the conventional RF, a testing sample follows one path from the root to leaf, based on the decisions made at each splitting node. For the ambiguous testing sam-ples, which often locate near the splitting boundaries, they can arrive at a wrong leaf node due to the wrong assignment made in any of the splitting nodes. To overcome this problem, we propose a *"soft split"* strategy to handle this problem. Specifically, in each split, we take a probabilistic view and allow each sample to go *both* left *and* right nodes with their certain probabilities, which are determined according to the distance of this sample to the splitting decision boundary. Finally, the probability for each leaf is the multiplication of all probabilities along the path, and the prediction of a sample is the weighted average over all non-zero leaf nodes. By using this strategy, we can relieve the problem caused by the mis-assignment in any of the splitting nodes. Experimental results show significant improvement by using SSRF, compared to the conventional RF. Besides, to further refine the labeling result, Haar-features based context model (HCM) is proposed to iteratively construct a sequence of classification forests by updating the context features from the newly-estimated label maps for training. Validated on two public datasets, ADNI and Head & Neck datasets, our proposed method consistently outperforms the conventional RF (using the hard split function).

2   Random Forest

Random Forest (RF) is an ensemble learner, which consists of multiple decision trees. Each tree is independently trained in a randomized fashion. Since the RF classifier is able to handle a high-dimension feature space efficiently and is inherently multi-class, it has recently gained popularity on anatomy labeling. As similar to the common learning techniques, random forest consists of *training* and *testing* stages.

RF Training: Given a set of training data $\mathbf{D} = \{(\mathbf{h}_i, l_i)|i = 1, ..., N\}$, where $\mathbf{h}_i$ and l_i are the feature vector and class label of the i-th training sample, RF aims to learn a non-linear mapping from the feature vector $\mathbf{h}$ of a sample to the corresponding class label l by constructing multiple decision trees. In RF classification, each decision tree is independently trained based on one subset of samples randomly extracted from the training set $\mathbf{D}$. In terms of the tree structure, a decision tree consists of two types of nodes, namely split nodes and leaf nodes. Each split node links two child nodes (left and right child nodes). In order to build a decision tree for classification, a split function is learned at each split node, which optimally splits the samples into two child nodes. A standard split function (decision stump function) is defined as follows:

$$f(\mathbf{h}|j, \tau) = \begin{cases} 0, & h(j) \leq \tau \\ 1, & h(j) > \tau \end{cases} \tag{1}$$

where j is the element index of $\mathbf{h}$, $h(j)$ is the j-th feature of $\mathbf{h}$, and τ is a threshold. If $h(j) \leq \tau$, $f(\mathbf{h}|j, \tau)$ is set zero, indicating that the sample $\mathbf{h}$ is assigned to left-child node; otherwise, if $f(\mathbf{h}|j, \tau)$ is one, the sample $\mathbf{h}$ is assigned to right-child node. To determine the optimal combination of feature and threshold, a random subset of features and the corresponding thresholds are sampled and tested. The one that offers the maximum entropy reduction is regarded as the optimal pair for this split function. After learning the split function, the samples are split and passed to two child nodes for recursive splitting. The training of a decision tree starts with finding the optimal split at the root node, and then recursively proceeds on child nodes until *either* the maximum tree depth is reached *or* the number of training samples is too small to split. Finally, the leaf node stores the class label distribution $p(l)$ of all training samples falling into this leaf node.

RF Testing: For a new testing sample, RF pushes it through each learned decision tree, starting at the root node. At each split node, the testing sample is assigned to one of child nodes by applying the corresponding decision stump function. If the function response is zero, the testing sample is assigned to the left child node; if the function response is one, it is assigned to the right child node. When the testing sample reaches a leaf node, the class label distribution $p(l)$ stored in that leaf node is used as the output of the decision tree and assigned as the probability of the testing sample belonging to class label l. For the entire forest, the final probability $\bar{p}(l)$ of the testing sample assigned to class label l is the average of outputs from all decision trees, i.e. $\bar{p}(l) = \frac{1}{T}\sum_{l=1}^{T} p(l)$, where T is the number of decision trees.

3   Proposed Method

3.1   Soft-Split Random Forest

In the testing stage, the conventional random forest makes *"hard split"* (i.e., either left or right) at each split node and thus assigns each sample with only one path from the root to a leaf node. This splitting strategy is effective when there exist a clear boundary among samples of different class labels. However, there may exist ambiguous samples, which lie near (or even lie on) splitting boundaries (Fig. 1(a)), which could lead to wrong assignment. Specifically, training samples may highly overlap in the feature space (Fig. 1(b)), which makes it difficult to find a clear separation/split. That is, there will be many "hard-to-split" samples close to the splitting hyper-plane, which are ambiguous in some sense. For those samples, even though they locate on one side of the hyper-plane, they are also likely belonging to the other side due to small noise. The conventional way of hard split tends to ignore this fact, and may misclassify sample to wrong side, thus leading to inaccurate prediction.

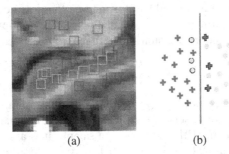

(a)   (b)

Fig. 1. Feature space distribution of voxels inside and outside hippocampus. Red and yellow boxes in (a) represent local patches of voxels outside and inside the hippocampus, respectively. Red crosses and yellow circles in (b) represent feature distributions of voxels outside and inside the hippocampus, respectively. Blue vertical line in (b) denotes a splitting decision boundary.

To solve this problem, we propose to use *"soft split"* strategy applied in the testing stage. The basic idea of *soft split* is that, when a new sample comes to a split node, instead of classifying it into only one child node in each split, we take a probabilistic view and allow each sample go to both left and right nodes with certain probabilities, which are determined by the distance of this sample to the learned splitting decision boundary. Finally, the probability of each leaf is the multiplication of all probabilities along the path from the root to the leaf, and the label probability of a testing sample is the weighted average of all leaf nodes of all trees visited with non-zero probability.

Specifically, in the testing stage of RF, for each split node, we define a *soft split* function based on the distance of the testing sample to the learned splitting decision boundary. Mathematically, the *soft split* function is defined as follows:

$$f_S(\mathbf{h}_t|j_0, \tau_0) = \frac{1}{1+e^{-\sigma d}}, \quad d = \begin{cases} \frac{h_t(j_0)-\tau_0}{r_{max}-\tau_0} & h_t(j) \geq \tau_0 \\ \frac{h_t(j_0)-\tau_0}{\tau_0-r_{min}} & h_t(j) \leq \tau_0 \end{cases} \tag{2}$$

where $\mathbf{h}_t$ is the feature vector of the testing sample, j_0 and τ_0 are the optimal feature index and threshold of the hard split function learned in the training stage, r_{min} and r_{max} are the minimum and maximum feature responses of training samples arrived in this split node, respectively, and σ is the tuning parameter that controls the slop of the function. To avoid the problem caused by different feature scales, the distance d is normalized to [0,1] by using r_{min} and r_{max}. Based on the *soft split* function, we use $p_R = f_S$ and $p_L = 1 - f_S$ for indicating the probabilities of the testing sample assigned to the right child node and the left child node, respectively. It can be clearly seen from f_S that when $h_t(j) \gg \tau_0$, $p_R \rightarrow 1$ and when $h_t(j) \ll \tau_0$, $p_R \rightarrow 0$; e.g., the larger distance between feature response $h_t(j_0)$ and the boundary τ_0 is, the more extreme the probabilities are. To improve the testing, when the feature response $h_t(j_0)$ is far from the boundary τ_0, the soft split function becomes hard split, and the sample is assigned to either left or right child node as follows:

$$f_S' = \begin{cases} 0 & f_S < c \\ f_S & c \leq f_S \leq 1 - c \\ 1 & f_S > 1 - c \end{cases} \tag{3}$$

where $c \in [0,0.5]$ is the cutting parameter.

Thus, using the soft split, a new sample will be split into both left and right nodes at each split node with certain probabilities. Finally, for each leaf node, its weight is computed as the multiplication of all probabilities along the path from the root node to itself. The estimated label probability of this new sample is weighted average of label probabilities of all leaf nodes across all different trees.

3.2   Haar-Features Based Context Model (HCM)

In the section, we present a Haar-features based context model (HCM) to iteratively improve the labeling accuracy by using both low-level appearance features (computed from the target image) and high-level context features (computed from tentative labeling probability maps of the target image). Specifically, at each iteration, random forest outputs a tentative labeling probability map of the target image, from which we can compute Haar-like features. These features are called context features and can be used together with the intensity features to refine the labeling results. In the following paragraphs, we detail the *training* and *testing* stages of our HCM.

Training: In the initial iteration, we first use the simple multi-atlas based majority voting to initialize the labeling probability maps of the training images. Specifically, for each training image, we linearly align all other images onto this image and then adopt the majority voting to obtain an initial labeling map by propagating labels from all aligned images to this image. In the second iteration, for each training voxel x in the training image, we extract Haar-like features from both training image and the initial labeling probability maps. The Haar-like features extracted from training image are called intensity features, and those extracted from probability maps are called context features. They can be combined as input features to train next random forest classifier. During the training of each split node, the minimum and maximum feature responses (r_{min} and r_{max}) are saved, in order to normalize the sample-to-boundary distance for the testing samples (Eq. 2). After the current RF classifier is trained, we can apply it to each training image for estimating the new labeling probability maps by combining local appearance and context information. Since the new labeling probability maps are often better than those obtained by majority voting, as shown in Fig. 2, we can use these new maps to replace those obtained by majority voting and compute the new context features. Once the context features have been updated, a new random forest classifier can be learned. This procedure is iterated until we obtain O sets of RF classifiers, each set containing one random forest classifier for each anatomical structure.

Testing: Given a new testing image, the labeling probability of each voxel is iteratively updated similarly as done in the training stage. Specifically, all the training images (atlases) are first linearly aligned onto the testing image, and majority voting is further used to fuse the label maps of all aligned atlases to initialize the probability map of the testing image. Then, Haar-like features are extracted from both testing image and the estimated probability map to serve as intensity and context features, respectively. Based on both features, with the learned RF, we can obtain new labeling probability maps, which can be fed into the next learned RF to further refine the labeling probability maps. This iterative procedure continues until all learned RF classifiers have been applied. Fig. 2 demonstrates this process of labeling hippocampus on a typical target image.

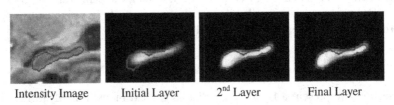

Intensity Image   Initial Layer   2nd Layer   Final Layer

Intensity Image   Initial Layer 2nd Layer   Final Layer

Fig. 2. The labeling probability map of hippocampus at each iterative layer of HCM. Red contours denote the ground-truth boundary of hippocampus.

4   Experiments

In this section, we perform experimental validation of our proposed method on the ADNI[1] dataset and the Head & Neck[2] dataset for evaluating its performance. In ADNI

---

[1] http://www.adni-info.org/
[2] http://www.imagenglab.com/pddca_18.html

dataset, we apply our method to segment the hippocampus from MRI images. In Head & Neck dataset, we apply our method to segment parotid glands and brain stem from CT images. To demonstrate the superiority of *soft-split* over *hard-split* RF, we compare our method to the *hard-split* RF without (HSRF) and with HCM (HSRF+HCM), respectively. To quantitatively evaluate the labeling accuracy, we use the Dice Similarity Coefficient (DSC) to measure the overlap degree between automatic and manual labeling results. In the experiments, we use five-fold cross-validation to evaluate the performance of our method, as well as the comparison methods.

Parameters: In the training stage, we train 20 trees for each RF. The maximum tree depth is set to 20, and the minimum number of samples in each leaf node is set to 4. In the training of each tree node, 1000 random Haar-like features are extracted from intensity image, and 100 random Haar-like features are extracted from the labeling probability map. σ and c in the *soft-split* random forest (SSRF) are set to 0.1 and 0.1, respectively.

ADNI Dataset: The ADNI dataset contains the segmentations of the left and right hippocampi (LH and RH) of brain MRIs, which have been manually labeled by expert. The size of each MR image is $256 \times 256 \times 256$. We randomly selected 64 subjects to evaluate both performances of our method and the comparison methods. The selected subset of ADNI includes 16 normal control (NC), 32 MCI (Mild Cognitive Impairment) subjects, and 16 AD (Alzheimer Disease) subjects. The middle columns of Table 1 list the results for the labeling of left and right hippocampi. We can see that *soft-split* random forest improves over the *hard-split* random forest. With the inclusion of Haar-features based context information, the performance is further boosted. Fig. 3 demonstrates a qualitative comparison.

Head & Neck Dataset: The Head & Neck dataset consists of 40 CT images. Each image contains manually labeled left and right parotid glands (LP and RP), and brain stem (BS). The spatial resolution of 40 CT images ranges over $[0.76 - 2.34] \times [0.76 - 2.34] \times [1.25 - 3]$ mm. The right columns of Table 1 show the labeling results for the left and right parotid glands, and brain stem, which also indicates the advantages of our proposed *soft-splitting* and HCM. Fig. 4 provides a qualitative comparison. To provide some comparisons, we cite recent results from [8]. In [8], the authors proposed a segmentation method based on multiple atlases, statistical appearance models and geodesic active contours (MABSInShape), which obtains average DSC 81% for LP, 84% for RP, and 86% for BS. It is worth noting that this method is evaluated on a subset of our dataset with only 18 high-resolution CT images, while we use 40 CT images containing both low- and high- resolution CT Images. Specifically, for high-resolution CT image set, SSRF and SSRF+HCM methods respectively obtain the average DSC 82% and 83% for LP, 85% and 86% for RP, and 88% and 89% for BS. By comparing our methods with MABSInShape, our methods also obtain better results.

Table 1. The mean and standard deviation of DSC and (%) by HSRF, HSRF+HCM, SSRF, and SSRF+HCM on ADNI and Head & Neck datasets, respectively.

Method	ADNI		Head & Neck		
	LH	RH	LP	RP	BS
HSRF	82.5±4.1	81.3±4.1	77.0±6.8	78.8±5.0	83.7±4.6
HSRF+HCM	85.5±3.2	85.2±3.5	80.5±7.0	81.4±5.1	84.8±4.7
SSRF	83.9±3.5	83.8±3.2	80.4±6.7	81.7±4.7	86.1±4.3
SSRF+HCM	**86.9±2.6**	**86.6±3.1**	**81.3±6.8**	**82.1±5.2**	**87.1±4.3**

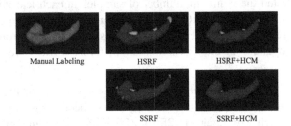

Fig. 3. Qualitative comparison of the labeling results of hippocampus for one subject using 4 different methods (red: manual labeling result; green: automated labeling results; blue: overlap between manual and automated labeling results).

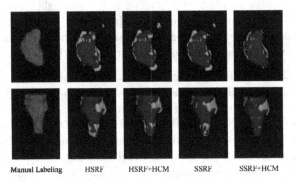

Fig. 4. Qualitative comparison of labeling results of LP (top) and BS (bottom) for one subject using 4 different methods (red: manual labeling results; green: automated labeling results; blue: overlap between manual and automated labeling results).

5   Conclusion

In this paper, we propose a *soft-split* random forest (SSRF) to effectively improve the reliability of the conventional random forest. Besides, the Haar-features based context model (HCM) is also proposed to improve the labeling performance by utilizing the context information of the target image. Specifically, we use Haar-like features to iteratively extract context information from the tentatively-estimated labeling probability maps of the target image. Our method shows more accurate labeling results than the conventional RF, on both ADNI and Head & Neck datasets.

References

1. Wang, H., et al.: Multi-atlas segmentation with joint label fusion. IEEE Transactions on Pattern Analysis and Machine Intelligence **35**(3), 611–623 (2013)
2. Freund, Y., et al.: A decision-theoretic generalization of on-line learning and an application to boosting. In: Vitányi, P.M. (ed.) EuroCOLT 1995. LNCS, vol. 904. Springer, Heidelberg (1995)
3. Breiman, L.: Random forests. Machine learning **45**(1), 5–32 (2001)
4. Magnotta, V.A., et al.: Measurement of Brain Structures with Artificial Neural Networks: Two-and Three-dimensional Applications 1. Radiology **211**(3), 781–790 (1999)
5. Zikic, D., Glocker, B., Criminisi, A.: Atlas encoding by randomized forests for efficient label propagation. In: Mori, K., Sakuma, I., Sato, Y., Barillot, C., Navab, N. (eds.) MICCAI 2013, Part III. LNCS, vol. 8151, pp. 66–73. Springer, Heidelberg (2013)
6. Tu, Z., et al.: Auto-context and its application to high-level vision tasks and 3d brain image segmentation. IEEE Transactions on Pattern Analysis and Machine Intelligence **32**(10), 1744–1757 (2010)
7. Kim, M., et al.: Automatic hippocampus segmentation of 7.0 Tesla MR images by combining multiple atlases and auto-context models. NeuroImage **83**, 335–345 (2013)
8. Fritscher, K.D., et al.: Automatic segmentation of head and neck CT images for radiotherapy treatment planning using multiple atlases, statistical appearance models, and geodesic active contours. Medical Physics **41**(5) (2014)

A New Image Data Set and Benchmark for Cervical Dysplasia Classification Evaluation

Tao Xu[1]([✉]), Cheng Xin[1], L. Rodney Long[2], Sameer Antani[2], Zhiyun Xue[2], Edward Kim[3], and Xiaolei Huang[1]

[1] Computer Science & Engineering Department, Lehigh University,
Bethlehem, PA, USA
tax313@lehigh.edu
[2] Communications Engineering Branch, NLM, Bethesda, MD, USA
[3] Computing Sciences Department, Villanova University, Villanova, PA, USA

Abstract. Cervical cancer is one of the most common types of cancer in women worldwide. Most deaths of cervical cancer occur in less developed areas of the world. In this work, we introduce a new image dataset along with ground truth diagnosis for evaluating image-based cervical disease classification algorithms. We collect a large number of cervigram images from a database provided by the US National Cancer Institute. From these images, we extract three types of complementary image features, including Pyramid histogram in L*A*B* color space (PLAB), Pyramid Histogram of Oriented Gradients (PHOG), and Pyramid histogram of Local Binary Patterns (PLBP). PLAB captures color information, PHOG encodes edges and gradient information, and PLBP extracts texture information. Using these features, we run seven classic machine-learning algorithms to differentiate images of high-risk patient visits from those of low-risk patient visits. Extensive experiments are conducted on both balanced and imbalanced subsets of the data to compare the seven classifiers. These results can serve as a baseline for future research in cervical dysplasia classification using images. The image-based classifiers also outperform results of several other screening tests on the same datasets.

1 Introduction

Cervical cancer ranks as the second most common type of cancer in women aged 15 to 44 years worldwide [1]. Among death cases caused by cervical cancer, over 80% occurred in less developed regions. Therefore, there is a need for lower cost and more automated screening methods for early detection of cervical cancer, especially those applicable in low-resource regions. Screening procedures can help prevent cervical cancer by detecting cervical intraepithelial neoplasia (CIN), which is the potentially precancerous change and abnormal growth of squamous cells on the surface of the cervix. According to the WHO system [1], CIN is divided into three grades: CIN1 (mild), CIN2 (moderate), and CIN3 (severe).

C. Xin—Co-first author

© Springer International Publishing Switzerland 2015
L. Zhou et al. (Eds.): MLMI 2015, LNCS 9352, pp. 26–35, 2015.
DOI: 10.1007/978-3-319-24888-2_4

Lesions in CIN2/3+ require treatment, whereas mild dysplasia in CIN1 only needs conservative observation because it will typically be cleared by an immune response in a year. Thus, in clinical practice one important goal of screening is to differentiate CIN1 from CIN2/3 or cancer (denoted as CIN2/3+ [2]).

The most widely used cervical cancer screening methods today include the Pap test, HPV testing, and visual examination. Digital Cervicography, a non-invasive visual examination method that takes a photograph of the cervix (called a cervigram) after the application of 5% acetic acid to the cervix epithelium, has great potential to be a primary or adjunctive screening tool in developing countries because of its low cost and accessibility in resource-poor regions. However, one concern with Cervicography is that the overall effectiveness of Cervicography has been questioned by reports of poor correlation between visual lesion recognition and high-grade disease as well as disagreement among experts when grading visual findings. To address the concern and investigate the feasibility of using images as a screening method for cervical cancer, we conjecture that computer algorithms can be developed to improve the accuracy in grading lesions using visual (and image) information. This conjecture is inspired and encouraged by recent successes in computer-assisted Pap tests such as the ThinPrep Imaging System (TIS) [3], FocalPoint [4], and the work by Zhang et al. [5]; these computer-assisted Pap tests apply multi-feature Pap smear image classification using SVM and other machine learning algorithms, and they have been shown to be statistically more sensitive than manual methods with equivalent specificity.

In this work, we describe our efforts of building a dataset of multiple features extracted from cervigram images along with patient diagnosis ground truth based on worst histology. We also present some baseline results of applying seven classic machine-learning algorithms to differentiate patient visits that are high-risk from those visits that are low-risk, using cervigrams. We train binary classifiers to separate CIN1/Normal and CIN2/3+ images. All the classifiers are trained and tested on the same datasets, with a uniform parameter optimization strategy. They are then compared by ROC curves and other evaluation measures. Moreover, we compare the performance of cervigram based classifiers with Pap tests and HPV tests results on the same datasets.

2 The Image Data Set for CIN Classification

Here we introduce a dataset for image-based CIN classification, built from a large medical data archive collected by the National Cancer Institute (NCI) in the Guanacaste project [6]. The archive consists of data from 10,000 anonymized women, and the data is stored in the Multimedia Database Tool (MDT) developed by the National Library of Medicine [7]. In the archive, each patient typically had multiple visits at different ages. During each visit, multiple cervical screening tests including Cervicography were performed. The Cervicography test produced two cervigram images for a patient during her visit and the images were later sent to an expert for interpretation.

In our dataset, we collected 345 positive (CIN2/3/cancer) patient visits and 767 negative (CIN1/Normal) patient visits from NLM's MDT. The ground truth diagnosis (i.e. the CIN grade) for each patient visit is based on the Worst Histology result of the visit. Multiple expert histology interpretations were done on each biopsy; the most severe interpretation is labeled the Worst Histology for that visit in the database. Then, for each patient visit, we take the pair of cervigram images for that visit, and extract three types of features from the images: the Pyramid histogram in L*A*B* color space (PLAB) feature, the Pyramid Histogram of Oriented Gradients (PHOG) feature, and the Pyramid histogram of Local Binary Patterns (PLBP) feature. The PLAB feature captures color information; the PHOG feature encodes edges and gradient information; and the PLBP feature extracts texture information. More details about the PLAB-PHOG-PLBP features and their extraction process can be found in [8]. For each image, after feature extraction, the total length of the concatenated PLAB-PHOG-PLBP feature is 2,538. Note that there are two images from each patient visit, which are visually similar but not identical. We have to avoid using one image for training while the other image is being used for testing. Thus we construct two separate image datasets, D1 and D2, and randomly assign one image of a visit to D1 and assign the other image from the same visit to D2. D1 and D2 are used separately in experiments, and each set contains 345 images from positive visits and 767 images from negative visits.

Our image dataset along with the ground truth diagnosis for each image can be used as a new image feature benchmark to evaluate automated cervical dysplasia (i.e. CIN) grading or classification algorithms.

3   Seven Classifiers for Comparison

On the cervigram image benchmark datasets introduced above, we compare seven classic machine learning methods, including random forest (RF), gradient boosting decision tree (GBDT), AdaBoost, support vector machines (SVM), logistic regression (LR), multilayer perceptron (MLP), and k-Nearest Neighbors (kNN). Some of them, such as SVM, have been widely used in the field of medical image analysis [9–12], while others, like random forest and GBDT, are witnessing applications only in the recent few years [13]. In the literature, there have been other works that aim to compare classifier performances on benchmark datasets. Morra et al. [9] compared AdaBoost with SVM while Osareh et al. [10] compared SVM with neural networks. In both papers, the comparisons were done between two classifiers. In the work by Wei et al. [11], more classifiers were studied, but excellent ensemble methods like RF and GBDT were not included. In this paper, we conduct a comprehensive comparison of seven popular classifiers. Next, we will briefly introduce each of them.

Random Forest (RF) is an increasingly popular machine learning method [14]. It builds an ensemble of many decision trees trained separately on a bootstrapped sample set of the original data. Each decision tree grows by randomly selecting a subset of candidate attributes for splitting at each node. We optimize parameters for RF by searching the number of trees in {10, 100, 200, 500, 1000, 2000} and searching the subset size of features for node splitting among {'sqrt', 100, 200, 500, 1000, 2000} where 'sqrt' is the square root of the whole feature size.

Gradient Boosting Decision Tree (GBDT) is a kind of additive boosting model which, in general, can be expressed as function (1)

$$f(x) = \sum_{m=1}^{M} \beta_m b(x; \gamma_m) \tag{1}$$

where β is called expansion coefficient, serving as the weight of the tree in each iteration, and $b(x; \gamma)$ are usually simple basic functions, e.g. decision tree, characterized by parameters γ. Details for the training process of GBDT can be found in [14]. We optimize the parameters for GBDT by searching the number of trees among {10, 100, 200, 500, 1000, 2000} and the learning rate in {1, 0.1, 0.01, 0.001, 0.0001}.

Adaboost is a classic boosting tree model [15]. It has the form $H(x) = \sum_t \alpha_t h_t(x)$, which can be trained by minimizing the loss function in a greedy fashion. An optimal weak classifier h_t is selected for each training iteration t. We use shallow decision trees (i.e. stumps) as the weak learners. In the final strong classifier $H(x)$, the weight of the weak classifier $h_t(x)$ is α_t, which is inversely proportional to the classification error of $h_t(x)$. To optimize parameters for AdaBoost, we search the depth (d) of each decision tree in {1, 2, 3, 4} and the number of weak classifiers from 10 to the whole feature size with an increment of 120/d.

Multilayer Perceptron (MLP) is a feedforward neural network. MLP uses layerwise connected nodes to build the architecture of the model. Each node(except for the input nodes) can be viewed as a neuron with a nonlinear activation function. In this paper, we use the sigmoid function(2) as the activation function,

$$\sigma(x) = \frac{1}{1 + exp(-(w * x + b))} \tag{2}$$

where the weight vector w and bias vector b in each layer pair are trained by the Back Propagation algorithm. We also introduce L2 regularization weight decay to prevent overfitting. We optimize hyperparameters for MLP by searching the hidden layer size in {2, 3}, the hidden unit size in {0.0625*m, 0.125*m, 0.25*m} where m is the feature size 2538, and searching the weight decay strength among {0.0005, 0.0001, 0.00001, 0.0}.

Logistic Regression is a type of probabilistic statistical classification model. For the binary classification problem, with labeled sample set $\{(x_i, y_i)\}_{i=1}^{N}$, it computes the positive probability by (3) and the model parameter θ is trained to minimize the cost function(4).

$$P_1(x_i) = \frac{1}{1 + exp(-\theta^T * x_i)} \qquad (3)$$

$$L(\theta) = -\frac{1}{N}[\sum_{i=1}^{N} y_i log P_1(x_i) + (1 - y_i) log(1 - P_1(x_i))] \qquad (4)$$

In our experiments, we use the batch gradient descent algorithm with L2 regularization to train the model. The strength of regularization is searched from 10^{-5} to 10^5, with an increment of 1 for the exponent.

Support Vector Machines (SVM) is one of the most widely used classifiers in medical image analysis [2,5,9,10]. It performs classification by constructing a hyperplane in a high-dimensional feature space. It can use either linear or non-linear kernels, and its effectiveness depends on the selection of kernel, the kernel's parameters, and the soft margin parameter C. Linear SVM is widely used because it has good performance and fast speed in many tasks. In this paper, we also choose to use the linear SVM; we did try nonlinear kernels such as the radial basis functions (RBF) but they are time consuming and did not improve performance in our task. For linear SVM, we need to optimize the parameter C. Let $C = 2^m$, we search m in the range [-8, 9] with a step increment of 1.

k-Nearest Neighbors (kNN) is one of the simplest classifiers, which classifies a new instance by a majority vote of its k nearest neighbors. In this paper, we use the Euclidean distance metric to find the k nearest neighbors. We search the optimal k value for our task in the range [1, 50] with a step increment of 1.

4 Experiments

In Section 2, we described the construction of two cervigram image datasets, D1 and D2, where each one contains 345 images from positive (CIN2/3+) patient visits and 767 images from negative (CIN1/normal) patient visits. Note that the datasets are imbalanced, i.e. they contain more negative cases than positive cases. Since many classification methods assume a balanced distribution of classes and require additional strategies to handle imbalanced data, we apply undersampling to the negative visits and randomly choose 345 negative visits from each dataset. The resulting two balanced datasets, D_1^{bal} and D_2^{bal}, use all 345 positive visits and the randomly selected 345 negative visits.

We conduct experiments to compare the seven classifiers described in Section 3, on the two balanced datasets D_1^{bal} and D_2^{bal}, and on the two larger imbalanced datasets, D_1 and D_2. The classifier implementations we use are from well known open source libraries. Our Random Forest, GBDT, and LR classifiers are implemented with scikit-learn [16]; the MLP classifier is provided by pylearn2 [17]; the SVM is offered by Libsvm [18]; the AdaBoost is provided by Appel et. al. [15]; and the kNN classifier is provided by the implementation in MATLAB.

We perform the same ten-round ten-fold cross validation using these seven classifiers. On each dataset, we randomly divide the samples (cervigrams) into

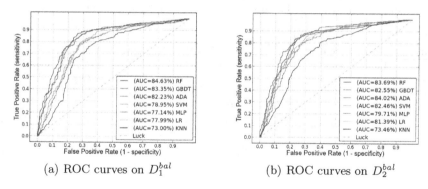

(a) ROC curves on D_1^{bal} (b) ROC curves on D_2^{bal}

Fig. 1. ROC curves on balanced datasets D_1^{bal} and D_2^{bal}.

ten folds. In the ten rounds, we rotationally use one fold for testing and nine folds for training. On the training set, we use a uniform strategy, Exhaustive Grid Search [18], to search for the optimal parameters of each classifier. Three cross validations are used in the parameter searching process. The exact parameters and search ranges for each classifier are discussed in the Section 3.

The results of the ten rounds are used to draw ROC curves. We compare different classifiers by analyzing their ROC curves, areas under ROC curves (AUC), and accuracy, sensitivity and specificity values at the point where the probability threshold is 0.5. We also compare the results of our image-based classifiers with several other screening tests results, obtained for the same visits that are used to construct our datasets.

4.1 Results on Balanced Datasets

In our first set of experiments, we compare seven classifiers on the balanced dataset D_1^{bal} and D_2^{bal}. The comparison results are shown in Fig. 1 as ROC curves and in Table 1 with overall AUCs, and accuracy, sensitivity and specificity values at the default probability threshold 0.5. The ROC curves illustrate that the three ensemble-tree models— RandomForest (RF), GBDT, and AdaBoost— outperform other classifiers. AUCs in Table 1 also show that the ensemble-tree models have a better overall performance. At the 5% significance level, there is no difference between RandomForest, GBDT and AdaBoost. On D_1^{bal}, for instance, the p value is 0.0708 by paired t-test between RF (1st rank) and AdaBoost (3rd rank). However, these three ensemble-tree classifiers are significantly better than all other classifiers. On D_1^{bal}, the p value is 0.0062 and $1.7191 * 10^{-4}$, by paired t-test between RF (1st rank) and SVM (4th rank), and between RF and kNN (lowest rank), respectively. We conjecture that the ensemble-tree models perform best because they are more robust to over-fitting than other models such as SVM and MLP when dealing with scalar data sets that are not too large.

Table 1. Overall AUC and accuracy (accu), sensitivity (sensi) and specificity (speci) at the default threshold on the balanced dataset D_1^{bal} and the imbalanced dataset D_1

Classifier	D_1^{bal}				D_1			
	AUC(%)	accu(%)	sensi(%)	speci(%)	AUC(%)	accu(%)	sensi(%)	speci(%)
RF	**84.63**	**80.00**	**84.06**	**75.94**	**84.83**	**78.24**	**67.54**	**83.05**
GBDT	83.35	78.55	82.03	75.07	82.28	77.07	62.61	83.57
AdaBoost	82.23	76.81	77.68	75.94	82.53	76.44	57.97	84.75
SVM	78.95	74.78	76.52	73.04	79.82	74.37	46.67	86.83
LR	77.99	74.20	76.23	72.17	79.99	75.45	54.20	85.01
MLP	77.14	75.27	77.78	72.75	78.60	76.53	59.13	84.35
kNN	73.00	70.87	75.07	66.67	74.38	71.67	48.12	82.27

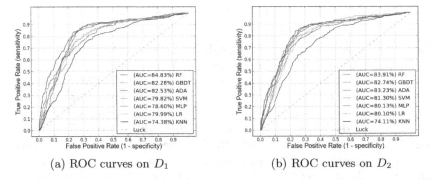

(a) ROC curves on D_1 (b) ROC curves on D_2

Fig. 2. ROC curves on imbalanced datasets D1 and D2.

4.2 Results on Imbalanced Datasets

We also conduct the same ten-round ten-fold experiments on the imbalanced datasets D1 and D2. The results are shown in Fig. 2 and Table 1. One clear difference between results on the imbalanced datasets and those on the balanced datasets is that, at the same default threshold, all seven classifiers give higher specificity values and lower sensitivity values on the imbalanced dataset (see Table 1, right column). This is expected since in the imbalanced datasets, there are more negative samples than positive samples, thus when penalizing equally errors on samples from any class and training to minimize the overall classification error, the classifiers trained on the imbalanced data become biased to the class with a majority of samples. Interestingly, since higher specificity is a desired property for a clinical test meant for screening, training classifiers on the imbalanced dataset (which more closely reflect the true underlying patient distribution) can be beneficial.

Moreover, Fig. 2 shows that the overall ROC curves and AUCs on the imbalanced datasets are similar to that on the balanced datasets. Although more samples are used to train classifiers on the imbalanced datasets, the overall performance by the classifiers did not seem to improve.

4.3   Cervigram Based RandomForest (RF) vs. Pap and HPV Tests

In this experiment, we first compute the average result of our image-based classifier RF to represent its visit-level performance on balanced and imbalanced datasets, respectively. We then compare the visit-level result of RF with Pap and HPV tests results, which are available for the same visits that are used to construct our datasets. As illustrated in Table 2, on both datasets the image-based RF classifier outperforms every single Pap test or HPV test at specificity around 90%.

Table 2. Comparing visit-level sensitivity (sensi) and specificity (speci) of image-based RF classifier with that of Pap tests and HPV tests.

Method	Balanced dataset		Imbalanced dataset	
	sensi(%)	speci(%)	sensi(%)	speci(%)
Alfaro ThinPrep	20.69	81.82	20.69	85.27
Cytyc ThinPrep	49.55	88.46	49.55	89.77
Costa Rica Pap	39.42	88.12	39.42	89.31
Hopkins Pap	36.00	97.11	36.00	97.13
HPV16	33.82	94.19	33.82	92.94
HPV18	08.16	97.97	08.16	98.17
Cervigram based RF	51.00	90.00	49.00	90.00

5   Conclusions

In this paper, we present a new benchmark dataset for evaluating cervical dysplasia classification or grading algorithms. Both image features and ground truth diagnosis are included in the dataset. It is our intention to publish[1] the original datasets D1 and D2, sample images and the source code for PLAB-PHOG-PLBP image feature extraction. We will also add information from other screening tests such as Pap and HPV and expand the size of the dataset in the future.

In our experiments, we adopt a uniform experimentation and parameter optimization framework to compare seven classic machine learning algorithms in terms of their performance in classifying an image into either CIN1/Normal (i.e. low-grade lesion/healthy) or CIN2/3+ (i.e. high-grade lesion/cancer). The reported results can serve as a baseline for future comparisons of automated cervical dysplasia classification methods. From the results, we find that ensemble-tree models—Random Forest, Gradient Boosting Decision Tree, and AdaBoost—outperform other classifiers such as multi-layer perceptron, SVM, logistic regression and kNN, on this task. This finding is consistent with the conclusion in other works [19]. Another finding is that, training and testing on the larger imbalanced dataset (containing more negative samples) give similar overall performance (measured by AUC and accuracy) to that on the balanced dataset (with equal

---

[1] Download from http://www.cse.lehigh.edu/~idealab/cervitor

number of negative and positive samples). However, the results on the imbalanced dataset have higher specificity than sensitivity whereas the results on the balanced dataset have higher sensitivity.

References

1. WHO: Human papillomavirus and related cancers in world. In: ICO Information Centre on HPV and Cancer Summary Report, August 2014
2. Kim, E., Huang, X.: A data driven approach to cervigram image analysis and classification. In: Color Medical Image analysis, Lecture Notes in Computational Vision and Biomechanics, vol. 6, pp. 1–13 (2013)
3. Biscotti, C.V., Dawson, A.E., et al.: Assisted primary screening using the automated thinprep imaging system. AJCP **123**(2), 281–287 (2005)
4. Wilbur, D.C., Black-Schaffer, W.S., Luff, R.D., et al.: The becton dickinson focalpoint gs imaging system: Clinical trials demonstrate significantly improved sensitivity for the detection of important cervical lesions. AJCP **132**(5), 767–775 (2009)
5. Zhang, J., Liu, Y.: Cervical cancer detection using SVM based feature screening. In: Barillot, C., Haynor, D.R., Hellier, P. (eds.) MICCAI 2004. LNCS, vol. 3217, pp. 873–880. Springer, Heidelberg (2004)
6. Herrero, R., Schiffman, M., Bratti, C., et al.: Design and methods of a population-based natural history study of cervical neoplasia in a rural province of costa rica: the guanacaste project. Rev. Panam. Salud Publica **1**, 362–375 (1997)
7. Jeronimo, J., Long, L.R., Neve, L., et al.: Digital tools for collecting data from cervigrams for research and training in colposcopy. Journal of Lower Genital Tract Disease **10**(1), 16–25 (2006)
8. Xu, T., Kim, E., Huang, X.: Adjustable adaboost classifier and pyramid features for image-based cervical cancer diagnosis. In: International Symposium on Biomedical Imaging (ISBI) (2015)
9. Morra, J.H., Tu, Z., Apostolova, L.G., et al.: Comparison of adaboost and support vector machines for detecting alzheimer's disease through automated hippocampal segmentation. Medical Imaging **29**, 30–43 (2010)
10. Osareh, A., Mirmehdi, M., Thomas, B., Markham, R.: Comparative exudate classification using support vector machines and neural networks. In: Dohi, T., Kikinis, R. (eds.) MICCAI 2002, Part II. LNCS, vol. 2489, pp. 413–420. Springer, Heidelberg (2002)
11. Wei, L., Yang, Y., Nishikawa, R.M., Jiang, Y.: A study on several machine-learning methods for classification of malignant and benign clustered microcalcifications. Medical Imaging **24**, 371–380 (2005)
12. Timoner, S.J., Golland, P., Kikinis, R., Shenton, M.E., Grimson, W.E.L., Wells III, W.M.: Performance issues in shape classification. In: Dohi, T., Kikinis, R. (eds.) MICCAI 2002, Part I. LNCS, vol. 2488, pp. 355–362. Springer, Heidelberg (2002)
13. Alexander, D.C., Zikic, D., Zhang, J., Zhang, H., Criminisi, A.: Image quality transfer via random forest regression: applications in diffusion MRI. In: Golland, P., Hata, N., Barillot, C., Hornegger, J., Howe, R. (eds.) MICCAI 2014, Part III. LNCS, vol. 8675, pp. 225–232. Springer, Heidelberg (2014)
14. Hastie, T., Tibshirani, R., Friedman, J., et al.: The elements of statistical learning, vol. 2. Springer (2009)

15. Appel, R., Fuchs, T., Dollr, P., Perona, P.: Quickly boosting decision trees pruning underachieving features early. In: ICML (2013)
16. Pedregosa, F., Varoquaux, G., Gramfort, A., et al.: Scikit-learn: Machine learning in Python. Journal of Machine Learning Research **12**, 2825–2830 (2011)
17. Goodfellow, I.J., Warde-Farley, D., Lamblin, P., et al.: Pylearn2: a machine learning research library (2013). arXiv:1308.4214
18. Chang, C., Lin, C.: LIBSVM: a library for support vector machines (2001)
19. Fernández-Delgado, M., Cernadas, E., Barro, S., Amorim, D.: Do we need hundreds of classifiers to solve real world classification problems? The Journal of Machine Learning Research **15**(1), 3133–3181 (2014)

Machine Learning on High Dimensional Shape Data from Subcortical Brain Surfaces: A Comparison of Feature Selection and Classification Methods

Benjamin S.C. Wade[1], Shantanu H. Joshi[2], Boris A. Gutman[1],
and Paul M. Thompson[1(✉)]

[1] Imaging Genetics Center, USC, Marina del Rey, CA, USA
{Benjamin.SC.Wade,Boris.Gutman,Paul.Thompson}@ini.usc.edu
[2] Ahmanson-Lovelace Brain Mapping Center, UCLA, Los Angeles, CA, USA
S.Joshi@ucla.edu

Abstract. Recently, high-dimensional shape data (HDSD) has been demonstrated to be informative in describing subcortical brain morphometry in several disorders. While HDSD may serve as a biomarker of disease, its high dimensionality may require careful treatment in its application to machine learning. Here, we compare several possible approaches for feature selection and pattern classification using HDSD. We explore the efficacy of three candidate feature selection (FS) methods: Guided Random Forest (GRF), LASSO and no feature selection (NFS). Each feature set was applied to three classifiers: Random Forest (RF), Support Vector Machines (SVM) and Naïve Bayes (NB). Each model was cross-validated using two diagnostic contrasts: Alzheimer's Disease and mild cognitive impairment; each relative to matched controls. GRF and NFS outperformed LASSO as FS methods and were comparably competitive. NB underperformed relative to RF and SVM, which were comparable in performance. Our results advocate the NFS-RF approach for its speed, simplicity and interpretability.

1   Introduction

Shape analysis is most commonly used for registering individual subcortical anatomies to a given template. The template itself could either be created using unbiased registration of individual shapes or by choosing a characteristic anatomical shape from the population. The registration step is followed by statistical analysis, which localizes differences in the geometric shape features at the population level. Different representations of shapes and surfaces give rise to diverse geometric features.

Several recent studies have reported on the advantages of including local shape descriptions of subcortical brain morphometry in mapping profiles of healthy or abnormal cohorts [1, 2]. Shape features are commonly defined vertex-wise on parameterized mesh surfaces of the brain region and thus be considered high dimensional, to various degrees. In many cases, high-dimensional shape data (HDSD) is advantageous beyond standard volumetric descriptions of a brain region in that it is

© Springer International Publishing Switzerland 2015
L. Zhou et al. (Eds.): MLMI 2015, LNCS 9352, pp. 36–43, 2015.
DOI: 10.1007/978-3-319-24888-2_5

descriptive of local, rather than global, morphometry; however, both levels of description are mutually complementary.

Our main contribution in this paper is a systematic evaluation of candidate frameworks for using HDSD as biomarkers within a machine learning context with an application to disease classification. However, because HDSD are, by definition, high dimensional they may require careful treatment in their application to machine learning to avoid common pitfalls associated with high-dimensional data, such as overfitting. Specifically, we compare the efficacy of several joint feature selection and classification methods to handle HDSD as a biomarker for brain disorders. We assess each approach using 2-fold cross-validation on two diagnostic contrasts: Alzheimer's Disease (AD) vs. normal controls (NC) and mild cognitive impairment (MCI) vs. NC. Classification of each contrast was based on two separate classes of HDSD: 1) the radial distance (RD), a proxy for the structure's local thickness and 2) the log of the Jacobian determinant (JD), a measure of local surface area dilation or contraction.

2   Methods

2.1   Subjects

We analyzed AD, MCI and respectively matched NC participants that underwent 1.5T T1-weighted structural brain MRI scans (MPRAGE, repetition time/echo time = 2400/1000 ms, flip angle = 8°, slice thickness = 1.2 mm, final voxel resolution = 0.9375 x 0.9375 x 1.2 mm^3) as part of phase 1 of the Alzheimer's Disease Neuroimaging Initiative (ADNI-1). Our sample included N=72 AD, N=169 MCI and N=101 NC participants scanned at one-year follow-up.

ADNI was launched in 2004 by the National Institutes of Health, the Food and Drug Administration, private pharmaceutical companies, and nonprofit organizations to identify and evaluate biomarkers of AD for use in multisite studies. All ADNI data are publicly available at adni.loni.usc.edu. All ADNI studies are conducted in compliance with the Good Clinical Practice guidelines, the Declaration of Helsinki, and the US 21 CFR Part 50 - Protection of Human Subjects, and Part 56 - Institutional Review Boards. Written informed consent was obtained from all ADNI participants before the study. ADNI is a multisite longitudinal study of patients with AD, MCI, and healthy older adult control [3].

2.2   High Dimensional Shape Features

Previously validated FreeSurfer [4] workflows, including non-brain tissue removal, intensity normalization and automated volumetric parcellation based on probabilistic information from manually labeled training sets, were used to segment the bilateral thalamus, putamen, pallidum, amygdala, accumbens, caudate and hippocampus from the raw brain MRIs. Each segmented volume was visually inspected to ensure its quality.

A parameterization of each surface was obtained using the Medial Demons method detailed in [1, 5]. Briefly, each surface was conformally mapped to the spherical domain. The spherical maps were rigidly rotated to a probabilistic atlas. Next, the

Spherical Demons (SD) [6] algorithm was used to non-linearly register the spherical maps on the basis of curvature. Two surface-based functions were defined at this stage; first, the global orientation function, defining the direction of the surface and, secondly, the local thickness of the surface with respect to a skeletonized medial core. Finally, SD was implemented again using both the newly defined medial core in conjunction with surface-based curvature to match each surface to the atlas.

From this process, shape features are defined at each vertex: 1) radial distance (RD), a proxy for thickness and 2) the log of the Jacobian determinant (JD) which indicates surface dilation when JD > 1 or atrophy when JD < 1. Among all 14 brain region surfaces, there were a total of 27,120 vertices; the RD and JD were defined at each.

2.3   Feature Selection

Classification using high-dimensional feature sets is often aided by prior feature subset selection. This is done to mitigate both the "curse of dimensionality", in which data sparsity scales exponentially with its dimensionality, and the potential for overfitting to training data. FS is distinguished from dimensionality reduction methods in that the former retains original values of features considered important by a given criterion while dimensionality reduction most often seeks to represent the original features by linear combinations of their original values in a lower subspace. We implemented two FS algorithms: 1) the guided random forest (GRF) [7] and 2) the least absolute shrinkage and selection operator (LASSO) [8]. We later compare the performance of classifiers using these subsets as well as classifiers using the full set of features. Feature selection was performed independently on RD and JD sets.

Guided Random Forest Feature Selection. GRF-FS is a recent extension of the random forest (RF) [9] framework in which importance scores from a standard RF are used to adjust the gain of the Gini index in the tree nodes in a subsequent RF. GRF has been shown to select a highly reduced subset of features and is detailed in [7] however we briefly outline it here. GRF is essentially a two-stage RF in which the importance scores derived from an initial RF are used to augment the splitting of nodes in a subsequent RF. Allowing $Gain(X_i)$ to be the gain of the Gini impurity index resulting from using feature X_i to split a node in a given tree, GRF weights $Gain(X_i)$ by the homologous importance score from a previous RF. That is,

$$Gain_G(X_i) = \lambda_i \, Gain(X_i) \qquad (1)$$

where λ_i is defined as $\lambda_i = 1 - \gamma + \gamma \frac{Imp_i}{Imp^*}$. Here, Imp_i is simply the importance score associated with variable X_i in the initial RF and Imp_* is the maximum importance score. $\frac{Imp_i}{Imp^*}$ is then the normalization of each importance score to the range [0,1]. Here $\gamma \in [0,1]$ is the weighting of importance scores from the initial RF. In the GRF framework, features having smaller importance scores are proportionately more highly penalized and therefore less likely to split a node – the criterion for feature selection. We use the maximum penalty, $\gamma = 1$, in order to select a small feature set.

Each forest was composed of 5,000 trees. GRF-FS was implemented in the R package RRF [7].

LASSO Feature Selection. The LASSO is a well-known procedure used to regularize the coefficients, β_j, of a linear regression model subject to an l_1-penalty. Provided a set of standardized features x_{ij} along with centered outcomes, y_i, for i in [1, N] and j in [1, p], the LASSO seeks to minimize,

$$\sum_{i=1}^{N}(y_i - \sum_{j} x_{ij}\beta_j)^2 + \lambda \sum_{j=1}^{p} |\beta_j| \, . \tag{2}$$

This process is the same as minimizing the sum of squares with the added constraint of $\sum |\beta_j| \leq s$. Due to the l_1-penalty, LASSO has the desirable quality of setting the coefficients of unimportant or redundant features to zero. This provides a natural framework for FS in which models are constructed using only features with non-zero coefficients. For our purposes the constraint, s, was determined empirically using 10-fold cross-validation on the training data; the s affording the minimal cross-validation error was chosen.

2.4   Classifiers

Each of the three feature sets was used as inputs to each of three widely-used classifiers. We briefly outline the attributes of the classifiers here.

Random Forest. RFs are a type of supervised classifier constructed from an ensemble of classification and regression trees (CART) that use the majority vote of its constituent terminal nodes to predict the class of a given observation. Each CART was provided a bootstrapped sample of 63% of the observations along with a random subset of $\sqrt{m}$ features at each node, where m is the number of features. The Gini index is calculated for each feature at the present node, v. Gini(v) is given by,

$$\text{Gini}(v) = \sum_{C=1}^{C} \hat{p}_c^v (1 - \hat{p}_c^v) \tag{3}$$

where $\hat{p}_c^v$ is the proportion of observations belonging to class C at node v. The RF algorithm aims to split each CART node by the feature X_i which maximizes the class purity of the resultant child nodes.

Support Vector Machines. We implemented an SVM with a radial basis kernel function where the optimal hyperplane is found by,

$$\underset{w}{\text{argmin}}(\frac{1}{2}w^t w + C\sum_{i=1}^{N}\xi_i) \tag{4}$$

subject to $y_i(w^t\,\phi(x_i) + b) \geq 1 - \xi_i$ and $\xi_i \geq 0, i = 1, \dots, N$. where C is the cost factor that penalizes misclassifications in training examples, w is a vector of coefficients, b is the constant intercept term, ξ_i controls the allowable (functional) margins on either side of the hyperplane, and ϕ is a radial basis kernel.

Naïve Bayes. The foundation of the NB classifier is Bayes rule which assumes conditional independence of the constituent features of X, $\{X_1, X_2,\dots,X_n\}$, with respect to each other, given the outcome. Given an outcome, $Y \in \{0,1\}$ and the set of continuous predictive features, X, a Gaussian NB framework is used in which the class probability estimate is,

$$P(Y = 1|X) = \frac{1}{1 + \exp\left(w_0 + \sum_{i=1}^{n} w_i x_i\right)} \tag{5}$$

where w_i in $w_1 \dots w_n$ are weightings given by, $w_i = \frac{\mu_{i0} - \mu_{i1}}{\sigma_i^2}$ and

$$w_0 = \ln\frac{P(Y=0)}{P(Y=1)} + \sum_i \frac{\mu_{i1}^2 - \mu_{i0}^2}{2\sigma_i^2}$$

where μ_i and σ_i are the mean and standard deviation of feature X_i.

3   Results

3.1   Feature Selection Subsets

Table 1 outlines the number of features retained by the GRF and LASSO methods grouped by the original metric feature set and diagnostic contrast. While both GRF and LASSO are shown to disregard the vast majority of the surfaces, LASSO-FS tended towards higher levels of sparsity relative to GRF-FS.

Table 1. Feature subset sizes from GRF and LASSO.

Method	Metric	AD	MCI
GRF	RD	1185	1360
GRF	JD	1225	1366
LASSO	RD	41	49
LASSO	JD	44	39

3.2   Classification Results

Figure 1 plots receiver operating characteristic (ROC) curves for each diagnostic contrast grouped by shape feature; a separate curve is given for each FS-method-classifier combination. The lower triangles within each plot provide pairwise results of DeLong's test [10] for differences in area under the curve (AUC). On average, AD was most easily separable from its respective NCs, followed by MCI. Several pairwise comparisons remained significantly different following false discovery rate (FDR) correction for multiple comparisons. Generally, NB-based classifiers underperformed relative to RF and SVM. RF and SVM-based classifiers were competitive with one another over the given feature subsets and across diagnostic contrasts. The SVM model based on the GRF-FS managed to significantly outperform related RF-based models in classifying AD on the JD data. The RF-NFS and SVM-NFS methods were the most accurate classifiers of AD based on the RD feature set and significantly outperformed NB-based methods. In the classification of MCI vs. NC, RF was the most accurate classifier in RD and JD feature sets. The RF-LASSO significantly outperformed the SVM-LASSO in the RD set. See Table 2 for exact AUC values.

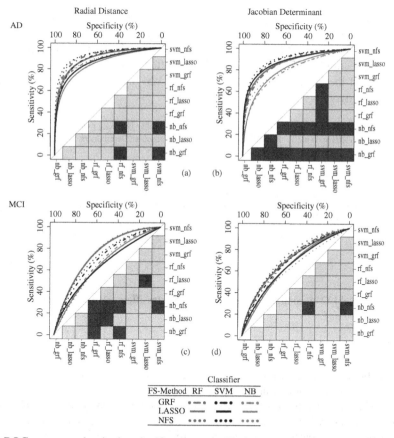

Fig. 1. ROC curves and pairwise significance tests. Each row contains ROCs by diagnostic contrast with shape descriptors column wise. The lower triangle of each figure is the pairwise Delong's test for difference in AUC. Black intersections indicate significant differences in AUC following FDR.

Table 2. AUC values for FS-classifier pairings by shape metric and contrast.

		Radial Distance		Jacobian Determinant	
Classifier	Selection	AD	MCI	AD	MCI
NB	GRF	88.15	66.36	78.72	68.4
NB	LASSO	84.89	64.8	80.54	64.95
NB	NFS	88.66	64.12	80.94	62.78
RF	GRF	91.99	74.67	85.86	70.78
RF	LASSO	90.13	74.73	86.7	69.93
RF	NFS	92.96	74.81	86.84	72.77
SVM	GRF	89.93	69.77	89.17	68.77
SVM	LASSO	86.83	64.02	87.95	65.18
SVM	NFS	93.51	71.98	90.51	71.07

In Figure 2 we average the AUC for each contrast-specific FS method (Figure 2a) and classifier (Figure 2b) in order to explore the general effects of FS and classifiers in this setting. Figure 2a indicates that LASSO underperformed relative to GRF and NFS FS. Interestingly, NFS outperformed GRF often. Figure 2b confirms the under-performance of the NB classifier. Here, RF and SVM are shown to have comparable performances, overall.

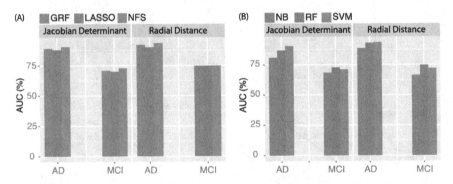

Fig. 2. AUC by contrast averaged across (A) classifiers and (B) FS method.

4   Discussion

In this study, we compared the efficacy of feature selection methods for HDSD derived from subcortical brain surfaces in combination with commonly used classifiers with interesting results. Specifically, the optimized LASSO chose feature subsets that were highly sparse when compared to GRF-based FS. This is notable since LASSO-FS was generally outperformed by the more retentive GRF method as well as use of the full feature space, NFS. It was similarly interesting that NFS tended to outperform GRF-FS. This may reflect a degree of over-specification to the training data proportionate to the sparsity of the selected subspace. Notably, we see from Figure 1 that, while differences between FS methods within the same classifier are present, most statistically significant differences in AUC stem from the difference of classifier itself.

It is admittedly possible that a feature space in $\mathbb{R}^{27,120}$ may not be large enough to push the limits of RFs or SVMs. However, since this is an adequate resolution for shape descriptors of subcortical surfaces we need only to address the efficacy of these methods within this extent. While both are fast, and the extra time needed to perform GRF-FS or LASSO-FS does not amount to any noticeable performance gains, our results suggest to avoid FS in this setting.

While only marginal differences were observed for FS methods, several significant differences emerged across diagnostic contrasts that stemmed from choice of classifier. In the contrasts of AD vs. NC and MCI vs. NC, RF and SVM consistently outperformed NB to a significant degree. SVM and RF offered competitive performances overall. In classifying AD based on JD descriptors, SVM-GRF was significantly more accurate than RF across feature subsets. However, in classifying MCI based on RD features, RF-LASSO outperformed SVM-LASSO.

Acknowledgements. This study was funded by award number R01MH092301 from the NIMH, the NIH 'Big Data to Knowledge' (BD2K) Center of Excellence grant U54 EB020403, funded by a cross-NIH consortium including NIBIB and NCI.

References

1. Gutman, B., Jahanshad, N., Ching, C., Wang, Y., Kochunov, P., Nichols, T., Thompson, P.: Medial demons registration localizes the degree of genetic influence over subcortical shape variability: an N = 1480 meta-analysis. In: International Symposium on Biomedical Imaging (2015)
2. Wade, B., Valcour, V., Busovaca, E., Esmaeili-Firidouni, P., Joshi, S., Wang, Y., Thompson, P.: Subcortical shape and volume abnormalities in an elderly HIV+ cohort. In: Proceedings of SPIE International Society of Optical Engineering (2015)
3. Mueller, S.G., Weiner, M.W., Thal, L.J., Petersen, R.C., Jack, C.R., Jagust, W., Trojanowski, J.Q., Toga, A.W., Beckett, L.: Ways toward an early diagnosis in Alzheimer's disease: The Alzheimer's Disease Neuroimaging Initiative (ADNI). Alzheimer's & Dementia : The Journal of the Alzheimer's Association **1**, 55–66 (2005)
4. Dale, A.M., Fischl, B., Sereno, M.I.: Cortical surface-based analysis. I. Segmentation and surface reconstruction. NeuroImage **9**, 179–194 (1999)
5. Gutman, B., Wang, Y., Rajagopalan, P., Toga, A., Thompson, P.: Shape matching with medial curves and 1-D group-wise registration. In: International Symposium on Biomedical Imaging, vol. 9, pp. 716–719 (2012)
6. Yeo, B.T.T., Sabuncu, M.R., Vercauteren, T., Ayache, N., Fischl, B., Golland, P.: Spherical Demons: Fast Diffeomorphic Landmark-Free Surface Registration. IEEE Transactions on Medical Imaging **29**, 650–668 (2010)
7. Deng, H.: Guided Random Forest in the RRF Package (2013). arXiv:1306.0237 1-2
8. Tibshirani, R.: Regression Shrinkage and Selection Via the Lasso. Journal of the Royal Statistical Society, Series B 267–288 (1996)
9. Breiman, L.: Random Forests. Machine Learning **45**, 5–32 (2001)
10. DeLong, E.R., DeLong, D.M., Clarke-Pearson, D.L.: Comparing the Areas under Two or More Correlated Receiver Operating Characteristic Curves: A Nonparametric Approach. Biometrics **44**, 837–845 (1988)

Node-Based Gaussian Graphical Model for Identifying Discriminative Brain Regions from Connectivity Graphs

Bernard Ng[1,2(✉)], Anna-Clare Milazzo[1], and Andre Altmann[1]

[1] FIND Lab, Stanford University, Stanford, CA, USA
[2] Parietal Team, Neurospin, INRIA Saclay, Paris, France
bernardyng@gmail.com

Abstract. Despite that the bulk of our knowledge on brain function is established around brain regions, current methods for comparing connectivity graphs largely take an edge-based approach with the aim of identifying discriminative connections. In this paper, we explore a node-based Gaussian Graphical Model (NBGGM) that facilitates identification of brain regions attributing to connectivity differences seen between a pair of graphs. To enable group analysis, we propose an extension of NBGGM via incorporation of stability selection. We evaluate NBGGM on two functional magnetic resonance imaging (fMRI) datasets pertaining to within and between-group studies. We show that NBGGM more consistently selects the same brain regions over random data splits than using node-based graph measures. Importantly, the regions found by NBGGM correspond well to those known to be involved for the investigated conditions.

Keywords: Brain · Connectivity · fMRI · Node-Based Gaussian Graphical Model

1 Introduction

Brain function is known to be largely mediated via the interactions between brain regions. Disruptions of these brain connections can result in severe consequences. Functional magnetic resonance imaging (fMRI) provides a non-invasive means for studying functional connectivity. The standard approach for analyzing brain connectivity estimated from fMRI data is to perform univariate test on each connection [1]. However, the bulk of our knowledge on brain function originates from lesion studies and task-based functional imaging studies [2], and hence, is organized around brain regions, e.g. hippocampus is involved in memory processes. Further, how to design treatments to target a specific brain connection is unclear. Devising methods for identifying brain regions that give rise to altered connection patterns is thus beneficial.

A modeling perspective that aids identification of discriminative brain regions is to treat the brain as a graph and characterize each brain region with a set of graph measures [3]. Under this perspective, brain regions are abstracted as graph nodes with connectivity modeled by graph edges. Graph measures, such as node degree (ND), clustering coefficient (CC), and betweenness centrality (BC), are widely employed, but only capture very specific attributes of the graphs, and thus, might at times fail to

© Springer International Publishing Switzerland 2015
L. Zhou et al. (Eds.): MLMI 2015, LNCS 9352, pp. 44–51, 2015.
DOI: 10.1007/978-3-319-24888-2_6

isolate the discriminative nodes. A simple example illustrating this shortcoming is shown in Fig. 1. Despite that the connections to node 1 are different between the two graphs, ND, CC, and BC of node 1 are exactly the same. Recently, a probabilistic graphical model has been put forth that more fully exploits the connectivity information in the graphs for identifying discriminative brain regions [4]. Promising results have been shown in a schizophrenia study.

In this paper, we explore a node-based Gaussian graphical model (NBGGM) [5] for identifying brain nodes that drive differences between connectivity graphs. Compared to the model in [4], NBGGM has much fewer modeling assumptions. The classical GGM (Section 2.1) provides sparse inverse covariance estimates with zero elements reflecting conditional independence between node pairs. The output of GGM is thus a sparse set of edges. In contrast to GGM, NBGGM incorporates a row-column overlap norm (Section 2.2) that promotes selection of entire rows and columns, resulting in sparsity patterns similar to that in Fig. 1(d). Relevant nodes can hence be identified from the sparsity patterns. The original NBGGM (Section 2.3) is designed for finding relevant nodes from a pair of graphs (or multiple graphs), but not from two sets of graphs, which often arises in fMRI studies. For example, one might be interested in studying the differences between two experimental conditions within the same group of subjects, i.e. a within-group study. Alternatively, one might be interested in comparing two groups of subjects, e.g. Alzheimer's disease (AD) patients vs. healthy controls, i.e. a between-group study. Both types of studies entail comparing two sets of graphs in drawing group inference. To facilitate group analysis, we propose an extension of NBGGM (Section 2.4) via incorporation of stability selection [6]. The underlying idea is that if we subsample the subjects many times and apply NBGGM on the "average" graphs of each subsample, nodes that are truly discriminative are likely to be selected over a large fraction of subsamples, whereas false nodes are unlikely to be persistently selected. Also, stability selection has the property of being insensitive to the choice of regularization parameters [6]. We evaluate NBGGM on two fMRI datasets pertaining to within and between-group studies, and compare its performance against using weighted ND, CC, and BC in identifying discriminative brain regions from functional connectivity graphs.

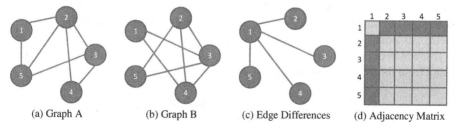

(a) Graph A   (b) Graph B   (c) Edge Differences   (d) Adjacency Matrix

Fig. 1. Motivation example. (a) Edges between nodes 1 and 2 as well as between nodes 1 and 5 in Graph A are absent in Graph B. (b) Edges between nodes 1 and 3 as well as between nodes 1 and 4 in Graph B are absent in Graph A. (c) All edge differences are associated with node 1, but ND = 2, CC = 1, and BC = 0 for node 1 of both graphs. (d) Adjacency matrix encoding edge differences with non-zeros in dark blue. NBGGM promotes selection of entire rows and columns, which produces sparsity patterns similar to (d), hence enables node identification.

2   Methods

2.1   Gaussian Graphical Model

Let $\mathbf{X}$ be a $n{\times}d$ time series matrix with n being the number of time samples and d being the number of nodes. Assuming $\mathbf{X}$ follows a centered multivariate Gaussian distribution, $N(\mathbf{0}, \mathbf{\Sigma})$, a sparse estimate of $\mathbf{\Sigma}^{-1}$ can be obtained by minimizing the penalized negative log data likelihood over the space of positive definite matrices [5]:

$$\min_{\mathbf{\Theta}>0} tr(\mathbf{C\Theta}) - logdet(\mathbf{\Theta}) + \lambda_1 \|\mathbf{\Theta}\|_1 , \tag{1}$$

where $\mathbf{C}$ is the sample covariance of $\mathbf{X}$, $\|\mathbf{\Theta}\|_1 = \sum_{i,j} |\mathbf{\Theta}_{ij}|$ is the l_1 norm of $\mathbf{\Theta}$, and λ_1 controls the level of sparsity. The key property of (1) is that 0's in its solution indicate the corresponding node pairs are estimated to be conditionally independent given the other nodes. $\|\mathbf{\Theta}\|_1$ promotes a sparse estimate of $\mathbf{\Sigma}^{-1}$, but does not impose any structure on the sparsity pattern. Constraining the sparsity pattern to be similar to Fig. 1(d) is useful for identifying relevant nodes. How to exert such a constraint is discussed next.

2.2   Row-Column Overlap Norm

A widely-used approach to impose structure on the sparsity patterns is to employ the group least absolute shrinkage and selection operator (LASSO) penalty [7]:

$$\|\mathbf{W}\|_{2,1} = \sum_{g=1}^{G} \|\mathbf{W}_g\|_2 , \tag{2}$$

where $\mathbf{W}_g$ is a vector with elements predefined to be in group g and G is the number of non-overlapping groups. Minimizing (2) promotes all elements within each group g to be jointly selected (or jointly set to 0). To select entire rows and columns, i.e. impose a sparsity pattern similar to Fig. 1(d), one might be tempted to predefine each column of $\mathbf{\Theta}$ as a group and apply (2). However, due to the symmetric constraint on $\mathbf{\Theta}$, selecting the entire column j of $\mathbf{\Theta}$, i.e. $\mathbf{\Theta}_{ij}$ for all i, requires $\mathbf{\Theta}_{ji}$ for all i to also be selected. Since all elements of each column are enforced to be jointly selected, the entire $\mathbf{\Theta}$ would be selected in theory. This problem is due to overlaps between groups. In practice, assuming nodes a and b are relevant, (2) would only select $\mathbf{\Theta}_{aa}$, $\mathbf{\Theta}_{ab}$, $\mathbf{\Theta}_{ba}$, and $\mathbf{\Theta}_{bb}$ [5], which does not help node identification. One way to deal with group overlaps arising from the symmetry of $\mathbf{\Theta}$ is to use a row-column overlap norm [5]:

$$\Omega(\mathbf{\Theta}) = \min_{\mathbf{V}} \sum_{j=1}^{d} \|\mathbf{V}_j\|_2 \quad s.t. \quad \mathbf{\Theta} = \mathbf{V} + \mathbf{V}^T , \tag{3}$$

where $\mathbf{V}$ is a $d{\times}d$ matrix and $\mathbf{V}_j$ is its jth column. Defining $\mathbf{V}_j$ as a group enforces entire columns to be selected, while imposing $\mathbf{\Theta} = \mathbf{V} + \mathbf{V}^T$ ensures $\mathbf{\Theta}$ is symmetric. Hence, adding (3) to (1) would produce the desired effect of generating sparse symmetric estimates of $\mathbf{\Sigma}^{-1}$ with entire rows and columns selected. How to adapt (1) and (3) for identifying discriminative nodes from a pair of graphs is discussed next.

2.3   Node-Based Gaussian Graphical Model

To identify nodes that give rise to differences between a pair of weighted graphs, one can combine (1) and (3) as follows [5], which we refer to as NBGGM:

$$\min_{\Theta^1 > 0, \Theta^2 > 0} \sum_{k=1}^{2} \left(tr(\mathbf{C}^k \Theta^k) - logdet(\Theta^k) \right) + \lambda_1 \sum_{k=1}^{2} \left\| \Theta^k \right\|_1 + \lambda_2 \Omega \left(\Theta^1 - \Theta^2 \right). \tag{4}$$

Penalizing $\Theta^1 - \Theta^2$ encourages Θ^1 and Θ^2 to be similar, while enforcing sparsity highlights their key distinctions. Importantly, $\Omega(\Theta^1 - \Theta^2)$ imposes structured sparsity such that entire rows and columns of $\Theta^1 - \Theta^2$ are jointly selected, which aids node identification. Given weighted graphs, all edges associated with any node will always display some differences between graphs (let it be small). Thus, in effect, $\Omega(\Theta^1 - \Theta^2)$ helps find nodes with edges displaying larger differences in edge weights. Jointly minimizing all terms in (4) is non-trivial. A widely-used strategy is to introduce auxiliary variables to decouple the objective into sub-problems that are easily solvable. This strategy is the core of alternating direction method of multipliers [5], which can efficiently solve (4). With the implementation in [5], we observed that the selected nodes are sometimes not visually apparent from $\Theta^1 - \Theta^2$. We instead recommend determining the selected nodes based on non-zero columns in $\mathbf{V}$, which we found to provide an unambiguous answer. For the choice of λ_1 and λ_2, we bypass selecting a specific combination by using stability selection, as discussed next. Note that NBGGM can also be used for finding co-hubs between a pair of graphs by applying (3) on $[\Theta^1; \Theta^2]$, i.e. Θ^1 and Θ^2 concatenated column-wise [5]. Also, (4) can be extended for multi-graphs [5].

2.4   Group Analysis with NBGGM

In fMRI connectivity studies, the task of comparing two sets of graphs, $\{\mathbf{C}^1(p)\}$ and $\{\mathbf{C}^2(q)\}$, is often encountered. Here, p and q denote subject indices. For within-group studies, $p = q$ and the analysis of interest is comparing conditions 1 and 2. In the case of between-group studies, $p \neq q$ and the analysis of interest is comparing two groups of subjects. A natural way to employ (4) in finding discriminative nodes is to apply it on the subject averages of $\{\mathbf{C}^1(p)\}$ and $\{\mathbf{C}^2(q)\}$. However, declaring the selected nodes as significant can be dangerous, since sparse methods tend to be unstable, i.e. perturbations to the data can easily result in a different set of nodes being selected [6]. To obtain a stable set of nodes, one strategy is to employ stability selection [6]:

1. Randomly subsample $\{\mathbf{C}^1(p)\}$ and $\{\mathbf{C}^2(q)\}$ by half, and compute their respective averages. For within-group analysis, choose the same set of subjects.
2. For each (λ_1, λ_2) combination in $[\lambda_1^{max}, \lambda_1^{min}] \times [\lambda_2^{max}, \lambda_2^{min}]$, apply (4) to the two average sample covariance matrices. Let $\mathbf{Z}^m(\lambda_1, \lambda_2)$ be a $d \times 1$ vector with elements corresponding to the nodes selected for subsample m set to 1.
3. Repeat steps 1 and 2 for $M = 1000$ times.
4. Compute the proportion of subsamples, $\pi_i(\lambda_1, \lambda_2)$, that node i is selected for each (λ_1, λ_2) combination.
5. Declare node i as significant if $max_{(\lambda_1, \lambda_2)} \pi_i(\lambda_1, \lambda_2) \geq \pi_{th}$.

A π_{th} that controls the expected number of false positives, $E(F)$, is given by [6]:

$$E(F) \le \frac{1}{2\pi_{th} - 1} \frac{\gamma^2}{d} , \tag{5}$$

where F is the number of false positives and γ is the expected number of selected nodes, which can be approximated by: $1/M \cdot \sum_m \sum_i (\mathbf{U}_{(\lambda 1, \lambda 2)} \mathbf{Z}_i^m (\lambda_1, \lambda_2))$. $\mathbf{U}_{(\lambda 1, \lambda 2)}$ denotes the union over all (λ_1, λ_2) combinations. We highlight two insights on (5) that have major implications on applying stability selection. First, (5) is a conservative bound on the family-wise error rate (FWER) = $P(F \ge 1)$, since $E(F) = \sum_{f=1}^{\infty} P(F \ge f) > P(F \ge 1)$. To control FWER at $\alpha = 0.05$ with multiple comparison correction, i.e. $P(F \ge 1) \le \alpha/d$, even for $\gamma = 1$, π_{th} based on (5) is >1. In [6], π_{th} is recommended to be set between 0.6 and 0.9. In this work, we set π_{th} to 0.8. Second, although stability selection does not require choosing a specific (λ_1, λ_2) pair, for $n/2 > d$, a "small enough" $(\lambda_1^{min}, \lambda_2^{min})$ pair could lead to all nodes being selected for all subsamples, thus $max_{(\lambda 1, \lambda 2)} \pi_i(\lambda_1, \lambda_2) = 1$. Hence, all nodes would be declared as significant. Since averaging the sample covariance matrices is equivalent to computing the sample covariance of their associated time series concatenated together, even with e.g. 20 subjects, $n/2$ would be in the thousands range, whereas d is typically in the hundreds range. Thus, to mitigate declaring all nodes as relevant, we set λ_1^{min} and λ_2^{min} such that <50% of the nodes would be selected by (4). λ_1^{max} and λ_2^{max} are set such that only ~1% of the nodes are selected.

3   Materials

Two fMRI datasets from a within-group and a between-group study were used for method evaluation. For the within-group case, fMRI data were collected from 19 healthy subjects as they think about joyful events (happy state) and sad events (ruminative state) in a self-driven manner without external stimulus. The data of the two mental states were acquired at two separate scan sessions, each lasting 8 min. Data acquisition was performed on a 3T GE scanner with TR = 2 s, TE = 30 ms, and flip angle = 77°. For each mental state, the fMRI data of each subject were motion corrected, normalized to MNI space, and spatially smoothed with at 6 mm FWHM Gaussian kernel using FSL. Motion artifacts, white matter and cerebrospinal fluid confounds, and average global signals were regressed out from the voxel time series. A highpass filter at 0.01 Hz was subsequently applied to remove scanner drifts. To define brain nodes, we employed the atlas in [8], which comprises 90 functionally-defined regions that span 14 widely-observed networks. Regions in the cerebellum were excluded due to incomplete coverage. Voxel time series within each region were averaged to generate brain region time series. Pearson's correlation matrices were then computed from these regional time series, which served as input to NBGGM and the contrasted graph measures. For the between-group case, resting state fMRI data of 6 min duration were collected from 20 AD subjects and 20 matched healthy controls (HC) with a similar acquisition protocol. The same preprocessing steps were performed except a bandpass filter at 0.01 to 0.1 Hz was employed. Also, all 90 regions in [8] were used to generate brain region time series.

4   Results and Discussion

In this work, we focused on method assessments with real fMRI data since substantive synthetic experiments had been performed in [5]. To quantitatively evaluate NBGGM on real data, we randomly split the subjects into two halves (S_1 and S_2) in 20 different ways for each dataset, and examined the consistency of the identified brain regions between S_1 and S_2. Consistency was estimated using the Dice coefficient (DC) $= 2|\mathbf{z}_1 \cap \mathbf{z}_2|/(|\mathbf{z}_1| + |\mathbf{z}_2|)$, where $\mathbf{z}_1$ and $\mathbf{z}_2$ are $d \times 1$ vectors with 1 indicating the corresponding brain regions were selected for S_1 and S_2, respectively, and 0 otherwise. Here, $\cap$ is the intersection operator and $| \cdot |$ denotes cardinality. For comparisons, we computed weighted versions of ND, CC, and BC [3] with negative Pearson's correlations set to 0, as required for computing these graph measures. These measures are widely used for node characterization. Specifically, ND is the number of edges connected to a node, CC is the fraction of neighbors of a node being neighbors of each other, and BC is the fraction of all shortest paths that contain a given node [3]. To identify discriminative brain regions with each graph measure, we applied a paired t-test and a two-sample test, respectively, in contrasting happy vs. ruminative and AD vs. HC. No brain regions were found to be significant at $p < 0.05$ with false discovery rate (FDR) correction [9] for S_1 and S_2 of all 20 random splits. To permit comparisons with NBGGM, we took the top regions for each graph measure based on the magnitude of the t-values, with the number of regions matching that found with NBGGM on S_1 and S_2 of each split, and computed the DC. We also tried applying stability selection to the graph measures, but the selection frequency was <0.8 (threshold used for NBGGM) for almost all regions, resulting in DC being close to 0, hence not presented here.

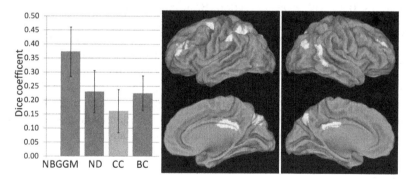

Fig. 2. Happy vs ruminative. NBGGM provided significantly higher consistency in the identified brain regions than the contrasted methods. Regions found by NBGGM shown in yellow.

Within-Group Analysis. The average DC over the 20 splits for happy vs. ruminative are shown in Fig. 2. Comparing NBGGM against each graph measure in a pairwise fashion, NBGGM's average DC is significantly higher based on a Wilcoxon signed rank test at $p < 0.05$ with Bonferroni correction. Applying NBGGM on all subjects detected brain regions associated with emotion processing (Fig. 2), whereas no brain regions were significant using the contrasted graph measures at $p < 0.05$ with FDR correction.

In particular, the left frontal pole is associated with happiness and sadness, and the right frontal pole tends to react to sadness, anger, and fear [10]. The cingulate cortex is involved with processing of anger, fear, sadness, and happiness [11], with the posterior division mainly involved with happy emotions. NBGGM also detected the precuneus, which is responsible for emotional judgment of self and others [12].

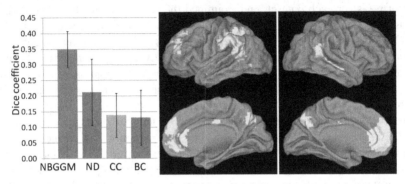

Fig. 3. AD vs HC. NBGGM provided significantly higher consistency in the identified brain regions than the contrasted methods. Regions found by NBGGM shown in yellow.

Between-Group Analysis. The average DC over the 20 splits for AD vs. HC are shown in Fig. 3. NBGGM's average DC is again significantly higher than the contrasted graph measures based on a Wilcoxon signed rank test at $p < 0.05$ with Bonferroni correction. Applying NBGGM on all subjects detected brain regions associated with AD (Fig. 3), whereas none of the graph measures found any significant brain regions at $p < 0.05$ with FDR correction. Brain regions found by NBGGM included the precuneus, the posterior cingulate cortex, and the medial prefrontal cortex, which are known to be affected in AD [13], with memory decline being the primary symptom. Other brain regions included the bilateral angular gyri, which are involved with memory retrieval [14]. The bilateral angular gyri, in addition, belong to the language network, and their detection along with the lateral occipital cortex as well as the supramarginal gyrus, which are part of the visuospatial network, might be linked to specific cognitive impairments in AD beyond the predominant amnestic variant, namely primary progressive aphasia and posterior cortical atrophy, respectively [15].

5   Conclusions

We proposed incorporating stability selection into NBGGM to extend its application to the identification of discriminative nodes from two sets of weighted graphs. A key advantage of NBGGM is that it does not require thresholding the weighted graphs and more holistically uses the connectivity information than popular node-based graph measures, such as weighted ND, CC, and BC that capture only local graph information. We showed on real fMRI data that NBGGM provides significantly higher consistency in discriminative node identification than ND, CC, and BC. Further, the regions identified by NBGGM conformed well to prior neuroscience knowledge.

Acknowledgements. Bernard Ng is supported by the Lucile Packard Foundation for Children's Health, Stanford NIH-NCATS-CTSA UL1 TR001085 and Child Health Research Institute of Stanford University.

References

1. Li, K., Guo, L., Nie, J., Li, G., Liu, T.: Review of methods for functional brain connectivity detection using fMRI. Comput. Med. Imaging Graph. **33**, 131–139 (2009)
2. Friston, K., Holmes, A., Worsley, K., Poline, J.B., Frith, C., Frackowiak, R.: Statistical parametric maps in functional imaging: A general linear approach. Human Brain Mapp. **2**, 189–210 (1995)
3. Rubinov, M., Sporns, O.: Complex network measures of brain connectivity: uses and interpretations. NeuroImage **52**, 1059–1069 (2010)
4. Venkataraman, A., Kubicki, M., Golland, P.: From connectivity models to region labels: identifying foci of a neurological disorder. IEEE Trans. Med. Imaging **32**, 2078–2098 (2013)
5. Mohan, K., London, P., Fazel, M., Witten, D., Lee, S.: Node-based learning of multiple Gaussian graphical models. J. Mach. Learn. Research **15**, 445–488 (2014)
6. Meinshausen, N., Bühlmann, P.: Stability Selection. J. Roy. Statist. Soc. Ser. B **72**, 417–473 (2010)
7. Yuan, M., Lin, Y.: Model selection and estimation in regression with grouped variables. J. Royal Stat. Soc. Series B **68**, 49–67 (2006)
8. Shirer, W.R., Ryali, S., Rykhlevskaia, E., Menon, V., Greicius, M.D.: Decoding subject-driven cognitive states with whole-brain connectivity patterns. Cereb. Cortex **22**, 158–165 (2012)
9. Nichols, T., Hayasaka, S.: Controlling the familywise error rate in functional neuroimaging: A comparative review. Stat. Methods Med. Research **12**, 419–446 (2003)
10. Damasio, A.R., Grabowski, T.J., Bechara, A., Damasio, H., Ponto, L.L., Parvizi, J., Hichwa, R.D.: Subcortical and cortical brain activity during the feeling of self-generated emotions. Nat. Neurosci. **3**, 1049–1056 (2000)
11. Vogt, B.A.: Pain and emotion interactions in subregions of the cingulate gyrus. Nat. Rev. Neurosci. **6**, 533–544 (2005)
12. Ochsner, K.N., Knierim, K., Ludlow, D.H., Hanelin, J., Ramachandran, T., Glover, G., Mackey, S.C.: Reflecting upon feelings: an fMRI study of neural systems supporting the attribution of emotion to self and other. J. Cogn. Neurosci. **16**, 1746–1772 (2004)
13. Greicius, M.D., Srivastava, G., Reiss, A.L., Menon, V.: Default-mode network activity distinguishes Alzheimer's disease from healthy aging: evidence from functional MRI. Proc. Natl. Acad. Sci. USA **101**, 4637–4642 (2004)
14. Seghier, M.L.: The angular gyrus: Multiple functions and multiple subdivisions. Neuroscientist **19**, 43–61 (2013)
15. Ranasinghe, K.G., Hinkley, L.B., Beagle, A.J., Mizuiri, D., Dowling, A.F., Honma, S.M., Finucane, M.M., Scherling, C., Miller, B.L., Nagarajan, S.S., Vossel, K.A.: Regional functional connectivity predicts distinct cognitive impairments in Alzheimer's disease spectrum. Neuroimage Clin. **23**, 385–395 (2014)

BundleMAP: Anatomically Localized Features from dMRI for Detection of Disease

Mohammad Khatami[1], Tobias Schmidt-Wilcke[2], Pia C. Sundgren[3,4],
Amin Abbasloo[1], Bernhard Schölkopf[5], and Thomas Schultz[1(✉)]

[1] Department of Computer Science, University of Bonn, Bonn, Germany
schultz@cs.uni-bonn.de
[2] Department of Neurology, Bergmannsheil University Hospital Bochum,
Bochum, Germany
[3] Department of Radiology, Department of Clinical Sciences, Lund University,
Lund, Sweden
[4] Department of Radiology, University of Michigan, Ann Arbor, MI, USA
[5] Max Planck Institute for Intelligent Systems, Tübingen, Germany

Abstract. We present BundleMAP, a novel method for extracting features from diffusion MRI (dMRI), which can be used to detect disease with supervised classification. BundleMAP uses manifold learning to aggregate measurements over localized segments of nerve fiber bundles, which are natural anatomical units in this data. We obtain a fully integrated machine learning pipeline by combining this idea with mechanisms for outlier removal and feature selection. We demonstrate that it increases accuracy on a clinical dataset for which classification results have been reported previously, and that it pinpoints the anatomical locations relevant to the classification.

1 Introduction

Diffusion MRI (dMRI) provides rich information on brain tissue microstructure, which is known to undergo characteristic changes in many neurological and psychiatric diseases. Recently, there has been increasing interest in making this information available to supervised machine learning techniques, in order to predict quantities such as disease status or severity [6]. An important challenge in achieving this goal is to extract suitable features from dMRI. Ideally, they should not only encode the relevant information, but they should also be interpretable, indicating which anatomical structures are particularly relevant.

In this work, we present BundleMAP, a novel integrated system for tract-based supervised learning based on dMRI data. Its name is derived from the fact that it combines manifold learning using ISOMAP [12] with registration and clustering to achieve a joint parametrization of the fiber bundles in a group

T. Schultz acknowledges DFG grant SCHU 3040/1-1. P.C. Sundgren acknowledges MICHR-02075, Alfred Osterlunds Research Foundation, and Skane Univ. Research Funding, Sweden.

© Springer International Publishing Switzerland 2015
L. Zhou et al. (Eds.): MLMI 2015, LNCS 9352, pp. 52–60, 2015.
DOI: 10.1007/978-3-319-24888-2_7

of subjects. We integrate this idea with methods for outlier removal and feature selection, and demonstrate that this allows us to detect disease, and to pinpoint specific segments on fiber bundles that contribute to the classification. A direct comparison to a previously reported result on patients with systemic lupus erythematosus [8] suggests that our system improves classification accuracy.

2 Related Work

A key ingredient of our method is the use of manifold learning to achieve a consistent parametrization of fiber bundles. Previous approaches to bundle parametrization have been presented outside the context of supervised classification. Many have required manual specification of start and end points [4,5] or manual alignment of a cutting plane [16]. Correspondences were achieved by fitting deformable models [15] or matching to a prototype fiber [7]. To our knowledge, we are the first to treat the joint parametrization of fiber bundles in a population as a manifold learning problem. We believe that this is quite natural, and we demonstrate that it leads to automated and robust results.

3 BundleMAP for Tract-Based Feature Extraction

3.1 Tracking the Bundles

In the initial step, tract-based feature extraction requires us to track the relevant fiber bundles. We demonstrate our method with a diffusion tensor based analysis [2], which is the most widely used model in clinical studies. When suitable data is available, it would be easy to extend it for multi-fiber tractography [13].

Rules for placing seed points for major fiber bundles have been established in the literature [14]. We aim for an automated pipeline that can easily be applied to large groups, without requiring separate user input for each subject. Therefore, we define the seed regions only once, in standard MNI space, and automatically warp them to each subject's individual space using a nonlinear transformation obtained from volumetric registration of Fractional Anisotropy maps, using an established image registration method [11]. Afterwards, the streamlines from all subjects are warped into the common MNI space using the inverse transformation. Performing tractography in the original scanner space allows us to sidestep the difficult problem of correctly adjusting local fiber directions while spatially transforming dMRI data [1].

Even though image registration is widely used in dMRI analysis, it is known to suffer from inaccuracies, the effects of which need to be carefully controlled [11]. Our approach includes two mechanisms that make it robust against inaccuracies in the registration: We eliminate outliers that arise if the warped seed region overlaps adjacent tracts (Sec. 3.2), and we use manifold learning to achieve the final correspondences (Sec. 3.3).

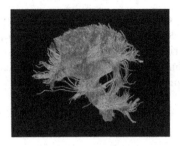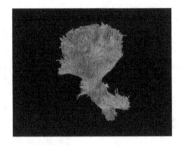

Fig. 1. Fibers from the *corticospinal tract* in all subjects in MNI space, before (left) and after (right) removal of erroneous fibers using a one-class SVM with $\nu = 0.15$.

3.2   Eliminating Fibers from Adjacent Bundles

Due to inevitable imperfections in image registration, which we use to place the seed regions in the individual subjects, we sometimes accidentally include fibers that do not belong to the bundle of interest. We perform two types of outlier elimination to remove them. First, many bundles allow for natural, anatomically motivated filters. For example, bundles that are known to connect ipsilateral regions should not cross the mid-sagittal plane.

Second, in the set of remaining fibers from all subjects, it is often quite obvious which of them are erroneous, since they follow trajectories that differ substantially from the majority of all reconstructed fibers. We use a one-class support vector machine (SVM) [9] to separate out those atypical fibers.

To this end, we employ the feature vector representation by Brun et al. [3], which summarizes streamlines using the mean and covariance of their vertices. The task of identifying the atypical fibers can now be formalized by considering fibers as samples of a probability distribution in that feature space, and estimating the support of that distribution. In other words, we are looking for a "small" region in feature space that should contain most fibers, and we discard all fibers outside of this core region.

A key tuning parameter in one-class SVM is $\nu \in (0, 1]$, which steers the fraction of fibers that will be discarded. In our experiments, we found that values around $\nu = 0.1$ worked well. In order to ensure that results are anatomically meaningful, we allow a human analyst to visually confirm the overall tracking result, and to adjust the exact setting of ν (cf. Fig. 1).

3.3   Manifold Learning of BundleMAP Coordinates

In our framework, image registration provides an initial alignment of the fibers, which is sufficient to eliminate the need to manually specify their start- and end-points. However, it does not yet establish a joint parametrization of the bundles from different subjects, which is required for tract-based feature extraction.

Section 2 reviews approaches that have used such a parametrization for statistical analysis. Similar to them, we assume that the core of fiber bundles forms

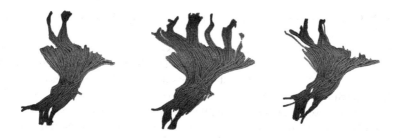

Fig. 2. These anatomical correspondences in three different subjects have been achieved using BundleMAP; same color indicates same position on the manifold.

a one- or two-dimensional manifold, on which data can be projected for further analysis. For example, in tract based morphometry, one of the fibers is selected to represent that manifold, and a parametrization is achieved by matching all other fibers to it [7].

Rather than selecting a distinguished fiber, we follow a more "democratic" approach, in which manifold learning is applied to infer the parametrization from a set of fibers which are all treated equally. This allows for noise and imperfections in all individual fibers, as long as their joint overall shape still indicates the bundle manifold. We focus on the one-dimensional case, since most bundles have a clear principal axis. We deal with the *corpus callosum,* an important bundle that connects the two brain hemispheres and is distinctly two-dimensional, by breaking it down into smaller segments along the front-to-back dimension.

Our implementaton is based on a modified ISOMAP algorithm [12]: We first build a k nearest neighbor graph ($k = 12$) on all streamline vertices. The weights of edges that connect points on the same streamline are set to the arc-length distance between them. For edges that connect vertices $\mathbf{v}_{1,2}$ on different streamlines, we average the projected distances onto the respective tangents $\mathbf{t}_{1,2}$, to eliminate the component orthogonal to the underlying manifold:

$$d(\mathbf{v}_1, \mathbf{v}_2) := \frac{1}{2} \sum_{i=1}^{2} \left| \frac{\mathbf{t}_i \cdot (\mathbf{v}_2 - \mathbf{v}_1)}{\|\mathbf{t}_i\|} \right| \tag{1}$$

Computing all-pairs shortest path distances on this graph and performing multidimensional scaling on the resulting distance matrix provides us with the desired parametrization: It assigns scalars to streamline vertices so that differences between them approximate geodesic distances on the underlying manifold.

Tract-based feature extraction requires a *joint* parametrization for all subjects. Unfortunately, the need to build an $\mathcal{O}(|\mathcal{V}|^2)$ distance matrix makes it prohibitive to simply use the union of all fibers as an input to ISOMAP. We use clustering and interpolation to provide a solution to this: First, based on ℓ_2 distances between the same feature vectors as in Sec. 3.2, k means selects a set of representative fibers on which ISOMAP is applied. Note that the clustering operates on the streamlines, which are much fewer than the number of all vertices, $|\mathcal{S}| \ll |\mathcal{V}|$.

For each vertex that was not part of the ISOMAP computation, the parameter value is found by localizing the k vertices that lie on representative bundles and are closest in MNI space. We then assign the weighted average of their BundleMAP parameter values, with inverse distance weights. At this stage, individual vertices are removed as outliers if their distance to the k-th nearest representative exceeds a threshold. An example that shows the resulting correspondences between three subjects is shown in Fig. 2.

3.4   Feature Extraction and Selection

A straightforward way to derive a feature vector from a set of n fiber bundles would be to average the four widely used diffusion MR measures Fractional Anisotropy (FA), and Mean, Axial and Radial Diffusivity (MD/AD/RD) along each of the bundles, leading to a feature vector of size $4 \times n$. However, if a disease only affects a small section of an elongated bundle, averaging over the full bundle will dilute its effect, leading to a weak feature.

Our BundleMAP parametrization allows us to avoid this by subdividing bundles into shorter segments, and averaging only over those. To this end, we normalize the BundleMAP coordinates to the $[0, 1]$ interval, which we subdivide uniformly into b bins, and only average data for streamline vertices whose position along the manifold falls into the same bin.

The bins should be chosen small enough that some of them are dominated by the disease, yet large enough to introduce some amount of tolerance against imperfect between-subject correspondences. Since it is difficult to guess a good tradeoff *a priori,* and it might differ between bundles, we precompute features that correspond to different binnings, and we use feature selection to decide on the optimal bin width for each bundle as part of the training.

Based on the training data, we determine the Fisher score (i.e., the ratio of the between-class variance to the within-class variance) of each precomputed feature. For each bundle, we then identify the binning that has led to the feature with the largest Fisher score. In the final feature vector, we include all features that correspond to the selected number of bins. It has been demonstrated that, when cross-validation is used, performing feature selection as a pre-process can lead to a drastic overestimation of accuracy [6]. To avoid this, we select the number of bins as part of the cross-validation loop.

4   Results

We applied our method to a cohort of 56 subjects, of which 38 were patients with systemic lupus erythematosus (SLE), 19 with neuropsychiatric symptoms (NPSLE), 19 without (non-NPSLE). The task was to reliably distinguish them from 18 age-matched healthy controls (HC) using supervised classification, based on dMRI data with 15 gradient directions at $b = 800\,s/mm^2$. Details on the cohort and protocol are given in [8].

We included 15 different fiber bundles: *Inferior longitudinal fasciculus* (ILF l/r), *superior longitudinal fasciculus* (SLF l/r), *cingulum bundle* (CING l/r), *fornix* (FOR l/r), *anterior thalamic radiation* (ATR l/r), *corticospinal tract* (CST l/r), as well as *splenium, body,* and *genu* of the *corpus callosum* (SPLE / BODY / GENU). We note that this selection includes fanning and curved bundles, which were adequately parameterized by our method.

4.1 Classification Accuracy

Since the different diffusion measures have vastly different scales, all features were normalized through a z transformation. Similar to [8], the confounding effect of age was reduced by age correcting features using linear regression. After performing feature extraction and selection as described in Sec. 3.4, a linear support vector machine [9] (soft margin, with default $C = 1$) achieved a leave-one-out classification accuracy of 84% (HC vs. non-NPSLE) and 78% (HC vs. NPSLE), respectively. In agreement with previous work [8], we were not able to reliably distinguish non-NPSLE from NPSLE based on the dMRI data (55% accuracy).

For comparison, we also tried classification based on averaging measures over the full bundles, i.e., without using the parametrization provided by our novel method. The resulting accuracy was only 59% (HC vs. non-NPSLE) and 54% (HC vs. NPSLE), indicating that the anatomical localization enabled by our BundleMAP coordinates clearly improves accuracy.

Similarly, our method improves upon a previous work, which has reported an accuracy of 70% for both cases on the same data [8]. This previous work has used a feature vector consisting of all voxels on the white matter skeleton, which is defined as part of the widely used Tract-Based Spatial Statistics (TBSS) [11]. This does not involve any spatial averaging, which makes it more sensitive to imaging noise and misalignments in the registration. It also leads to a much larger number of features ($> 120,000$), which increases the risk of overfitting. In order not to increase this number even more, only Fractional Anisotropy was considered for classification in the previous work, while our approach also uses mean, axial, and radial diffusivities.

4.2 Anatomical Interpretability

Apart from achieving good accuracy, an additional benefit of our newly derived features lies in their anatomical interpretability. As explained in Sec. 3.4, our method computes a Fisher score for each bundle, which is large if the bundle is discriminative, i.e., along some part of the bundle, at least one diffusion measure differs greatly between groups, but exhibits low variance within each group.

For both conditions, Table 1 lists the five highest ranking bundles. Since Fisher scores were slightly different in each cross-validation fold, their average over all folds was used to create the ranking. The results for NPSLE agree well

Table 1. The top five features for each classification task indicate in which fiber bundles FA, MD, AD, or RD are particularly affected by each subtype of the disease.

	Rank 1	Rank 2	Rank 3	Rank 4	Rank 5
HC vs. NPSLE	ILF l	ATR r	SLF l	GENU	CING l
HC vs. non-NPSLE	FOR l	CING l	FOR r	ATR r	SPLE

Table 2. The number of bins that is selected as optimal by our method depends on the bundle and condition, and is chosen in a stable manner.

HC vs.	ILF l	ILF r	SLF l	SLF r	CING l	CING r	FOR l	FOR r
NPSLE	6 (100%)	3 (81%)	6 (59%)	3 (70%)	7 (100%)	5 (86%)	3 (70%)	3 (97%)
non-NPSLE	6 (86%)	5 (51%)	6 (95%)	7 (68%)	6 (100%)	5 (95%)	5 (92%)	5 (73%)

HC vs.	ATR l	ATR r	CST l	CST r	SPLE	BODY	GENU	
NPSLE	2 (100%)	7 (100%)	7 (84%)	7 (95%)	3 (68%)	5 (100%)	7 (100%)	
non-NPSLE	2 (97%)	3 (68%)	6 (49%)	7 (97%)	4 (100%)	6 (84%)	7 (100%)	

with the statistical maps shown in [8]: Four out of the five listed bundles are part of the prefrontal white matter region in which a statistically significant reduction in Fractional Anisotropy was reported previously.

In contrast, the top rated bundles in the non-NPSLE cohort differ from those in NPSLE, and there is almost no overlap with the regions in which Fractional Anisotropy (FA) was found to be significantly affected in the same cohort. This might be explained by the fact that, in addition to FA, our features also account for three other diffusion measures (MD, AD, RD) that have not been considered in [8]. Results from our BundleMAP approach suggest that white matter integrity in the fornix and cingulum might have a special role to play in the assessment of SLE patients; this should be investigated further in future studies.

4.3   Selecting the Number of Bins

In Section 3.4, we discussed a mechanism for selecting the exact number of bins into which diffusion measures along each fiber bundle should be aggregated. In our experiments, we set the maximum number the algorithm could select to seven; we also tried six and eight, and found that it had little effect on accuracy.

For each bundle, Table 2 reports the number of bins that was most frequently selected by our algorithm, along with the percentage of cross-validation folds that selected that exact number. In most cases, the number of bins is chosen in a stable manner. This is reassuring, since stability has been highlighted as a necessary and sufficient condition for learnability [10].

The numbers in Table 2 vary between two and seven, confirming the need to adaptively set the number of bins. The numbers for many homologous bundles (left/right) are correlated. If symmetry is broken, this may indicate that disease affects the two hemispheres differently.

5   Conclusion

In order to use neuroimaging data in systems for disease detection, feature extraction is needed to make the rich information provided by diffusion MRI available to machine learning. In this work, we have proposed BundleMAP, an integrated framework to derive a novel feature vector from dMRI, using a carefully designed combination of image registration, fiber tractography, manifold learning, outlier removal, and feature selection. Our features outperform a previously published result, and can be interpreted in terms of brain anatomy.

In the future, we plan to apply our framework to a greater variety of diffusion MR studies, including ones that involve modern HARDI or multi-shell dMRI data, and to fuse our features with ones from other modalities, such as fMRI.

References

1. Alexander, D.C., Pierpaoli, C., Basser, P.J., Gee, J.C.: Spatial transformations of diffusion tensor magnetic resonance images. IEEE Trans. on Medical Imaging **20**(11), 1131–1139 (2001)
2. Basser, P.J., Pajevic, S., Pierpaoli, C., Duda, J., Aldroubi, A.: In vivo fiber tractography using DT-MRI data. Magnetic Resonance in Medicine **44**, 625–632 (2000)
3. Brun, A., Knutsson, H., Park, H.-J., Shenton, M.E., Westin, C.-F.: Clustering fiber traces using normalized cuts. In: Barillot, C., Haynor, D.R., Hellier, P. (eds.) MICCAI 2004. LNCS, vol. 3216, pp. 368–375. Springer, Heidelberg (2004)
4. Colby, J.B., Soderberg, L., Lebel, C., Dinov, I.D., Thompson, P.M., Sowell, E.R.: Along-tract statistics allow for enhanced tractography analysis. NeuroImage **59**, 3227–42 (2012)
5. Corouge, I., Fletcher, P.T., Joshi, S., Gouttard, S., Gerig, G.: Fiber tract-oriented statistics for quantitative diffusion tensor MRI analysis. Medical Image Analysis **10**, 786–798 (2006)
6. O'Donnell, L., Schultz, T.: Statistical and machine learning methods for neuroimaging: examples, challenges, and extensions to diffusion imaging data. In: Hotz, I., Schultz, T. (eds.) Visualization and Processing of Higher Order Descriptors for Multi-Valued Data, pp. 293–313. Springer (2015)
7. O'Donnell, L.J., Westin, C.F., Golby, A.J.: Tract-based morphometry for white matter group analysis. NeuroImage **45**, 832–844 (2009)
8. Schmidt-Wilcke, T., Cagnoli, P., Schultz, T., Lotz, A., Mccune, W.J., Sundgren, P.C.: Diminished white matter integrity in patients with systemic lupus erythematosus. NeuroImage: Clinical **5**, 291–297 (2014)
9. Schölkopf, B., Smola, A.J.: Learning with Kernels. MIT Press (2002)
10. Shalev-Shwartz, S., Shamir, O., Srebro, N., Sridharan, K.: Learnability, stability and uniform convergence. J. of Machine Learning Research **11**, 2635–70 (2010)
11. Smith, S.M., Jenkinson, M., Johansen-Berg, H., Rueckert, D., Nichols, T.E., Mackay, C.E., Watkins, K.E., Ciccarelli, O., Cader, M.Z., Matthews, P.M., Behrens, T.E.J.: Tract-based spatial statistics: Voxelwise analysis of multi-subject diffusion data. NeuroImage **31**(4), 1487–1505 (2006)

12. Tenenbaum, J.B., de Silva, V., Langford, J.C.: A global geometric framework for nonlinear dimensionality reduction. Science **290**(5500), 2319–23 (2000)
13. Tournier, J.D., Calamante, F., Connelly, A.: Robust determination of the fibre orientation distribution in diffusion MRI: Non-negativity constrained super-resolved spherical deconvolution. NeuroImage **35**, 1459–1472 (2007)
14. Wakana, S., Caprihan, A., Panzenboeck, M.M., Fallon, J.H., Perry, M., Gollub, R.L., Hua, K., Zhang, J., Jiang, H., Dubey, P., Blitz, A., van Zijl, P., Mori, S.: Reproducibility of quantitative tractography methods applied to cerebral white matter. NeuroImage **36**, 630–644 (2007)
15. Yushkevich, P.A., Zhang, H., Simon, T.J., Gee, J.C.: Structure-specific statistical mapping of white matter tracts. NeuroImage **41**, 448–461 (2008)
16. Zhu, H., Styner, M., Tang, N., Liu, Z., Lin, W., Gilmore, J.H.: FRATS: functional regression analysis of DTI tract statistics. IEEE Trans. on Medical Imaging **29**(4), 1039–1049 (2010)

FADR: Functional-Anatomical Discriminative Regions for Rest fMRI Characterization

Marta Nuñez-Garcia[1,2]([✉]), Sonja Simpraga[1], Maria Angeles Jurado[3], Maite Garolera[4], Roser Pueyo[3], and Laura Igual[1]

[1] Department of Applied Mathematics and Analysis, University of Barcelona, Barcelona, Spain
marta.nunez@upf.edu
[2] Physense, DTIC, Universitat Pompeu Fabra, Barcelona, Spain
[3] Department of Psychiatry and Clinical Psicobiology, IR3C, University of Barcelona, Barcelona, Spain
[4] Neuropsychology Unit,Clinical Research of Brain, Cognition and Behavior, Consorci Sanitari de Terrassa, Barcelona, Spain

Abstract. Resting state fMRI is a powerful method of functional brain imaging, which can reveal information of functional connectivity between regions during rest. In this paper, we present a novel method, called Functional-Anatomical Discriminative Regions (FADR), for selecting a discriminative subset of functional-anatomical regions of the brain in order to characterize functional connectivity abnormalities in mental disorders. FADR integrates Independent Component Analysis with a sparse feature selection strategy, namely Elastic Net, in a supervised framework to extract a new sparse representation. In particular, ICA is used for obtaining group Resting State Networks and functional information is extracted from the subject-specific spatial maps. Anatomical information is incorporated to localize the discriminative regions. Thus, functional-anatomical information is combined in the new descriptor, which characterizes areas of different networks and carries discriminative power. Experimental results on the public database ADHD-200 validate the method being able to automatically extract discriminative areas and extending results from previous studies. The classification ability is evaluated showing that our method performs better than the average of the teams in the ADHD-200 Global Competition while giving relevant information about the disease by selecting the most discriminative regions at the same time.

Keywords: Resting-state fMRI · Independent Component Analysis · Elastic Net · Feature selection · Classification

1 Introduction

Brain connectivity is a promising source for diagnosis, characterization and prediction of pathologies, which are linked to abnormal functional organization of

© Springer International Publishing Switzerland 2015
L. Zhou et al. (Eds.): MLMI 2015, LNCS 9352, pp. 61–68, 2015.
DOI: 10.1007/978-3-319-24888-2_8

the brain. The brain functional connectivity can be estimated through resting-state fMRI (rs-fMRI) [1], which reveals patterns of synchronous activity within distant regions of the brain during rest.

Precursor methods for identifying distinctive patterns are mostly seed-based approaches [1]. The main limitation of these methods is the fact that they are model-dependent methods, i.e. they need prior assumptions about the seeds or region of interest (ROI) to study. Currently, Independent Component Analysis (ICA) [2] is used as a reference method for identifying functional networks. ICA is an unsupervised method, which defines distributed functional connectivity networks named Resting State Networks (RSN). This approach does not need previous hypotheses about ROIs, and networks are not limited to a priori selected regions. Moreover, the Probabilistic version of ICA (PICA) [2] includes noise into the model estimate and, therefore, diminishes the effects of noise such as artifacts. More recently, graph-based approaches have been proposed to build predictive modeling based on properties of brain graphs describing the brain function [3], [4]. Graphs are commonly built using anatomical regions as vertices and edges are defined by correlation measures of the regional time courses. However the graph-based approach has been shown successful in diagnosis and predictive modeling [4], but is less used for characterization, because it lacks interpretability in terms of discriminative anatomical regions.

Defining regions in a data-driven way using ICA is beneficial in that it captures the connectivity better than anatomically-defined atlases. Nevertheless, if we seek for a brain parcellation that also takes the anatomical aspect into account, it would require combining the functional and anatomical information, and there is no unified way of achieving this, yet [5]. The benefit of a *functional-anatomical representation* is that it retains the anatomical interpretability, while allowing for each anatomical region to exhibit more than one distributed function. In this paper, we propose a method for finding functional-anatomical regions, that discriminate the abnormal patterns of patients vs. healthy subjects. The presented method takes advantage of the decomposition resulting from ICA in spatial maps and it defines a novel descriptor by combining the spatial connectivity information with anatomical atlas for the parcellation. The approach is based on feature selection [6] to select the set of the most discriminative regions. Many of the feature selection methods fail to do grouped selection and tend to select one variable from a group and ignore the others. This is beneficial if a sparse representation is sought, e.g. in predictive modeling, where adding a correlated variable does not contribute to the model predictive performance. However, in the case of characterizing a disorder, the whole group of discriminative regions is of clinical interest. For this reason, we consider for the selection stage, the Elastic Net (EN) method [6], which provides a sparse representation, while encouraging grouping effect. The method outputs anatomical regions that represent subnetworks within the networks singled out using ICA. A similar scheme was defined in [7], where the Recursive Feature Elimination is used to eliminate irrelevant voxels and estimate spatial patterns. However, authors proposed a univariate data processing and voxel-based representation. Thus, in contrast to our method, they do not decompose the signal, losing the opportunity to define

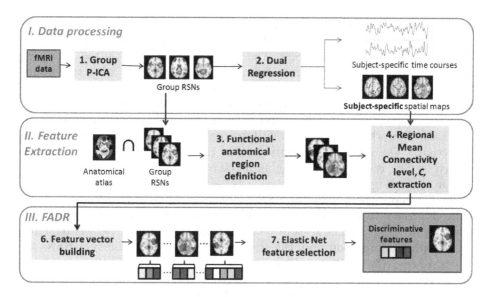

Fig. 1. Flowchart of FADR based on three main stages: I. Data processing: it takes as input the fMRI data from all subjects, it obtains the group RSN and after performing Dual Regression it acquires subject specific information (time courses and associated spatial maps); II. Feature extraction: Definition of functional-anatomical regions by intersecting an anatomical atlas and all the group RSN. For each subject, regional mean connectivity level estimation; III. FADR: it builds the feature vector by concatenating all the features extracted in the previous stage. Note that different anatomical regions can appear several times due to its presence in several RSNs. Feature selection based on Elastic Net. The output of the framework is the set of most discriminative features.

functionally specific spatial maps. The analysis on a dataset of Attention-Deficit and Hyperactive Disorder (ADHD) shows that our proposal is able to extend the results from previous studies and point to discriminative pathological regions.

In the following Section 2 we present the proposed approach for selecting functional-anatomical discriminant regions, in Section 3 we show experiments and results, and in Section 4 we finish with conclusions and future work.

2   Functional-Anatomical Discriminative Regions Method

The framework of FADR standing for Functional-Anatomical Discriminative Regions and illustrated in Figure 1, proceeds as follows:

I. Data Processing. Data processing is performed based on PICA. Group RSNs are obtained and are subsequently thresholded discarding in that way the voxels which are more likely to belong to noise rather than the real signal modeled with a mixture of Gaussian and Gamma distributions (the corresponding threshold here is the standard 50%) [2]. Subsequent dual regression [2] allows to obtain subject-specific spatial maps and the corresponding subject-specific time courses.

II. Feature Extraction. Having acquired the group RSNs, the aim is extracting a functional-anatomical representation useful for the joint comparison of all the areas in the different RSNs. The potential regions within the networks are defined by intersecting regions from an anatomical atlas with the group RSNs.The feature value for each region is then obtained in the following way. Voxel-wise values in a given subject-specific spatial map represent the extent to which a voxel follows the temporal pattern linked to the belonging component. Each network follows a different temporal pattern, which implies distinct connectivity. The mean connectivity level of the i-th region of the r-th RSN, denoted by $C_{r,i}$, is computed averaging voxels of the r-th subject-specific spatial maps in the i-th region.

Let m denote the number of RSNs, n_r the number of anatomical regions involved in the r-th RSN, R_r, and n the total number of extracted anatomical regions, $n = \sum_{r=1}^{m} n_r$. The feature vector for the k-th subject (V^k) is built by concatenating information from the regions belonging to the different RSNs as follows: $V^k = \{R_1^k, \ldots, R_r^k, \ldots, R_m^k\}, R_r^k = \{C_{r,1}^k, \ldots, C_{r,n_r}^k\}, k = 1, \ldots, s$, where s is the total number of subjects.

Observe that, as there are regions which are involved in several networks, the same region is considered several times inside the feature vector. This is not redundant, since a region may be discriminative specially as a part of a certain network (following a particular temporal pattern) but not within another.

III. FADR. Variables in our feature vector can carry considerable correlation among them, since they are formed in terms of parts of RSNs. Thus, we base our selection stage on EN [6], because of its main properties: sparsity and grouping of correlated features. EN is a feature selection method that bridges the gap between lasso and ridge regression by combining their penalties [6]. Similar to lasso, it performs automatic variable selection and continuous shrinkage, by employing L_1 penalty. Combining this with L_2 penalty, it promotes the selection of groups of correlated variables.

Let us denote the set of subject labels with $Y = (l_1, l_2 \ldots, l_s)^T, l_k \in \{0, 1\}, k = 1, \ldots, s$, and $X = (V^1, \ldots, V^s)^T \in \mathbb{R}^{s \times n}$ be the set of n features. Considering the linear regression model: $\hat{Y} = \sum_{j=1}^{n} \mathbf{x}_j \hat{\beta}_j$, $\hat{\beta}$ coefficients are estimated by fitting the model. The criterion function to be minimized is formulated as:

$$L(\lambda_1, \lambda_2, \beta) = \|Y - X\beta\|_2^2 + \lambda_1\|\beta\|_1 + \lambda_2\|\beta\|_2^2, \tag{1}$$

with λ_1 and λ_2 are positive parameters that determine the weights of the terms forming the elastic net penalty function. If we denote $\alpha = \frac{\lambda_2}{\lambda_1 + \lambda_2}$, then the elastic net penalty can be formulated as $(1 - \alpha)\|\beta\|_1 + \alpha\|\beta\|_2^2$.

By minimizing the L function, we extract the set of discriminative features corresponding to the ones with highest $\hat{\beta}$ values. The size of the final set of selected features is estimated as the one which gives the maximum classification performance in the training set via Linear Support Vector Machines (SVMs) [8]. More precisely, we compared the accuracy of classifiers using the k best $\hat{\beta}$'s, with k ranging from 1 to the number of features n and selected the feature set with the best performance.

3   Experiments and Results

Data Sets. Our method was validated on the *ADHD-200* database from NITRC[1]. This dataset consists of separated training and test sets provided by the ADHD-200 consortium[2]. The training set is formed by a total of 765 rs-fMRIs (from 480 control and 285 ADHD patients), while the test set compiles 146 rs-fMRIs (from 80 control and 66 ADHD patients).

More detailed information about the dataset can be found in ADHD-200 Global Competition[2]. There exist different varieties of ADHD disorder and in the ADHD-200 Competition 4-classes were considered: Typically Developing Children, ADHD-Combined, ADHD-Hyperactive/Impulsive and ADHD-Inattentive. In our case, we propose a 2-class classification problem dealing with typically developing children and children with ADHD, considering all ADHD subtypes together, since our purpose is to characterize functional-anatomical abnormalities common to all ADHD subtypes. All the data were downloaded already pre-processed by the Athena Pipeline (NITRC)[1].

Validation of the Feature Selection. ICA was performed using MELODIC[3] and the subject-specific spatial maps were obtained through Dual Regression in FSL[3]. After that the whole framework was implemented in MATLAB and the anatomical regions were defined using the AAL atlas[4]. Feature selection was performed only using the training data to avoid biases in the evaluation of generalization performance. The search space for the l-SVM parameter c was $[0.0001 - 5]$ and we optimized the EN function parameter[5] [9] using 10-fold cross-validation. As explained before the final number of features was selected as the one given the highest accuracy in the training set.

Classification Comparison. We compared the classification performance of FADR method with the results of the methods presented by the 21 teams that participated in the ADHD-200 Competition[2]. Five of the seven sites (members of the Consortium) that provided data for testing gave open access to the status of the subjects (labels). The results of the competition were obtained using the whole test set (7 sites), but we present the results independently for the 5 sites, namely Kennedy Krieger Institute (KKI), New York University Child Study Center (NYU), Peking University, University of Pittsburgh and Oregon Health & Science University (OHSU). In order to stress the advantages of using EN, we also compared FADR with the classification obtained using the whole Functional-Anatomical Representation (FAR) without our proposed feature selection stage.

Results. ICA analysis was ran with automatic estimation of the number of ICs which resulted in 21 ICs. The initial feature vector of FADR method was formed

---

[1] http://www.nitrc.org/plugins/mwiki/index.php/neurobureau:AthenaPipeline

[2] http://fcon_1000.projects.nitrc.org/indi/adhd200/results.html

[3] MELODIC and DualRegression are part of FMRIB Software Library (FSL) (www.fmrib.ox.ac.uk/fsl).

[4] Automated Anatomical Labeling (AAL) www.gin.cnrs.fr/spip.php?article217.

[5] http://www.stanford.edu/~hastie/glmnet_matlab/

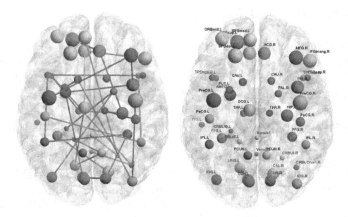

Fig. 2. Representation of the 59 selected regions (FADR method outcome). Regions belonging to the same RSN (functionally connected) share the same color and the size of the spheres correspond to the discriminative power assigned by FADR. On the left, functional connections among regions are also drawn as edges. Regions were visualized with BrainNet Viewer (Xia et al., 2013, http://www.nitrc.org/projects/bnv/)

by 1,259 regions, by concatenating the regions involved in the 21 ICs. The final set of 59 selected regions is listed in Table 1 and illustrated in Figure 2. Using these 59 features the accuracy in the training set was 79.84%. Observe that the impact of EN drastically reduced the final set of selected regions. These regions participate in different distributed functions, as is indicated in RSN columns in Table 1. This can be inspected by the experts for further characterization which is the principal advantage of our method. According to [10], [11], [12] and [13] most of the regions selected by our model are interpretable as related with ADHD: subnetwork #1 and #2 involve Basal Ganglia, together with Thalamus in subnetwork #21; subnetwork #3, #4 and #7 involve Frontal Gyrus; subnet-

Table 1. Set of the 59 selected regions (FADR outcome). ID is just an identifier of each particular feature. In the columns RSN we show to which RSN each anatomical region belongs. We have maintained the original labels (names) of the anatomical regions.

ID	RSN	Anatomical region	ID	RSN	Anatomical region	Feature	RSN	Anatomical region	ID	RSN	Anatomical region
1	7	Precuneus_L	16	7	Cerebelum_Crus1_R	31	6	Cingulum_Mid_L	46	7	Postcentral_L
2	3	Precuneus_R	17	4	Frontal_Sup_Medial_L	32	9	Vermis_3	47	7	Temporal_Pole_Sup_L
3	10	Thalamus_L	18	12	Temporal_Pole_Mid_R	33	13	Fusiform_R	48	21	Thalamus_R
4	21	Lingual_L	19	8	Cerebelum_6_R	34	14	Temporal_Pole_Sup_R	49	9	Temporal_Inf_L
5	7	Postcentral_R	20	7	Parietal_Inf_L	35	2	Frontal_Mid_Orb_L	50	5	Cuneus_L
6	19	Fusiform_L	21	16	Precuneus_R	36	3	Frontal_Inf_Tri_R	51	21	Calcarine_L
7	2	Caudate_L	22	10	Parietal_Inf_L	37	11	Insula_R	52	2	Caudate_R
8	10	Cingulum_Mid_L	23	2	Temporal_Pole_Mid_L	38	3	Frontal_Mid_R	53	10	Calcarine_R
9	2	Hippocampus_R	24	17	Cingulum_Ant_R	39	17	Precentral_L	54	4	Temporal_Pole_Sup_L
10	7	Parietal_Inf_R	25	3	Precentral_R	40	21	Occipital_Inf_L	55	17	Vermis_9
11	21	Cerebelum_4_5_L	26	4	Frontal_Sup_L	41	2	Postcentral_R	56	10	Frontal_Mid_Orb_L
12	2	Fusiform_R	27	7	Cuneus_R	42	14	Occipital_Inf_R	57	10	Rectus_L
13	13	Putamen_L	28	9	Occipital_Inf_R	43	19	Precentral_R	58	21	Cerebelum_10_L
14	7	Cerebelum_6_R	29	1	Amygdala_L	44	16	Cingulum_Mid_L	59	6	Precentral_R
15	16	Precuneus_L	30	7	Frontal_Sup_Orb_L	45	1	Pallidum_R			

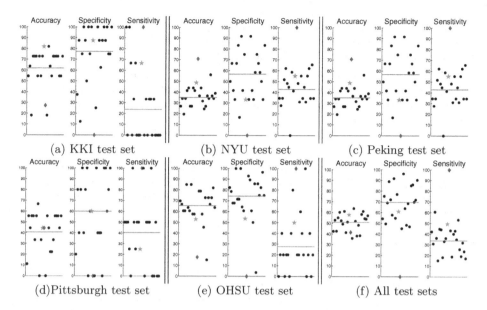

Fig. 3. Comparison of Accuracy, Sensitivity and Specificity for FAR, FADR and the 21 methods of the competition using the 5 different test sets independently (from (a) to (e)) and all together (f). The results of the 21 teams are shown in black circles, green star correspond to FADR and red diamond to FAR. The horizontal line represents the mean value of the 21 participants in the competition.

work #6, #10 and #17 involve cingulate cortex; and subnetwork #7 and #10 involve parietal lobule.

Fig. 3 shows the obtained Accuracy, Sensitivity and Specificity separately for each test set. As can be seen FADR is able to outperform the mean of the teams Accuracy except for the OHSU dataset. FADR gives the highest accuracy for the KKI test set, the second highest accuracy for NYU and the third highest accuracy for Peking. Moreover, it is important to note that our main objective was not the classification, but the characterization using rest fMRI providing the most discriminative regions. Finally, the poor results obtained with FAR proved the necessity of the feature selection stage.

4   Conclusions

In this paper, we presented the novel method FADR for selecting a discriminative subset of functional-anatomical regions of the brain in order to characterize functional connectivity abnormalities. For that, we proposed a supervised framework combining ICA with Elastic Net strategy and defined a new descriptor based on both functional and anatomical information. The proposed representation allowed to show that a certain anatomical region may be discriminative specifically according to one function, but not another. We showed the benefits of using EN for obtaining a good classification performance, while localizing the most discriminative regions, which is crucial in further clinical interpretations. This study was consistent with previous results in ADHD.

Future work will consist of studying the manner of using EN-based feature selection strategies on graphs, to combine the diagnostic power of graphs with the possibility to explicitly obtain and interpret important connectivity networks related to specific diseases.

Acknowledgments. This work was partly supported by the Spanish Ministry of Science and Innovation (TIN2012-38187-C03-01), by Catalan Government (2014-SGR-1219), and by the Vice-rectorship for Science and Teaching Policy, University of Barcelona.

References

1. Biswal, B.B., Mennes, M., Zuo, X.N., et al.: Toward discovery science of human brain function. PNAS **107**(10), 4734–4739 (2010)
2. Calhoun, V.D., Liu, J., Adali, T.: A review of group ICA for fMRI data and ICA for joint inference of imaging, genetic, and ERP data. NeuroImage **45**(1, Supplement 1), S163–S172 (2009). Mathematics in Brain Imaging
3. Bullmore, E., Sporns, O.: Complex brain networks: graph theoretical analysis of structural and functional systems. Nature Reviews Neuroscience **10**(3), 186–198 (2009)
4. Richiardi, J., Achard, S., Bunke, H., Van De Ville, D.: Machine learning with brain graphs: Predictive modeling approaches for functional imaging in systems neuroscience. IEEE Signal Process. Mag. **30**(3), 58–70 (2013)
5. Varoquaux, G., Craddock, R.C.: Learning and comparing functional connectomes across subjects. NeuroImage **80**, 405–415 (2013)
6. Zou, H., Hastie, T.: Regularization and variable selection via the elastic net. Journal of the Royal Statistical Society **67**(2), 301–320 (2005)
7. De Martino, F., Valente, G., Staeren, N., Ashburner, J., Goebel, R., Formisano, E.: Combining multivariate voxel selection and support vector machines for mapping and classification of fMRI spatial patterns. NeuroImage **43**(1), 44–58 (2008)
8. Pereira, F., Mitchell, T., Botvinick, M.: Machine learning classifiers and fMRI: a tutorial overview. NeuroImage **45**(1 Suppl.), S199–209 (2009)
9. Friedman, J., Hastie, T., Tibshirani, R.: Regularization paths for generalized linear models via coordinate descent. Journal of Statistical Software **33**(1), 1–22 (2010)
10. Posner, J., Park, C., Wang, Z.: Connecting the dots: A review of resting connectivity MRI studies in attention-deficit/hyperactivity disorder. Neuropsychology Review, 1–13 (2014)
11. Institute, A.: Adhd institute, January 2015. http://www.adhd-institute.com/burden-of-adhd/aetiology/neurobiology/
12. Wang, X., Jiao, Y., Tang, T., Wang, H., Lu, Z.: Altered regional homogeneity patterns in adults with attention-deficit hyperactivity disorder. European Journal of Radiology **82**(9), 1552–1557 (2013)
13. Morein-Zamir, S., Dodds, C., Hartevelt, T.J., Schwarzkopf, W., Sahakian, B., Müller, U., Robbins, T.: Hypoactivation in right inferior frontal cortex is specifically associated with motor response inhibition in adult adhd. Human Brain Mapping **35**(10), 5141–5152 (2014)

Craniomaxillofacial Deformity Correction via Sparse Representation in Coherent Space

Zuoyong Li[1,2], Le An[2], Jun Zhang[2], Li Wang[2], James J. Xia[3,4], and Dinggang Shen[2(✉)]

[1] Department of Computer Science, Minjiang University, Fuzhou, China
[2] Department of Radiology and BRIC, University of North Carolina at Chapel Hill, Chapel Hill, USA
dinggang_shen@med.unc.edu
[3] Department of Oral and Maxillofacial Surgery, Houston Methodist Research Institute, Weill Medical College of Cornell University, New York, USA
[4] Department of Oral and Craniomaxillofacial Science, Shanghai Ninth Hospital, Shanghai Jiao Tong University, School of Medicine, Shanghai, China

Abstract. Orthognathic surgery is popular for patients with craniomaxillofacial (CMF) deformity. For orthognathic surgical planning, it is critical to have a patient-specific jaw reference model as guidance. One way is to estimate a normal jaw shape for the patient, by first searching for a normal subject with similar midface and then borrowing his/her (normal) jaw shape as reference. Intuitively, we can search for multiple normal subjects with similar midface and then linearly combine them as final reference. The respective coefficients for linear combination can be estimated, i.e., by sparse representation of patient's midface by midfaces of all training normal subjects. However, this approach implicitly assumes that the representation of midface shapes is strongly correlated with the representation of jaw shapes, which is unfortunately difficult to meet in practice due to generally different data distributions of shapes of midfaces and jaws. To address this limitation, we propose to estimate the patient-specific jaw reference model in a coherent space. Specifically, we first employ canonical correlation analysis (CCA) to map the midface and jaw landmarks of training normal subjects into a coherent space, in which their correlation is maximized. Then, in the coherent space, the mapped midface landmarks of patient can be sparsely represented by the mapped midface landmarks of training normal subjects. Those learned sparse coefficients can now be used to combine the jaw landmarks of training normal subjects for estimating the normal jaw landmarks for patient and then building normal jaw shape reference model. Moreover, we also iteratively maximize the correlation between the midface and the jaw shapes in the new coherent space with a multi-layer mapping and refinement (MMR) process. Experimental results on real clinical data show that the proposed method can more accurately reconstruct the normal jaw shape for patient than the competing methods.

1   Introduction

Craniomaxillofacial (CMF) surgeries are required for a significant number of patients with CMF deformity in the United States [1]. Among different kinds of CMF surgeries,

© Springer International Publishing Switzerland 2015
L. Zhou et al. (Eds.): MLMI 2015, LNCS 9352, pp. 69–76, 2015.
DOI: 10.1007/978-3-319-24888-2_9

orthognathic surgery is one of the most performed procedures on *patients with normal midface but abnormal jaw*. The surgery repositions all the displaced bones to their normal positions, and replaces the missing skeletal parts with bone grafts or alloplasts if needed. The success of orthognathic surgery depends *not only* on the surgical techniques, *but also* on the accurate surgical plans. However, in practice, surgical planning is extremely challenging due to the complexity of patient-specific deformity. Conventional surgical planning is achieved in the following way: a surgeon first cuts a 3D model, and then moves and rotates the bony segments to a desired position based on the "averageness" of normal subjects.

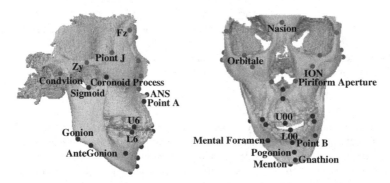

Fig. 1. Sample midface landmarks (red points) and jaw landmarks (blue points).

The conventional surgical planning is subjective and highly dependent on the surgeon's experience. For more accurate surgery planning, a patient-specific jaw reference model is desired. The patient-specific model should predict the normal jaw shape for a patient with CMF deformity, in order to help surgeons determine the difference between the original deformed shape and the reference shape for the development of a feasible surgical plan. To achieve this goal, Ren *et al.* [2] proposed a sparse representation (SR)-based method. Specifically, the bony landmarks on maxilla and mandible sub-models [3-4], divided from a 3D surface model [5], can be grouped into midface and jaw landmarks as shown in Fig. 1. After grouping, the landmarks of all normal subjects and all patients are first linearly aligned to a common landmark template, and then these aligned midface and jaw landmarks of all normal subjects are used to construct a pair of over-complete dictionaries for midface and jaw, respectively. Afterwards, the midface dictionary is used to sparsely represent the aligned midface landmarks of a patient, and the learned sparse coefficients can be directly applied to the normal jaw dictionary for predicting the patient-specific jaw reference shape, i.e., the estimated jaw landmarks after correction.

A basic assumption in the above SR-based approach [2] is that the midface and jaw landmarks have high correlation, such that the sparse coefficients learned from the midface landmarks can be directly applied to predict the jaw landmarks. However, in practice, the midface and jaw landmarks are not necessarily correlated well. As a result, directly applying the learned coefficients may lead to sub-optimal results. To cope with this issue, we first map both midface and jaw landmarks into a coherent space by using canonical correlation analysis (CCA) [6]. Since the midface and jaw landmarks can now be better correlated in the coherent space, the sparse coefficients learned from the mapped midface landmarks are applied to the mapped jaw landmarks with more confidence. In addition, we also introduce a multi-layer mapping scheme by first iteratively refining the subject samples of midface and jaw landmarks in the respective dictionaries and then refining the estimation result in a similar manner.

In the following, details of the proposed method are described in Section 2. Then, we report experimental results in Section 3 and draw conclusion in Section 4.

2   Method

The overview of the proposed method is given in Fig. 2. Specifically, the training data are used to learn the mappings to the coherent space via CCA, and also used to build the intermediate dictionaries in the respective coherent space during the multi-layer mapping process. Then, for the midface landmarks of a given patient, we can estimate a set of *corrected* jaw landmarks for the patient by using the learned sparse coefficients in the final coherent space. Before detailing our method, we discuss below a simple SR-based (baseline) method [2].

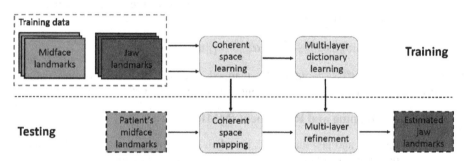

Fig. 2. Flowchart of the proposed method.

2.1   Sparse Representation (SR)-Based Jaw Prediction

Given the midface landmarks of a patient, denoted by a vector x^{mid}, the goal of SR [2] is to predict the desired normal jaw landmarks x^{jaw} after surgical correction, by using a coupled dictionary pair, D^{mid} and D^{jaw}, constructed from the midface and jaw landmarks of training normal subjects. Note that the landmarks of all subjects have been aligned to a common template before dictionary construction.

The reconstruction coefficients α for x^{mid} are learned by reconstructing x^{mid} using the midface dictionary D^{mid} in the following minimization problem:

$$\min_{\alpha} \left\| x^{mid} - D^{mid}\alpha \right\|_2^2 + \lambda_1 \|\alpha\|_1 + \lambda_2 \|\alpha\|_2^2, \tag{1}$$

where both L1 and L2 penalty terms are applied to α. Eq. (1) is referred to as Elastic Net [7]. As compared to the standard sparse coding in a Lasso problem [8], in which only the L1 penalty term is used, the introduction of the L2 penalty term encourages a grouping effect such that the correlated atoms in D^{mid} are more likely to be selected jointly. With the learned reconstruction coefficients α, the desired normal jaw landmarks for the patient can be estimated by

$$x^{jaw} = D^{jaw}\alpha. \tag{2}$$

2.2 Mapping-Based Sparse Representation for Jaw Prediction

- **Coherent Space Learning by CCA**

As mentioned, in practice, the correlation between the corresponding elements (midface and jaw) in the coupled dictionaries, D^{mid} and D^{jaw} (built from the training normal subjects), is not necessarily high. To maximize it, we first apply CCA [6] to find their respective mappings, W_{mid} and W_{jaw}, to the coherent space, so that the correlation between the mapped dictionary pair, $\tilde{D}^{mid}$ and $\tilde{D}^{jaw}$, can be maximized.

- **Jaw Prediction in Coherent Space**

In the coherent space, the sparse reconstruction of x^{mid} can be similarly performed as in Eq. (1). Specifically, the reconstruction coefficients α are obtained by using the following updated objective function:

$$\min_{\alpha} \left\| \tilde{x}^{mid} - \tilde{D}^{mid}\alpha \right\|_2^2 + \lambda_1 \|\alpha\|_1 + \lambda_2 \|\alpha\|_2^2, \tag{3}$$

where $\tilde{x}^{mid} = W_{mid}^T x^{mid}$ contains the mapped midface landmarks of the patient. The estimated jaw landmarks of the patient can be given by $x^{jaw} = D^{jaw}\alpha$.

- **Multi-layer Mapping and Refinement (MMR)**

Mapping the midface and jaw landmarks into their coherent space using CCA as stated above can improve the correlation between midface and jaw landmarks of training subjects. But there may still exist large gap between the distributions of midface landmarks and jaw landmarks. To further address this issue, inspired by multiple dictionary learning [9], we use a multi-layer mapping scheme to improve the estimation of normal jaw landmarks for the patient in a coarse-to-fine manner. Specifically, we learn multiple pairs of intermediate dictionaries in-between D^{mid} and D^{jaw} to gradually align the distribution of midface landmarks and the distribution of jaw landmarks.

In the training stage, the first intermediate dictionary is built by using a leave-one-out strategy from D^{mid}. Specifically, each atom d_i^{mid} in D^{mid} is sparsely represented by all other atoms in D^{mid}, which can be denoted as $D_{\sim i}^{mid}$ that is constructed from D^{mid} by removing d_i^{mid}. Then, the learned reconstruction coefficients can be applied to $D_{\sim i}^{jaw}$ that corresponds to $D_{\sim i}^{mid}$, and a new updated atom d_i^1 is obtained. By repeating on all atoms in D^{mid}, we can build an intermediate dictionary D^1, with all obtained d_i^1. Similarly, we can construct multiple intermediate dictionaries such as $D^1, D^2, ..., D^S$, from the original jaw dictionary D^{jaw}. The atoms in the intermediate dictionaries can be perceived as transitional states from midface landmarks to jaw landmarks.

During the testing, a patient's midface landmark set, $\tilde{x}^{mid}$, is first reconstructed by $\tilde{D}^{mid}$ and then the coefficients are applied to D^{jaw} for an intermediate estimation x^1. Then, x^1 is reconstructed by D^1 and, by applying the learned coefficients on D^{jaw} again, the estimation x^2 is obtained for the second intermediate layer. Similar process iterates and, at the last intermediate layer, the final output x^{jaw} is estimated from D^{jaw} by using the reconstruction coefficients learned from x^S and D^S. Fig. 3 illustrates this multi-layer refinement process. The iteration number of MMR is empirically set to 10.

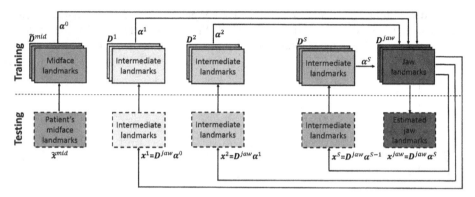

Fig. 3. Multi-layer mapping refinement for estimation.

3　Experiments

3.1　Dataset

Our dataset includes 30 normal subjects and 30 patients with CMF deformity who had already undergone double-jaw orthognathic surgery. They were randomly selected from our clinical archive database with computed tomography (CT) scans. Each subject has 58 manually annotated landmarks, including 31 midface landmarks and 27 jaw landmarks (some of the representative landmarks are shown in Fig.1).

3.2　Measurement

To quantitatively evaluate the proposed method, a measurement named "**normality score**" is introduced. It ranges from 0 to 1, denoting deformity to normality. Specifically, the score is calculated via sparse representation and a linear mapping as follows. 1) **Sparse representation:** Similar to the sparse representation introduced in Section 2, a dictionary is first constructed by all training normal subjects and also training patient subjects, which are already aligned to the common template. Note that the training normal subjects selected to build the patient-specific reference model are removed from this dictionary. Then, the built patient-specific reference model can be sparsely represented by this dictionary to obtain the sparse coefficient vector. 2) **Linear mapping:** In the above dictionary, each included normal subject is labeled with "1", while each included patient subject is labeled with "0". In this way, we can have a label vector for containing labels of all included (normal and patient) subjects in the dictionary at the same order. Thus, the score of the built patient-specific reference model can be determined as the dot product of the estimated sparse coefficient vector and the label vector (for the dictionary). Note that, before calculating the dot product, we normalized the estimated sparse coefficient vector by dividing its sum.

3.3   Quantitative Results

We conducted four experiments to calculate the normality score of the estimated patient-specific reference models using SR [2], SR+CCA, SR+MMR, and SR+CCA+MMR. As a comparison, we also give the normality scores of normal subjects and patients.

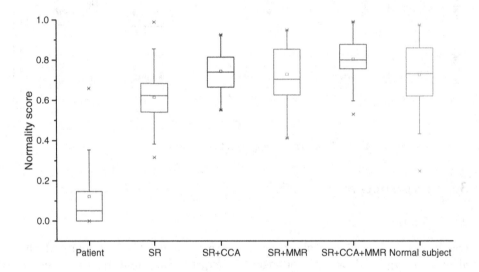

Fig. 4. Normality scores for patients, reference models, and normal subjects.

Fig. 4 shows the boxplot of normality scores. From this figure, we summarize the following conclusions. 1) The patients have very low scores, which mean there are large deformities among these subjects. 2) By simply using the SR [2] to get the reference model, the scores increase significantly. It demonstrates the effectiveness of the basic theory that the sparse coefficients of midface landmarks could be used to estimate jaw landmarks. 3) By adding the steps of CCA and/or MMR, the scores are further improved, and the highest scores are achieved by adding both CCA and MMR to SR. It means that the steps of using CCA and MMR indeed reduce the incoherence between midface and jaw landmarks, and these two steps could also facilitate each other to achieve better performance. 4) The scores of reference models are even higher than the scores of normal subjects. It is because that there are individual differences among normal subjects; but for a reference model, it is obtained by the linear combination of many normal subjects, which means the built reference model is even more normal than a specific normal subject.

3.4   Qualitative Comparison

To visually compare the patients' original jaw shapes and the estimated patient-specific reference models, examples from two patients are shown in Fig. 5. It can be clearly seen that by using our method, the desired jaw shapes are successfully recovered in the reference models (Fig. 5 (b)) as compared to the original deformed shapes (Fig. 5 (a)), with the help from the normal subjects in the training set (Fig. 5 (c)).

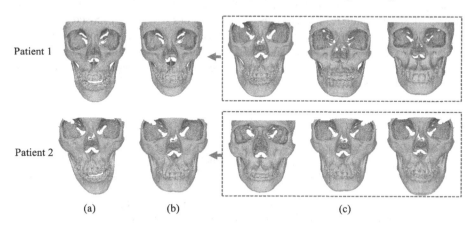

Fig. 5. Comparison of patients and the estimated reference models. (a) Patients' original jaw shapes. (b) Estimated patient-specific reference models by our method. (c) Normal subjects which are used to sparsely reconstruct the reference models.

Fig. 6 shows the comparison between some samples of normal subjects and patient-specific reference models. As can be seen, the normal subjects' jaw shapes are different from each other and do not strictly conform to a canonical "perfect" shape. On the other hand, the rectified jaw shapes of the patients look more rectified than the normal subjects since the estimated models are based on the "averageness" of the normal subjects. This observation also complies with the quantitative results in Fig. 4, in which the normality scores of the estimated reference models are higher than those of the normal subjects.

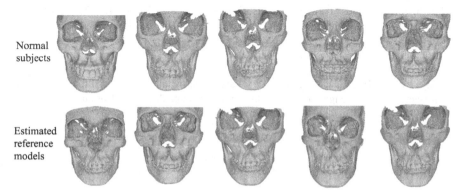

Fig. 6. Comparison of normal subjects and patient-specific reference models.

4   Conclusion

In this paper, we presented a novel method to estimate the patient-specific jaw reference model for patients with CMF deformity from their midface landmarks. Our estimation is performed in the data-coherent space, in which the midface landmarks and jaw landmarks are better correlated. This estimation scheme is further improved by learning the intermediate dictionaries and then refining the estimation in an iterative manner. Experimental results demonstrated superiority of the proposed method in comparison with the baseline SR-based methods. The estimated patient-specific jaw reference model by our method can serve as guidance for surgeons. Future work includes extension of our current framework for syndromic craniofacial deformities, where all cranial base, midface, and jaw are deformed.

References

1. Xia, J.J., Gateno, J., Teichgraeber, J.F.: New clinical protocol to evaluate craniomaxillofacial deformity and plan surgical correction. J. Oral Maxillofac. Surg. **67**(10), 2093–2106 (2009)
2. Ren, Y., Wang, L., Gao, Y., Tang, Z., Chen, K.C., Li, J., Shen, S.G., Yan, J., Lee, P.K., Chow, B., Xia, J.J., Shen, D.: Estimating anatomically-correct reference model for craniomaxillofacial deformity via sparse representation. In: Golland, P., Hata, N., Barillot, C., Hornegger, J., Howe, R. (eds.) MICCAI 2014, Part II. LNCS, vol. 8674, pp. 73–80. Springer, Heidelberg (2014)
3. Swennen, G.R., Schutyser, F.A., Hausamen, J.E.: Three-dimensional cephalometry: a color atlas and manual. Springer (2005)
4. Wang, L., Chen, K.C., Gao, Y., Shi, F., Liao, S., Li, G., Shen, S.G.F., Yan, J., Lee, P.K.M., Chow, B., Liu, N.X., Xia, J.J., Shen, D.: Automated bone segmentation from dental CBCT images using patch-based sparse representation and convex optimization. Medical Physics **41**(4), 043503 (2014)
5. Xia, J.J., McGrory, J.K., Gateno, J., Teichgraeber, J.F., Dawson, B.C., Kennedy, K.A., Lasky, R.E., English, J.D., Kau, C.H., McGrory, K.R.: A new method to orient 3-dimensional com-puted tomography models to the natural head position: a clinical feasibility study. J. Oral Maxillofac. Surg. **69**(3), 584–591 (2011)
6. Hotelling, H.: Relations between two sets of variates. Biometrika **28**, 312–377 (1936)
7. Zou, H., Hastie, T.: Regularization and variable selection via the Elastic Net. J. R. Stat. Soc. B **67**(2), 301–320 (2005)
8. Tibshirani, R.: Regression shrinkage and selection via the lasso. J. R. Stat. Soc. B, 267–288 (1996)
9. Jiang, J., Hu, R., Wang, Z., Han, Z.: Face super-resolution via multilayer locality-constrained iterative neighbor embedding and intermediate dictionary learning. IEEE Trans. Image Process. **23**(10), 4220–4231 (2014)

Nonlinear Graph Fusion for Multi-modal Classification of Alzheimer's Disease

Tong Tong[1]([✉]), Katherine Gray[1], Qinquan Gao[2], Liang Chen[1],
and Daniel Rueckert[1]

[1] Department of Computing, Imperial College London, London, UK
`t.tong11@imperial.ac.uk`
[2] Fujian Province Key Lab of MIPT, Fuzhou University, Fuzhou, China

Abstract. Recent studies have demonstrated that biomarkers from multiple modalities contain complementary information for the diagnosis of Alzheimer's disease (AD) and its prodromal stage mild cognitive impairment (MCI). In order to fuse data from multiple modalities, most previous approaches calculate a mixed kernel or a similarity matrix by linearly combining kernels or similarities from multiple modalities. However, the complementary information from multi-modal data are not necessarily linearly related. In addition, this linear combination is also sensitive to the weights assigned to each modality. In this paper, we propose a nonlinear graph fusion method to efficiently exploit the complementarity in the multi-modal data for the classification of AD. Specifically, a graph is first constructed for each modality individually. Afterwards, a single unified graph is obtained via a nonlinear combination of the graphs in an iterative cross diffusion process. Using the unified graphs, we achieved classification accuracies of 91.8% between AD subjects and normal controls (NC), 79.5% between MCI subjects and NC and 60.2% in a three-way classification, which are competitive with state-of-the-art results.

1 Introduction

Alzheimer's disease (AD), the most common cause of dementia, is a progressive neurodegerative disease that usually results in a gradual loss of intellectual and social skills, ultimately leading to death. The prevalence of AD is predicted to be almost double in the next 20 years [1]. To this end, there has been significant interest in developing different biomarkers for the diagnosis of AD and its early stage mild cognitive impairment (MCI). Different imaging modalities, such as magnetic resonance imaging (MRI) and fluorodeoxyglucose positron emission tomography (FDG-PET), and biological measures can reveal different aspects of pathological changes due to AD, thus may provide complementary information for diagnosis. It has been demonstrated that the fusion of information from different modalities can enhance the diagnostic performance [2–11].

In order to combine multi-modal data, the simplest way is to concatenate features obtained from different modalities. The different features are first normalized and concatenated into one vector for each subject. Then, a classifier is

© Springer International Publishing Switzerland 2015
L. Zhou et al. (Eds.): MLMI 2015, LNCS 9352, pp. 77–84, 2015.
DOI: 10.1007/978-3-319-24888-2_10

trained using the concatenated feature vectors. For example, in [2], a support vector machine (SVM) classifier was applied to the concatenated features from multiple modalities for the classification of AD. However, the simple concatenation has been shown not to optimally integrate multi-modal data and is bias to the single modality which provides a large number of features [7]. To avoid this, a common strategy is to analyze the features from each modality independently before the combination. In [3,4,8], an individual kernel matrix K_i is calculated for each modality, and a combined kernel matrix K_c is then obtained by a linear combination of multiple kernel matrices $K_c = \sum_{i=1}^{m} \alpha_i K_i$, where m is the number of modalities and α_i is the weight assigned to ith modality. A similar strategy was used in [7] to combine similarity matrices instead of kernel matrices. However, all these methods assumed that the complementary information are linearly provided, which may not necessarily be true. In addition, the combined kernel matrix or similarity matrix is sensitive to the weight α_i assigned to each modality, which need to be tuned using computationally expensive cross-validation loops.

In this paper, we present a nonlinear graph fusion (NGF) method to make full use of the complementary information across modalities. A graph is first built using the features from each modality. Then, a graph fusion step is carried out to obtain a unified graph for classification. The graph fusion step is a nonlinear approach based on message-passing theory [12] that iteratively updates every graph, making it more similar to the others after each iteration. NGF converges to a unified graph after a few iterations. It utilizes the local structure in graphs by reducing the weak connections in graphs and enhancing the strong connections present in one or more graphs. This can be used to fully exploit the complementary information across these graphs. In addition, NGF does not require assignment of weights to different modalities, thus avoiding the need of parameter tuning using cross-validation loops. In this work, we use four types of data including MRI and FDG-PET data, cerebrospinal fluid (CSF) biomarker measures, and categorical genetic information to evaluate the performance of the proposed NGF on the multi-modal classification of AD. The classification performance of NGF is compared with the classification performance obtained using features from each single modality and with the classification performance based on a linear combination of kernels [3] or similarity matrices [7].

2 Methods

There are three steps in the proposed method: (1) constructions of graphs using measurements from each individual modality; (2) calculation of a unified graph via an iterative cross diffusion process; (3) classification using the unified graph representation. In the following, we will present the details of these steps.

2.1 Graph Construction

Suppose we have n subjects and each subject has measurements from m modalities. Using measurements from ith modality, a graph $G^i = (V^i, E^i)$ can be constructed to model the relations among the n subjects, where the nodes V^i correspond to n subjects and the edges E^i are weighted by how similar the subjects are. Here, we denote the edge weights as a $n \times n$ similarity matrix W^i, in which $W^i(a, b)$ represent the similarity between subject a and subject b using measurements from ith modality. The similarity matrix W^i can be calculated using different methods. One common way is to calculate the pairwise Euclidean distance and transform it into a similarity matrix using an exponential kernel. Here, we use random forests as proposed in [7] to calculate the similarity between pairs of subjects. Specifically, measurements of subject a and b are passed down each tree in the forest. The similarity between them is then calculated using the number of trees in which both subjects end up in the same terminal node divided by the total number of trees in the forest.

2.2   Nonlinear Graph Fusion

After the graph construction step, we have m graphs with the same nodes V^i but with different edges E^i, which are represented by the similarity matrix W^i. In order to fuse these graphs, we need to fuse these similarity matrices. First, we apply a normalization step to all similarity matrices. One simple way to perform the normalization is $\tilde{W}^i = W^i / D^i$, where $D^i(a, a) = \sum_{b=1}^{n} W^i(a, b)$ is the diagonal matrix so that $\sum_{b=1}^{n} \tilde{W}^i(a, b) = 1$. However, since self-similarities in the diagonal entries of W^i are used, this normalization may not be numerical stable. Thus, we carried out the normalization over the similarity matrix W^i as follows:

$$\tilde{W}^i(a, b) = \begin{cases} \frac{W^i(a,b)}{2\sum_{b=1}^{n} W^i(a,b)}, b \neq a \\ \\ 1/2, b = a \end{cases} \tag{1}$$

Here $\sum_{b=1}^{n} \tilde{W}^i(a, b) = 1$ still holds, but avoids self-similarities in the diagonal entries of W^i. After normalization, $\tilde{W}^i$ is asymmetric. In order to reduce the noise in graphs, we calculate a sparse graph $\tilde{S}^i$ using k nearest neighbors (k-NN) to measure local affinity as:

$$\tilde{S}^i(a, b) = \begin{cases} \tilde{W}^i(a, b) \text{ if } b \in k\text{-NN}(a) \\ \\ 0 \text{ otherwise} \end{cases} \tag{2}$$

Here the similarities between non-neighboring subjects are set to zero. Then, the sparse matrix $\tilde{S}^i$ only keeps the strong connections between subjects and removes the weak connections, which can be robust to the noise of similarity measures. In contrast to $\tilde{S}^i$, the normalized matrix $\tilde{W}^i$ encodes the full information about the similarities between subjects.

Given measurements from m modalities, we can obtain m normalized matrices $\tilde{W}^i, i = 1, 2, ..., m$ and m sparse matrices $\tilde{S}^i, i = 1, 2, ..., m$ using eqs. (1) and (2) respectively. To calculate a single unified graph, the fusion step is an iterative cross diffusion process [13] which starts from $\tilde{W}^i$ as the initial state and uses

$\tilde{S}^i$ as the kernel matrix. Let $\tilde{W}^i_{t=0} = \tilde{W}^i$ represent the initial similarity matrix for ith modality. The similarity matrix can then be iteratively updated via the cross diffusion process as:

$$\tilde{W}^i_{t+1} = \tilde{S}^i \times \left(\frac{1}{m-1} \sum_{j=1,j\neq i}^{m} \tilde{W}^j_t \right) \times \left(\tilde{S}^i \right)^T \tag{3}$$

Here $i = 1, 2, ..., m$ generates m parallel interchanging diffusion processes at each iteration. After each iteration, the normalization step as in eq. (1) is applied to all the updated similarity matrices $\tilde{W}^i_{t+1}, i = 1, 2, ..., m$. This normalization step is carried out to ensure that the self similarity of a subject is always higher than the similarities between this subject and other subjects. It also ensures that the final graph is full rank, which can be important for classification. The proof of the convergence of this diffusion process can be found in [13]. Moreover, the normalization of similarity matrices after each iteration has been found to result in faster convergence of NGF [13]. The graph of a modality (i.e. MRI) then absorbs useful/complementary information from graphs of other modalities (PET;CSF;Genetic) after each iteration. In the end, this graph will have useful information from all other modalities. After T iterations, the final unified similarity matrix $\tilde{W}_u$ is calculated as:

$$\tilde{W}_u = \frac{1}{m} \sum_{i=1}^{m} \tilde{W}^i_T \tag{4}$$

Figure 1 shows examples of the similarity matrices using measurements from different modalities. The unified matrix $\tilde{W}_u$ using NGF is also compared with that using concatenated measurements from all modalities.

2.3 Classification

Based on the unified similarity matrix $\tilde{W}_u$, manifold learning techniques can be applied to find a coordinate embedding as in [7] so that a low-dimensional feature vector for each subject is calculated for classification. However, this will involve other parameters for tuning such as the dimensions of the coordinates kept for classification. To avoid this, we use the entries in the unified similarity matrix directly as features for classification as all the relationship information between subject are kept in this matrix. Then, traditional classification methods such as SVM can be used for classification. Here, we employ the random forest algorithm [14] for classification as it has been shown to be powerful in classification of AD [15].

3 Experiments and Results

The proposed NGF method was evaluated using data of 147 subjects from the Alzheimer's Disease Neuroimaging Initiative (ADNI) study (http://adni.loni.usc.edu/). Table 1 shows the demographic information for the study population.

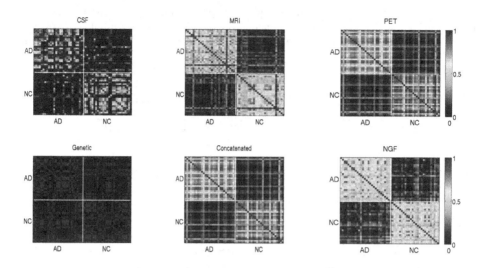

Fig. 1. Similarity matrices for the classification of AD vs NC. Each entry in the symmetric matrix represents the similarity between a pair of subjects. The similarity matrix based on concatenated measurements is very similar to the one based on measurements from PET. This is due to the fact that the features obtained from PET are high-dimensional and also the most discriminative for the classification of NC vs AD, thus dominating the similarity matrix using the concatenated measurements. In contrast to the concatenated measurements, the proposed NGF is not affected by this problem.

This subset was selected according to the subject exclusion rule as described in Appendix B in [7]. Imaging data from baseline MRI and FDG-PET of these 147 ADNI participants were used. The MR images were segmented into 83 anatomical regions using multi-atlas propagation [16]. The 83 grey matter volumes in these regions normalised by the intracranial volume were used as MR features. The FDG-PET images were first non-linearly registered to the MNI template space. Then, the intensity values of the smoothed and normalized images were directly used as features, resulting in 239,304 voxel-based measurements from FDG-PET. In addition, the CSF measures of $A\beta$, tau and phosphorylated tau, as well as ApoE genotype information were also included as additional features for classification. Finally, 239,391 features including 83 MR volumetric features, 239,304 FDG-PET intensity features, 3 CSF features and 1 genetic feature were used for classification.

The classification performance of the NGF method was validated in different scenarios, including AD vs normal controls (NC), MCI vs NC and multi-class classification of three diagnostic groups. Experiments were performed using leave-25%-out cross validation. The average classification accuracy (ACC), sensitivity (SEN) and specificity (SPE) over 100 runs were computed. There are two parameters in the proposed NGF method. The number of iterations T in NGF was set to 20 as the cross diffusion process has converged after 20 iterations in

Table 1. Demographic information for the study population. For each group, the total number of subjects, average age, average Mini-Mental State Examination (MMSE) score and average Clinical Dementia Rating-Sum of Boxes (CDR-SB) score are shown.

Group	Number	Age (mean ± std)	MMSE score (mean ± std)	CDR-SB score (mean ± std)
NC	35	74.5 ± 5.2	28.9 ± 1.2	0.04 ± 0.14
MCI	75	75.7 ± 6.8	27.6 ± 1.7	1.6 ± 0.89
AD	37	76.8 ± 6.6	23.5 ± 2.0	4.43 ± 1.77

our experiments. The effect of the other parameter k in eq. (2) is analyzed in the following section.

3.1   Influence of k

Experiments were conducted to investigate the influence of k on the classification performance of the proposed NGF method. Figure 2 shows the classification accuracies for AD vs NC, MCI vs NC and the three-way classification with varying settings of k. As can be seen from the figure, in different classification scenarios, the proposed NGF method is robust with respect to different settings of k in the range between 10 and 45.

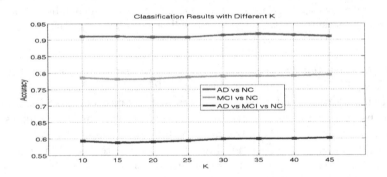

Fig. 2. Results of the proposed NGF method using different settings of k.

3.2   Comparison with Other Methods

Experiments were carried out to assess the classification performance using measurements from each single modality. A random forest classifier was applied to the original imaging or biological features, and the obtained single-modality classification results are presented in Table 2. In addition, we concatenated all the features from four modalities into a single feature vector for classification. The classification accuracies based on the concatenated feature set are not significantly different from that based on FDG-PET features alone. This is due to the fact that the high-dimensional features (239,304) from FDG-PET dominate the results of the concatenated feature set. In constrast to the concatenated features, the other three methods including multiple kernel learning (MKL) in [3], the combined embedding in [7] and the proposed NGF are not affected by this problem. The classification accuracies based on NGF are significantly higher ($p < 0.01$) than those based on individual modality and the concatenated measurements for all classification experiments using Wilcoxon signed-rank tests. Using the same dataset and the same cross validation, the classification accuracies of NGF are also significantly higher than the results using MKL as in [3] and the state-of-the-art results presented in [7], both of which are based on a linear combination of kernels [3] or similarity matrices [7], demonstrating the effectiveness of the proposed method. Also, it should be mentioned that the classification of AD vs MCI vs NC is more challenging than other classification scenarios. For example, in [17], 29 state-of-the-art algorithms were evaluated in the three-group classification but only one can achieve an accuracy over 60%.

Table 2. Comparison of classification results based on single-modality classification and multi-modality classification (Top group: single-modality classification results; Bottom group: multi-modality classification results).

	AD vs NC			MCI vs NC			AD vs MCI vs NC
	ACC	SEN	SPE	ACC	SEN	SPE	ACC
CSF	76.5%	73.0%	80.5%	63.1%	62.0%	65.5%	45.3%
MRI	81.6%	79.8%	83.8%	66.9%	63.7%	74.0%	56.6%
PET	86.0%	86.8%	85.1%	66.5%	65.7%	68.1%	54.4%
Genetic	72.6%	71.3%	74.1%	73.8%	94.7%	26.6%	53.7%
Concatenated features	86.2%	85.1%	86.1%	66.3%	68.5%	66.9%	54.1%
Multiple kernel learning in [3]	87.5%	85.5%	89.3%	75.5%	90.8%	41.1%	56.6%
Combined embedding in [7]	89.0%	87.9%	90.0%	74.6%	77.5%	67.9%	-
Proposed NGF	91.8%	88.9%	94.7%	79.5%	85.1%	67.1%	60.2%

4   Discussion and Conclusion

In this work, we proposed a novel method to fuse data from multiple modalities for the classification of AD. The nonlinearity in NGF allows the proposed method to make full use of local structures in the graphs obtained from each modality, thus integrating the complementary information across different modalities. Furthermore, the proposed method can avoid the tuning of the weights assigned to each modality as in the multiple kernel learning methods [3,4,8]. In our work, we utilized all the features for classification, some of which may not be related to the pathological changes due to AD. Future work will integrate feature selection into the proposed framework as this has been demonstrated to further improve performance in the classification of AD [3,11].

References

1. Brookmeyer, R., Johnson, E., Ziegler-Graham, K., Arrighi, H.M.: Forecasting the global burden of Alzheimer's disease. Alzheimer's and Dementia **3**(3), 186–191 (2007)
2. Kohannim, O., Hua, X., Hibar, D.P., Lee, S., Chou, Y.Y., Toga, A.W., Jack, C.R., Weiner, M.W., Thompson, P.M.: Boosting power for clinical trials using classifiers based on multiple biomarkers. Neurobiology of Aging **31**(8), 1429–1442 (2010)
3. Zhang, D., Wang, Y., Zhou, L., Yuan, H., Shen, D.: ADNI: Multimodal classification of Alzheimer's disease and mild cognitive impairment. NeuroImage **55**(3), 856–867 (2011)
4. Hinrichs, C., Singh, V., Xu, G., Johnson, S.C.: ADNI: Predictive markers for AD in a multi-modality framework: an analysis of MCI progression in the ADNI population. NeuroImage **55**(2), 574–589 (2011)
5. Zhang, D., Shen, D.: ADNI: Multi-modal multi-task learning for joint prediction of multiple regression and classification variables in Alzheimer's disease. Neuroimage **59**(2), 895–907 (2012)
6. Yuan, L., Wang, Y., Thompson, P.M., Narayan, V.A., Ye, J.: ADNI: Multi-source feature learning for joint analysis of incomplete multiple heterogeneous neuroimaging data. NeuroImage **61**(3), 622–632 (2012)
7. Gray, K.R., Aljabar, P., Heckemann, R.A., Hammers, A., Rueckert, D.: ADNI: Random forest-based similarity measures for multi-modal classification of Alzheimer's disease. NeuroImage **65**, 167–175 (2013)
8. Young, J., Modat, M., Cardoso, M.J., Mendelson, A., Cash, D., Ourselin, S.: ADNI: Accurate multimodal probabilistic prediction of conversion to Alzheimer's disease in patients with mild cognitive impairment. NeuroImage: Clinical **2**, 735–745 (2013)
9. Liu, F., Wee, C.Y., Chen, H., Shen, D.: Inter-modality relationship constrained multi-modality multi-task feature selection for Alzheimer's disease and mild cognitive impairment identification. NeuroImage **84**, 466–475 (2014)
10. Thung, K.H., Wee, C.Y., Yap, P.T., Shen, D.: ADNI: Neurodegenerative disease diagnosis using incomplete multi-modality data via matrix shrinkage and completion. NeuroImage **91**, 386–400 (2014)
11. Jie, B., Zhang, D., Cheng, B., Shen, D.: Manifold regularized multitask feature learning for multimodality disease classification. Human Brain Mapping **36**(2), 489–507 (2015)
12. Pearl, J.: Probabilistic reasoning in intelligent systems: networks of plausible inference. Morgan Kaufmann (1988)
13. Wang, B., Jiang, J., Wang, W., Zhou, Z.H., Tu, Z.: Unsupervised metric fusion by cross diffusion. In: IEEE Conference on CVPR, pp. 2997–3004. IEEE (2012)
14. Breiman, L.: Random Forests. Machine Learning **45**(1), 5–32 (2001)
15. Moradi, E., Pepe, A., Gaser, C., Huttunen, H., Tohka, J.: ADNI: Machine learning framework for early MRI-based Alzheimer's conversion prediction in MCI subjects. NeuroImage **104**, 398–412 (2015)
16. Heckemann, R.A., Keihaninejad, S., Aljabar, P., Gray, K.R., Nielsen, C., Rueckert, D., Hajnal, J.V., Hammers, A.: ADNI: Automatic morphometry in Alzheimer's disease and mild cognitive impairment. NeuroImage **56**(4), 2024–2037 (2011)
17. Bron, E.E., Smits, M., et al.: Standardized evaluation of algorithms for computer-aided diagnosis of dementia based on structural MRI: The CADDementia challenge. NeuroImage (2015)

HEp-2 Staining Pattern Recognition Using Stacked Fisher Network for Encoding Weber Local Descriptor

Xian-Hua Han$^{(\boxtimes)}$, Yen-Wei Chen, and Gang Xu

Ritsumeikan University, 1-1-1, NojiHigashi, Kusatsu, Shiga 525-8577, Japan
hanxhua@fc.ritsumei.ac.jp

Abstract. This study addresses the recognition problem of the HEp-2 cell using indirect immunofluorescent (IIF) image analysis, which can indicate the presence of autoimmune diseases by finding antibodies in the patient serum. Generally, the method used for IIF analysis remains subjective, and depends too heavily on the experience and expertise of the physician. This study aims to explore an automatic HEp-2 cell recognition system, in which how to extract highly discriminate visual features plays a key role in this recognition application. In order to realize this purpose, our main efforts include: (1) a transformed excitation domain instead of the raw image domain, which is based on the fact that human perception for disguising a pattern depends not only on the absolute intensity of the stimulus but also on the relative variance of the stimulus; (2) a simple but robust micro-texton without any quantization in the excitation domain, called as Weber local descriptor (WLD); (3) a data-driven coding strategy with a parametric probability process, and the extraction of not only low- but also high-order statistics for image representation called as Fisher vector; (4) the stacking of the Fisher network into deep learning framework for more discriminate feature. Experiments using the open HEp-2 cell dataset released in the ICIP2013 contest validate that the proposed strategy can achieve a much better performance than the state-of-the-art approaches, and that the achieved recognition error rate is even very significantly below the observed intra-laboratory variability.

1 Introduction

Indirect immunofluorescence (IIF) is widely used as a diagnostic tool via image analysis; it can reveal the presence of autoimmune diseases by finding antibodies in the patient sera. Since it is effective for diagnosing autoimmune diseases [1], the demand for applying IIF image analysis in diagnostic tests is increasing. One research area involving IIF image analysis lies in the identification of the HEp-2 staining cell patterns using progressive techniques developed in the computer vision and machine learning fields. Several attempts to achieve the automatic recognition of HEp-2 staining patterns have been made. Perner et al. [2] proposed the extraction of texture and statistical features for cell image representation and then combined the extraction with a decision tree model for HEp-2

© Springer International Publishing Switzerland 2015
L. Zhou et al. (Eds.): MLMI 2015, LNCS 9352, pp. 85–93, 2015.
DOI: 10.1007/978-3-319-24888-2_11

cell image classification. Soda et al. [3] investigated a multiple expert system (MES) in which an ensemble of classifiers was combined to label the patterns of single cells; however, research in the field of IIF image analysis is still in its early stages. There is still significant potential for improving the performance of HEp-2 staining cell recognition. Further, although several approaches have been proposed, they have usually been developed and tested on different private datasets under varying conditions, such as image acquisition according to different criteria and different staining patterns. Therefore, it is difficult to compare the effectiveness of these different approaches. In our study, we aim to achieve the automatic recognition of six HEp-2 staining patterns in an open HEp-2 dataset, which was recently released as part of the second HEp-2 cells classification contest at ICIP2013. In the first HEp-2 cells classification contest at ICIP2012, it was shown that the LBP-based descriptor, rotation invariant co-occurrence LBP (RICLBP) for cell image representation, achieved promising HEp-2 cell classification performance [4]. In the second HEp-2 cells classification contest at ICIP2013, it was further shown that the combination of another extended LBP version, pairwise rotation invariant co-occurrence LBP (PRICoLBP) [5] and Bag-of-Features (BOF) [6] with a Sift descriptor [7] achieved the best recognition results. LBP based descriptors [5] characterize each 3×3 local patch into a binary series by comparing the surrounding pixel intensity with that of the center pixel, which unfortunately leads to much information loss, and the generally applied histogram of binary patterns is restricted to the use of low-order statistics for image representation.

In contrast to previous studies, we explore a simple yet powerful local descriptor of HEp-2 cell images; we model it using a general probability process. Motivated by the fact that the human perception of a pattern depends on not only the absolute intensity but also the relative variance of the stimulus, we first transform the raw domain image data into a differential excitation-domain and then explore the local patch. This transformation was inspired by Weber's law, a psychological law, in which the noticeable change of a stimulus (such as sound or light) is a constant ratio of the changed stimulus to the original stimulus. The differential excitation domain can represent the local saliency pattern in the input image domain. In this transformed domain, we simply take an $l \times l$ local patch, called as Weber local descriptor (WLD), that has been proven to be powerful for discriminating texture patterns even in an original image domain. Several researchers have used Weber's law in computer vision, where for example in [8], Weber's law is used to directly concatenate a local descriptor in the excitation domain for image representation. This strategy first requires the normalization of the processed image into a uniform size, which therefore leads to very high-dimensional vectors for image representation. In this paper, to aggregate the large number of WLD in the excitation domain, we model them using a general probability process; more specifically, the process is a Gaussian mixture model (GMM) [9]. Through modeling with GMM, we can achieve a data driven partition of the WLD space by learning parameters using training data, and aggregate the deviations to the learned average GMM parameters of the extracted WLD from an arbitrary image; the deviation vectors consist of not only low-order but also high-order statistics, which is also called as Fisher vector or Fisher network. In order to explore high-level features for cell image representation, we further stack the Fisher network (called as stacked Fisher network: SFN) into deep learning framework. Unlike the single layer Fisher network that directly encodes and summarizes all WLD of an input cell image as Fisher vector for image representation, the proposed SFN first aggregates the divinations (Fisher vectors: FVs) to the learned GMM parameters in densely sampled sub-region based on WLD, and then de-correlate and compresses these subregion-level FVs, and finally employs another FV for encoding the compressed subregion-level FVs. Experiments using the open HEp-2 cell dataset released in the ICIP2013 contest validate that the proposed strategy can achieve a much better performance than the state-of-the-art approaches, and that the achieved recognition error rate is even very significantly below the observed intra-laboratory variability.

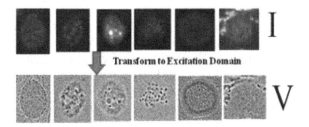

Fig. 1. Sample images in the excitation domain.

2 Materials

The open ICIP2013 HEp-2 dataset includes intermediate and positive intensity intensity types of HEp-2 cells; the purpose of the study involving this dataset is typically to develop a means to recognize the staining pattern given the intensity types. Staining patterns primarily include the following six classes, with available image numbers for positive and intermediate intensity types shown in parentheses, respectively, for each class: Homogeneous (1087, 1407); Speckled (1457, 1374); Nucleolar (934, 1664); Centromere(1387, 1364); Golgi(943, 1265); NuMem (347, 377) (see the detailed explanation in supplement materials). There are over 10000 images, each showing a single cell, obtained from 83 training IIF images by cropping the bounding box of the cell. Example images for all six staining patterns of the positive intensity type are shown in the upper portion of Fig. 1. Using the provided HEp-2 cell images and their corresponding patterns, we extract features that are effective for image representation, and learn a classifier (or a mapping function) using these extracted features of cell images and corresponding staining patterns. With the constructed classifier (the mapping function), the staining pattern can be automatically predicted given any HEp-2 cell image. In the next section, we describe our proposed feature extraction framework for cell image representation.

3 Methods

In this section, we describe our proposed framework for HEp-2 cell image representation, which is shown in Fig. 1. In the subsections that follow. we first introduce Weber's law, which motivates the transformed excitation domain for exploring local structures. Second, we describe our proposed data-driven model of the explored WLDs using GMM, and explore both low- and high-order statistics of the encoded WLDs for sub-region representation, also called the first layer Fisher network (FN). Finally, the second layer FN is introduced for modeling sub-region descriptor from the first layer FN.

3.1 Weber's Law

Weber's law states that the just noticeable difference (JND) is in constant proportion to the original stimulus magnitude, which corresponds to the perception excitation domain of a human being. To transform the original image domain to the differential excitation domain of human perception, we use intensity differences between a current focused pixel and its neighbors as the incremental threshold (i.e., changes). First we calculate the difference between a current pixel and its neighbors as

$$\nabla I_c = \sum_{i=0}^{p-1}(\nabla I_c^i) = \sum_{i=0}^{p-1}(I_c^i - I_c) \qquad (1)$$

where I_c denotes the stimulus magnitude at position x_c, I_c^i $(i = 0, 1, \cdots, p-1)$ is the ith neighbor of I_c, and p is the number of neighbors. As stated in Weber's law, the ratio of the difference to the stimulus (i.e., the intensity) of the current position would give directly affect human perception if activated or excitable. The ratio of the difference to the stimulus is expressed as $H_{ratio}(x_c) = \frac{\nabla I_c}{I_c}$. To calculate the differential excitation of the current pixel $\xi(x_c)$, denoted as v_c, we employ the arctangent function on H_{ratio} as

$$v_c = \xi(x_c) = \arctan[H_{ratio}(x_c)] = \arctan[\frac{\nabla I_c}{I_c}] = \arctan[\sum_{i=0}^{p-1}\frac{(I_c^i - I_c)}{I_c}] \qquad (2)$$

The differential excitation $\xi(x_c)$ has a magnitude range $[-\frac{\pi}{2}, \frac{\pi}{2}]$, which is directly applied for local pattern extraction in the excitation domain. Using this range, we can preserve more discriminating features than only using the absolute value of $\xi(x_c)$. Intuitively, a positive value of $\xi(x_c)$ simulates the case in which the surroundings are lighter than the current pixel, whereas a negative value of $\xi(x_c)$ simulates the case in which the surroundings are darker than the current pixel. Some example images (denoted as $\mathbf{I}$) from the ICIP2013 HEp-2 competition datasets and their corresponding transformed excitation images (denoted as $\mathbf{V}$) are shown in Fig. 1, which shows that saliency patterns in the transformed excitation domain have been successfully detected.

In the transformed differential excitation domain, we work with all possible $l \times l$ neighborhoods (with l set to $3, 5, \cdots$, among others) for micro structure representation (called as Weber local descriptor: WLD); i.e., $\mathbf{v}^c = \{v_c, v_c^1, v_c^2, \cdots v_c^{l \times l - 1}\}$, where v_c is the excitation magnitude of the center pixel and the rest are those of its $(l \times l - 1)$-neighbors. This WLD can capture the main salience pattern, which would activate human perception, and therefor be much discriminant for image representation. Aggregating the large amount of micro-structure vector into a compact and discriminant vector for image representation has a crucial impact on the post-performance of image classification applications. Motivated the studies on image feature extraction in generic image classification involving aggregate local descriptors extracted from the original image domain into a histogram, such as BOF, LBP, we propose to exploit the distribution $p(\mathbf{v}^c \mid \mathbf{I})$ of the WLD space for a given image to represent the image. The following subsection describes our adaptive modeling approach: Fisher network, regarding the WLD.

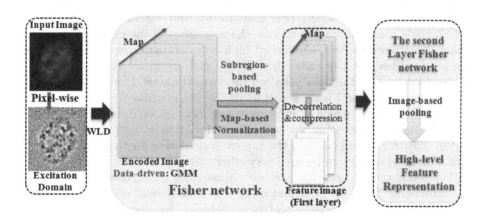

Fig. 2. The flowchart of the stacked Fisher network.

3.2   The First Layer FN

We denote the WLD space samples, which are randomly selected from training images, by $\mathbf{X} = [\mathbf{x}_1, \mathbf{x}_2, \cdots, \mathbf{x}_T]$, where $\mathbf{x}_i \in \mathbf{R}^D$; further T is the sample number and D is the dimension of the WLD. Assuming that the WLD space samples have probability distribution as in a GMM, we can formulate

$$P(\mathbf{X}/\lambda) = \sum_{k=1}^{K_1} w_k N(\mathbf{X}/\mu_k, \mathbf{\Sigma}_k) \tag{3}$$

where λ is the parameter for formulating the probability function in the GMM with K_1-components, denoted by $\lambda = \{w_k, \mu_k, \Sigma_k, k = 1, \cdots, K\}$. w_k, μ_k, and Σ_k are the mixture weight, mean vector, and covariance matrix of Gaussian k, respectively, and $N(\mathbf{X}/\mu_k, \Sigma_k)$ is the Gaussian distribution with mean and covariance μ_k and Σ_k, respectively.

Given the training WLD samples, we can adaptively learn the prior parameters $\lambda = \{w_k, \mu_k, \Sigma_k, k = 1, \cdots, K_1\}$ of the GMM using an expectation maximization (EM) strategy [10] by maximizing the likelihood of the GMM of the training samples, which is equivalent to minimizing the (negative) log-likelihood as

$$L(\lambda) = -\sum_{t=1}^{T} \ln \sum_{k=1}^{K_1} w_k N(\mathbf{x}_t/\mu_k, \Sigma_k) \qquad (4)$$

The EM strategy [9] iterates until it reaches a predefined iteration number or no (or minimal) change occurs in the above objective function. At that point, we identify the parameters $\lambda = \{w_k, \mu_k, \Sigma_k, k = 1, ..., K_1\}$ in the GMM that better fit the training texton samples.

The learned parameters (i.e., $\lambda = w_k, \mu_k, \Sigma_k, k = 1, \cdots, K_1$) of the data-driven model (GMM) can fit into a WLD ensemble from a subregion of any HEp-2 cell image. The deviation statistics to the parameters are then the weight w_k (the 0th order), mean μ_k (the first order), and variance Σ_k (the second order); these can manifest the specific characteristics of the explored ensemble. These deviation statistics, also called high-order statistics or a Fisher vector, can be described via the Fisher kernel [10], and are given by the gradient of the log-likelihood of the data based on the learned model. It was proven in [10] that the utility of the Fisher kernel as the kernel machine in a discriminative classification model, which is inherently nonlinear, is equivalent to that of a linear kernel machine using the normalized deviation statistics as the feature vector. Therefore, the benefit of the explicit formulation for the Fisher vector is that a linear classifier can be used very efficiently.

For computational convenience, we assume that the weights are subject to the constraint: $\sum_{k=1}^{K_1} w_k = 1$, and using a D-dimensional micro-texton space, we assume that the covariance matrix is diagonal, denoted by $\sigma_k = diag(\Sigma_k)$. Given any texton sample $\mathbf{x}_t$ in the dataset $\mathbf{X}$ of a cell image, the occupancy probability for the kth Gaussian component can be formulated as

$$\gamma_t(k) = \frac{w_k P(k/\mathbf{x}_t, \lambda)}{\sum_{k=1}^{K_1} w_k P(k/\mathbf{x}_t, \lambda)} \qquad (5)$$

To explicitly avoid enforcing the constraints of weights w_k, we take a new relative parameter α_k to adopt soft-max formalism to define $w_k = \frac{exp(\alpha_k)}{\sum_{j=1}^{K_1} exp(\alpha_j)}$. After re-parameterization using α_k and normalization with the Fisher information matrix $\mathbf{F}$ [11-12], the deviation for a WLD sample $\mathbf{x}_t$ from parameters $\lambda = \alpha_k, \mu_k, \Sigma_k, k = 1, \cdots, K_1$ can be formulated as

$$\check{G}^{\mathbf{X}}_{\alpha_k} = \frac{1}{\sqrt{w_k}} \sum_{t=1}^{T} [\gamma_t(k) - w_k], \quad \check{G}^{\mathbf{X}}_{\mu_k^d} = \frac{1}{\sqrt{w_k}} \sum_{t=1}^{T} \gamma_t(k) [\frac{x_t^d - \mu_k^d}{\sigma_k^d}]$$

$$\check{G}^{\mathbf{X}}_{\sigma_k^d} = \frac{1}{\sqrt{w_k}} \sum_{t=1}^{T} \gamma_t(k) \frac{1}{\sqrt{2}} [\frac{(x_t^d - \mu_k^d)^2}{(\sigma_k^d)^2} - 1]$$

(6)

where superscript d denotes the dth dimension of the input vector $\mathbf{x}_t$, and k reflects the kth Gaussian component in the learned model. Therefore, given a WLD ensemble $\mathbf{X}$, the aggregated deviation statistics from parameters α_k, μ_k, and Σ_k can be considered as 0th-order, first-order, and second-order statistics. The final feature for image or subregion representation is the concatenation of the deviation statistics with respect to all parameters, which can also be called as the Fisher vector (FV), and is of dimension $(2D + 1)K_1$.

To avoid dependence on the sample size, we normalize the resulting FV by the WLD sample size extracted from the given image or its subregion, i.e., $\check{\mathbf{G}}^{\mathbf{X}}_\lambda = \frac{1}{T} \check{\mathbf{G}}^{\mathbf{X}}_\lambda$.

3.3   The Second Layer FN

The single layer Fisher network aggregates (pools) all encoded WLDs in an image (pooling procedure), which only obtain the statistics (mid-level features) of the used WLDs (low-level features). In order to achieve much higher-level feature, we apply region-based pooling, which means achieving the statistics of the encoded WLD only from a sub-region by densely sampling image, and then normalize the pooled encoded vector for sub-region representation. Due to the high-dimension vector from the first Fisher network, we de-correlate them by principle component analysis (PCA) and compress by taking the PCs with accumulation contribution rate 90% for serving as the inputs of the 2nd FN layer. After learning a GMM with size of K_2, we apply another FN layer with these pre-processed subregion-based FVs and then extract the statistics of encoded subregion FVs over the entire image, which is prospected to have much higher-level vision than a single layer FN. The flowchart of our proposed stacked FN is shown in Fig. 2.

4   Experimental Results

Using the HEp-2 cell dataset, we validate the recognition performance of the two types of intensity (i.e., intermediate and positive) using the single FN (FN1: 32 Gaussian components, i.e. $K_1=32$) with local descriptors in raw images and the transformed excitation domains (denoted as FN1_Raw and FN1_WLD, respectively) and SIFT (denoted as FN1_SIFT); we compare our results with those of conventional LBP-based descriptors RICLBP [4] and PRICoLBP [5], which have been proven to achieve promising recognition performance. In the HEp-2 cell database, each pattern has a different available numbers of cell images as introduced in Section 2 above. We observe that the Golgi pattern has much less

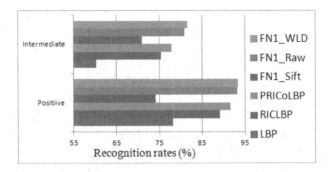

Fig. 3. Comparison of the recognition performances using the single layer FN with different descriptors and the state-of-the-art methods for both Positive and intermediate intensity types.

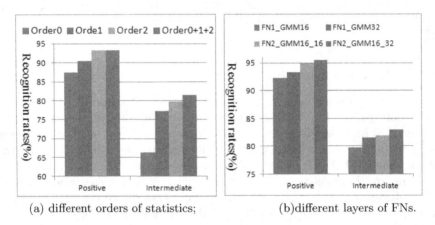

(a) different orders of statistics;   (b)different layers of FNs.

Fig. 4. Comparative results for (a)different orders of statistics from single layer FN (b)different layers of FNs.

available cell images than other patterns. Thus, in our experiment, we randomly select 600 cell images from the five patterns excluding Golgi and 300 cell images from Golgi as training data; the remaining images were used as test data for both positive and intermediate intensity types. We use a linear SVM as the classifier (which is much more efficient than a nonlinear SVM) on the features extracted with our proposed framework; the nonlinear approach was used on the LBP-based descriptors for obtaining higher accuracies. We repeat the above procedure 20 times, with final results calculated as the average recognition performance of the 20 runs, each calculating the percentages of properly classified cell images for all test samples. Fig. 3 shows results of comparative recognition performance; promising performance results (about $2-6\%$ improved) with the single FN of 32 ($K_1 = 32$ Gaussian components can be achieved compared with the conventional LBP-based descriptors RICLBP and PRICoLBP, which were the winners of the HEp-2 cell classification contests of 2012 and 2013, respectively.

As introduced in Section 3 above, the statistics from FN include not only low-order statistics (i.e., the 0th, denoted as Order0) but also high-order statistics (i.e., first- and second-order statistics, denoted as Order1 and Order2). Fig. 4 (a) presents the recognition performances with different orders of statistics using single layer FN with 32 Gaussian components, which manifests that the concatenated statistics of all orders achieve the best performance results for both positive and intermediate intensity types. Fig. 4(b) gives the compared recognition rates by stacking two layer FNs (denoted as FN2_GMM16_16 and FN2_GMM16_32 with K_1=16, K_2=16 and 32, respectively) and the single FNs (denoted as FN1_GMM16, and FN1_GMM32 with $K_1 = 16, 32$, respectively).

5   Conclusions

In this paper, we explored a robust local descriptor (called as WLD) inspired by Weber's law and its high-order statistics for HEp-2 cell image representation. Via modeling the WLDs with a parametric probability process, we can extract middle-level features for image sub-region representation, and further stack the above procedure into deep framework for high-level feature extraction, which is called as stacked Fisher network (SFN). Experiments on the HEp-2 cell dataset from ICIP2013 validated that our proposed strategy achieves the best recognition performance as compared with existing state-of-the-art approaches.

References

1. Conrad, K., Schoessler, W., Hiepe, F., Fritzler, M.J.: Utoantibodies in systemic autoimmune diseases. Pabst Science Publishers (2002)
2. Perner, P., Perner, H., Muller, B.: Mining knowledge for HEp-2 cell image classification. Journal Artificial Intelligence in Medicine **26**, 161–173 (2002)
3. Soda, P., Iannello, G.: Aggregation of classifiers for staining pattern recognition in antinuclear autoantibodies analysis. IEEE Transactions on Information Technology in Biomedicine **13**(3), 322–329 (2009)
4. Foggia, P., Percannella, G., Soda, P., Vento, M.: Benchmarking HEp-2 Cells Classification Methods. IEEE Transaction on Medical Imaging **32**(10), 1878–1889 (2013)
5. Qi, X., Xiao, R., Guo, J., Zhang, L.: Pairwise rotation invariant co-occurrence local binary pattern. In: Fitzgibbon, A., Lazebnik, S., Perona, P., Sato, Y., Schmid, C. (eds.) ECCV 2012, Part VI. LNCS, vol. 7577, pp. 158–171. Springer, Heidelberg (2012)
6. Lazebnik, S., Schmid, C., Ponce, J.: Beyond bags of features: spatial pyramid matching for recognizing natural scene categories. In: CVPR, pp. 2169–2178 (2006)
7. Lowe, D.: Distinctive image features from scale-invariant keypoint. International Journal of Computer Vision **60**(2), 91–110 (2004)
8. Chen, J., Shan, S., He, C., Zhao, G., Pietikainen, M., Chen, X., Gao, W.: WLD: A Robust Local Image Descriptor. IEEE Transactions on Pattern Analysis and Machine Intelligence **32**(9), 1705–1720 (2010)
9. Xu, L., Jordan, M.I.: On Convergence Properties of the EM Algorithm for Gaussian Mixtures. Neural Computation **9**(1), 129–151 (1996)
10. Dick, U., Kersting, K.: Fisher kernels for relational data. In: Fürnkranz, J., Scheffer, T., Spiliopoulou, M. (eds.) ECML 2006. LNCS (LNAI), vol. 4212, pp. 114–125. Springer, Heidelberg (2006)

Supervoxel Classification Forests for Estimating Pairwise Image Correspondences

Fahdi Kanavati[1]([✉]), Tong Tong[1], Kazunari Misawa[2], Michitaka Fujiwara[3], Kensaku Mori[4], Daniel Rueckert[1], and Ben Glocker[1]

[1] Biomedical Image Analysis Group, Department of Computing, Imperial College London, 180 Queen's Gate, London SW7 2AZ, UK
fk412@imperial.ac.uk
[2] Aichi Cancer Center, Nagoya 464-8681, Japan
[3] Nagoya University Hospital, Nagoya 466-0065, Japan
[4] Information and Communications, Nagoya University, Furo-cho, Chikusa-ku, Nagoya 464-8603, Japan

Abstract. This paper proposes a general method for establishing pairwise correspondences, which is a fundamental problem in image analysis. The method consists of over-segmenting a pair of images into supervoxels. A forest classifier is then trained on one of the images, the source, by using supervoxel indices as voxelwise class labels. Applying the forest on the other image, the target, yields a supervoxel labelling which is then regularized using majority voting within the boundaries of the target's supervoxels. This yields semi-dense correspondences in a fully automatic, efficient and robust manner. The advantage of our approach is that no prior information or manual annotations are required, making it suitable as a general initialisation component for various medical imaging tasks that require coarse correspondences, such as, atlas/patch-based segmentation, registration, and atlas construction. Our approach is evaluated on a set of 150 abdominal CT images. In this dataset we use manual organ segmentations for quantitative evaluation. In particular, the quality of the correspondences is determined in a label propagation setting. Comparison to other state-of-the-art methods demonstrate the potential of supervoxel classification forests for estimating image correspondences.

1 Introduction

Establishing correspondences between images is a fundamental and important problem in many medical image analysis tasks. To this end, dedicated image registration techniques have been developed and successfully employed in fully automated analysis pipelines [15]. Many of these techniques work best when applied on particular types of images, such as brain scans, where simple initialisation strategies work well. In general settings, however, the images to be registered might capture very different fields of view, as it is often the case in pre- and post-operative abdominal scans. In such settings, establishing an initial alignment can be quite challenging if no prior information is available. It can be beneficial to utilize anatomy recognition and landmark detection methods which

© Springer International Publishing Switzerland 2015
L. Zhou et al. (Eds.): MLMI 2015, LNCS 9352, pp. 94–101, 2015.
DOI: 10.1007/978-3-319-24888-2_12

provide spatial priors for registration [7]. However, this requires an annotated image database for training. Obtaining a large number of manually annotated images can be tedious, costly and time-consuming.

Contribution: We propose a general method for establishing initial pairwise correspondences which does not require any prior information or manual annotations. We employ classification forests [2], but in contrast to previous work class labels for training are generated automatically. Our method consists of over-segmenting a pair of images into supervoxels. We then train a forest classifier on one of the images – the source image – by using its supervoxels indices as voxelwise class labels. Applying the forest on the other image – the target image – yields a supervoxel label prediction for each of its voxels. Majority voting is then carried out within the supervoxels of the target image where each voxel casts a vote as to what the final supervoxel label should be. The final labelling yields correspondences between the supervoxels of the two images. Supervoxels are an ideal representation for semi-densely distributed correspondences relaxing the one-to-one matching assumption between images. Establishing supervoxel correspondences between two images solves the initialization problem for many image analysis tasks such as atlas/patch-based segmentation [4,8], registration, and atlas construction.

Related Work: Random forests [2], as a supervised machine learning technique, have found many successful applications in medical image analysis [5,6,10,14]; this is mainly due to their accuracy, robustness, and scalability. They rely on the availability of labelled images which is contrast to the approach taken here where labels are generated automatically. While traditionally, forests are trained on a database containing many images, recently, the idea of encoding a single labelled image (or atlas) as a forest [14] has been proposed in the context of multi-atlas label propagation. This has inspired our idea of using the atlas-forest approach for learning image correspondences from a single source image, which is labelled automatically via a supervoxelisation. Supervoxels – and their 2D counterpart, superpixels – have found many applications in computer vision [9,12]. They allow the grouping of voxels into locally consistent regions that have similar properties thereby reducing redundancy and computational complexity. Supervoxels are mainly used within segmentation pipelines. We are not aware of previous work that has used supervoxels as label entities in classification forests, in particular, with the aim of establishing image correspondences.

2   Methods

2.1   Problem Formulation

The aim of our method is to estimate correspondences between a set of image regions, i.e. supervoxels. Let I_i be an image that is over-segmented into an indexed set $\mathcal{SV}^i = (sv_k^i)_{k \in C^i}$ of distinct supervoxels sv_k^i. The image therefore consists of $|\mathcal{SV}^i|$ supervoxels with the index set $C^i = \{1, ..., |\mathcal{SV}^i|\}$ denoting the distinct labels of the supervoxels. Each supervoxel $sv_k^i = \{\mathbf{v}_l^i\}_1^{|sv_k^i|}$ in turn is a set of voxels $\mathbf{v}_l^i$. With N^i representing the total number of voxels in the image, we would have $\sum_k |sv_k^i| = N^i$.

Establishing correspondences from an image I_i to an image I_j consists of finding a mapping function g^i that maps each supervoxel $sv_k^j \in \mathcal{SV}^j$ to a value/label in the index set C^i so that $\forall k \in C^j, \exists c \in C^i \mid g^i(sv_k^j) = c$. We propose to use random classification forests to learn the mapping function g^i.

2.2 Random Forests

First we give a brief overview of random forests [2] when applied to a single 3D image. An excellent in depth review can be found at [5]. Random forests are a collection of binary decision trees. They involve two stages: training and testing. The data used for training the forest consists of all the voxels from a single image. We denote the training set as $\mathcal{S} = \{\mathbf{v}_k, c_k\}_1^N$ with $c_k \in C$ being the label of voxel $\mathbf{v}_k$. A tree consists of a set of nodes such that each node can either be a leaf node or has two child nodes.

Each mth node has a binary weak classifier $f(\mathbf{v}, \theta) = [\phi_m(\mathbf{v}) - \tau_m]$ with $\theta_m = \{\phi_m, \tau_m\}$; $\phi_m(\mathbf{v})$ is an appearance feature and τ_m is a threshold. The weak classifier serves as a split function that determines whether a given sample should go down the left or the right child node. For a set of samples S^m arriving at the mth node, different θ_m values yield different disjoint subsets S_L^m and S_R^m.

Training a tree involves finding at each mth node the optimal $\hat{\theta}_m$, via maximisation of an objective function $h(S^m, S_L^m, S_R^m, \theta^m)$. Each node has access to a limited number n_f of randomly generated values for θ^m. The randomness ensures that each tree ends up being unique. Starting from the root node, the samples are recursively split up into two subsets based on the optimal split, with a subset going down each child node. Once a stopping criteria is met – such as maximal depth or minimal sample count – the node becomes a leaf and the distribution of samples that reached it is stored as a posterior probability $p_t(c|\mathbf{v})$.

When *testing* on a new target image, its voxels are passed down the learnt tree going left or right, depending on their response to the split function found during training, until reaching a leaf node (Fig. 1). The outputs from all the T trees in the forest are then combined by averaging: $p(c|\mathbf{v}) = \frac{1}{T} \sum_t p_t(c|v)$. The final voxel label is obtained by selecting the maximum $\hat{c} = \arg\max_c p(c|\mathbf{v})$.

For a *classification forest*, the objective function h at a node with samples S is the information gain $H(S) - \sum_{i=\{L,R\}} \frac{|S_i|}{|S|} H(S_i)$, where $H(S)$ is the Shannon entropy $- \sum_{c \in C} p(c) \log p(c)$ and $p(c)$ is the normalised empirical histogram of the labels of the training samples in S.

A *regression forest*, unlike a classification forest, maps an input into a continuous output. To use a regression forest to output correspondences, each voxel $\mathbf{v}$ has its position assigned as its label $\mathbf{c} = (x, y, z)$. The objective function used

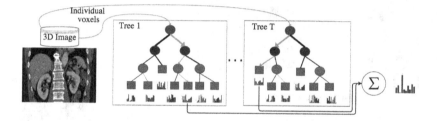

Fig. 1. An overview of random forests. All voxels of a single image are fully used to train each tree. During testing, a voxel starts at the root node and depending on its response to the binary split function at each node (circle), it is sent left or right until it reaches a leaf node (square). The posterior probability distributions from the reached leaf nodes are then averaged to obtain a final label posterior distribution.

in this case [3] is the error of the fit $\sum_{v \in S}(\mathbf{c} - \bar{\mathbf{c}})^2 - \sum_{i=\{L,R\}} \sum_{v \in S_i}(\mathbf{c} - \bar{\mathbf{c}})^2$ with $\bar{\mathbf{c}}$ being the mean position vector for all the points at a node with samples S.

Appearance Features. Similarly to [14], we use a set of context appearance features with offsets up to 200mm; large offsets have been found useful [6] for discriminating between organs. The features used consist of intensities and differences between intensities in two different regions. The feature function $\phi(\mathbf{v})$ mentioned in Sec. 2.2 is characterised by: an offset $\Delta \mathbf{x} \in \mathbb{R}^3$ and a 3D box $B_s(\mathbf{x})$ centred at $\mathbf{x}$ with a size parameter $s \in \mathbb{R}^3$. For a voxel with $\mathbf{v} \in \mathbb{R}^3$ representing its position, $\phi(\mathbf{v})$ can be any of the following:

1. Mean intensity of local box: $\langle I(B_s(\mathbf{v})) \rangle$
2. Difference of intensity of local point and mean intensity of offset box: $I(\mathbf{v}) - \langle I(B_s(\mathbf{v} + \Delta \mathbf{x})) \rangle$
3. Difference of mean intensity of local box and mean intensity of offset box: $\langle I(B_s(\mathbf{v})) \rangle - \langle I(B_s(\mathbf{v} + \Delta \mathbf{x})) \rangle$
4. Difference of a pair of offset box means $\langle I(B_s(\mathbf{v}_1 + \Delta \mathbf{x}_1)) \rangle - \langle I(B_r(\mathbf{v}_2 + \Delta \mathbf{x}_2)) \rangle$

Once the response $\phi(\mathbf{v})$ has been evaluated for all samples at a given node, the optimal value for the threshold τ is obtained by uniformly dividing the response space into $n_{\text{thresholds}}$ and choosing the value the maximises the information gain.

2.3 Supervoxel Classification Forest (SVF)

In our proposed method we encode a single image into a classification forest as in [14]; however, instead of using organ labels, the label of each voxel is the index of the *supervoxel it belongs to*. Random forests can easily handle a large number of labels making them suitable for this task.

To generate supervoxels, we use the efficient SLIC superpixel [1] algorithm. It performs k-means clustering using intensities balanced with the euclidean distance as a distance measure; it takes as input the size of the desired supervoxels

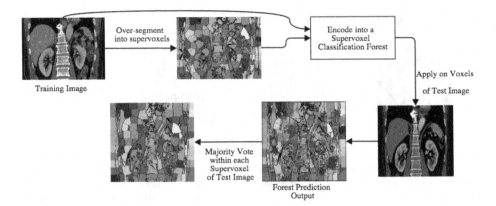

Fig. 2. Proposed method for establishing correspondences at a supervoxel level. First, the training image is segmented into supervoxels (randomly coloured) which are then used as labels to train a classification forest using all the voxels in the image. Applying the forest on a test image yields a supervoxel label prediction for each voxel that does not necessarily follow the test image's supervoxel boundaries. As a final step, the voxels within each supervoxel in the test image cast votes as to what its label should be. Same colour indicates a match between supervoxels in the training and the test image.

and a compactness parameter that enforces regularity in the supervoxel shape. The output is a set of approximately regularly spaced supervoxels that tend to follow intensity boundaries.

Given the training image I_i and its set of labels $|C^i|$ (or in this case supervoxel indices), a training set is constructed using all the voxels in the image $\{\mathbf{v}_k^i, c_k\}_1^N$ with $c_k \in C^i$ and we use it to train an SVF as described in Sec. 2.2.

When applying the forest on a test image, the label predictions from the forest tend to be noisy (Fig. 2); therefore, we perform as a final step a majority voting within each supervoxel of the test image based on the predicted labels of their voxels. Each supervoxel sv_k^j in the test image I_j receives votes from each one of its voxels as to what its label from C^i should be. The final supervoxel label of sv_k^j is obtained by selecting the label with the maximum votes $c_k^j = \arg\max_{c \in C^i} \sum_{\mathbf{v} \in sv_k^j} p(c|\mathbf{v})$.

3   Experiments and Results

Ground truth data for one-to-one correspondences between images is hard to obtain. Therefore, to quantitatively evaluate our method, we test it in a simple multi-atlas label propagation (MALP) setting. We do this as MALP is an application that inherently requires establishing correspondences between images in order to propagate labels. Most state-of-the-art methods in MALP such as in [11,13] use affine registration as a first step to give an initial set of dense correspondences between the atlases and the target image before proceeding with a more sophisticated label propagation scheme. Although affine registration is less accurate than doing non-rigid registration, it is used because it is more efficient. As random forests are quite efficient during test time, we compare our method against affine registration to evaluate the accuracy of the initial set of correspondences. Additionally we compare our method against a conventional organ label classification forest (LF) and a coordinate regression forest (RegF).

We use a dataset of 150 abdominal CT scans acquired from different subjects. The 3D scans have an in-plane resolution of 512×512 with a number of slices between 238 and 1061. Voxel sizes vary from 0.55 to 0.82 with a slice spacing ranging from 0.4 to 0.8 mm. Manual organ segmentations of the liver, spleen, kidneys, and pancreas are provided by clinical experts.

Given a test image that we would like to segment, we treat the remaining 149 images as atlases. The MALP setting would then be as follows:

– Select a subset of the most similar atlases as measured globally by SSD similarity between down-sampled versions of the atlases and the test image.
– The next step is obtaining a label prediction Lp_a from each atlas a. For **LF**, we simply apply the atlas forest on the test image to obtain Lp_a directly. For **affine registration**, all the images are affinely aligned to a template space. The labels from the atlas are then transferred to the test image based on the one-to-one voxel correspondences. For **RegF**, applying the atlas regression forest yields correspondences between the coordinates of the atlas and the test image. The labels are then transferred from the atlas to the test image. Lastly, applying an atlas **SVF** on the test image yields correspondences between the atlas and the test image on a supervoxel level. Each supervoxel from the atlas has an organ label which is obtained via majority voting from the organ labels of its voxels. The supervoxel-level organ labels are then transferred from the atlas to the supervoxels of the test image.
– The final labelling Lp of the test image is then obtained by fusing Lp_a from all the atlases via a voxel-wise majority vote.

To test whether using supervoxels can have an influence on the labelling obtained from RegFs and LFs, we apply a post-processing step – by assigning to each supervoxel the most frequent label of its voxels – either on the predictions Lp_a of each atlas before fusing (svpre) or directly on Lp after the fusion (svpost). We use 2000 supervoxels. In addition, for SVFs, we test with with 500, 1000, and 2000 supervoxels on average per image. Fig. 3 shows the Dice overlap from the different methods using the closest 20 atlases.

All the forests (LF, SVF, RegF) are trained with the same parameters: 5 trees –as not much difference has been observed from using 1 to 5 trees [14]–, maximum depth 32, minimum samples 4, $n_{\mathrm{thresholds}} = 15$, $n_f = 500$, and with the images down-sampled to a $2 \times 2 \times 2 mm^3$ spacing. With an implementation in C++, generating supervoxels on full resolution images takes around 30-50 seconds per image on a single machine with core i7 @ 3.40 GHz with 16 GB memory. For SVFs, training on a $160 \times 160 \times 93$ volume takes ~ 4 mins/tree while testing takes ~ 4s with a pre-processing time of ~ 10s.

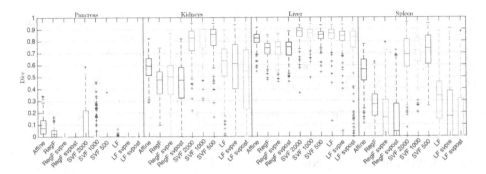

Fig. 3. Dice overlap using the 20 closests atlases to perform MALP. Results for affine registration (Affine), SVF, RegF, RegF svpre, RegF svpost, LF, LF svpre, and LF svpost. We see that SVF scores a higher dice overlap, especially for the kidneys and spleen. We also note that using supervoxels as a post-processing step with RegF and LF does not improve the prediction result.

4   Discussion and Conclusion

In this paper we propose a method for estimating correspondences between images on a supervoxel level using classification forests. The advantage of our approach is that it does not rely on the availability of prior organ annotations. Training a random forest using automatically generated supervoxels as class labels allows training on unlabelled images. Qualitative evaluation of the estimated correspondences in a simple multi-atlas propagation setting demonstrate the potential of using SVFs for estimating correspondences. We do not apply any further post-processing to improve the segmentation, such as graph-cuts, which is what is typically done in some state-of-the-art methods for segmenting abdominal datasets [11,13]. Random forests are extremely efficient during test time making them an attractive option to use for estimating correspondences in large datasets.

   In addition, results seem to indicate that using an SVF to propagate labels from an atlas to a target image yields a higher prediction accuracy than using traditional random forests, such as a LF or a RegF. One possible reason might be that LFs have difficulty learning features to distinguish between one organ vs another, if an organ, for example the liver, covers a wider span of contextual appearance features due its size. Whereas RegFs ignore organ boundaries and will mix voxels from organs with those of the background. On the other hand, SVFs offer a nice balance between locality and tissue type consistency via the use of supervoxels.

   The current supervoxel segmentation is not optimal when using a small number of supervoxels that do not adhere perfectly to the boundaries of the underlying ground truth segmentation. This is especially true for the pancreas. Computing Dice overlaps between the ground truth organ labels and the their supervoxelised version –obtained by assigning to each supervoxel the majority vote of the ground truth label of its voxels– yields for 150 images: pancreas 0.641 ± 0.138, kidneys 0.927 ± 0.061, liver 0.935 ± 0.022, and spleen 0.908 ± 0.054. Future work would include investigating more appropriate supervoxel segmentation and hierarchical representations. Moreover, it would be interesting to exploit mutual correspondences as it is possible to obtain them by training independently on both images, then testing on each other and keeping only the mutual correspondences. For purposes of evaluation such an approach would require a more sophisticated label propagation scheme which we do not adopt here.

References

1. Achanta, R., Shaji, A., Smith, K., Lucchi, A., Fua, P., Susstrunk, S.: SLIC superpixels. No. EPFL-REPORT-149300, p. 15, June 2010
2. Breiman, L.: Random forests. Machine learning, 5–32 (2001)
3. Breiman, L., Friedman, J., Stone, C.J., Olshen, R.A.: Classification and regression trees. CRC Press (1984)
4. Coupé, P., Manjón, J.V., Fonov, V., Pruessner, J., Robles, M., Collins, D.L.: Patch-based segmentation using expert priors: Application to hippocampus and ventricle segmentation. NeuroImage 54(2), 940–954 (2011)
5. Criminisi, A., Shotton, J., Konukoglu, E.: Decision forests for classification, regression, density estimation, manifold learning and semi-supervised learning. Learning 7, 81–227 (2011)
6. Criminisi, A., Shotton, J., Robertson, D., Konukoglu, E.: Regression forests for efficient anatomy detection and localization in CT studies. In: Menze, B., Langs, G., Tu, Z., Criminisi, A. (eds.) MICCAI 2010. LNCS, vol. 6533, pp. 106–117. Springer, Heidelberg (2011)
7. Glocker, B., Zikic, D., Haynor, D.R.: Robust registration of longitudinal spine CT. In: Golland, P., Hata, N., Barillot, C., Hornegger, J., Howe, R. (eds.) MICCAI 2014, Part I. LNCS, vol. 8673, pp. 251–258. Springer, Heidelberg (2014)
8. Heckemann, R.A., Hajnal, J.V., Aljabar, P., Rueckert, D., Hammers, A.: Automatic anatomical brain mri segmentation combining label propagation and decision fusion. NeuroImage 33(1), 115–126 (2006)
9. Lucchi, A., Smith, K., Achanta, R., Knott, G., Fua, P.: Supervoxel-based segmentation of mitochondria in em image stacks with learned shape features. IEEE Transactions on Medical Imaging 31(2), 474–486 (2012)
10. Montillo, A., Shotton, J., Winn, J., Iglesias, J.E., Metaxas, D., Criminisi, A.: Entangled decision forests and their application for semantic segmentation of CT images, pp. 184–196 (2011)
11. Tong, T., Wolz, R., Wang, Z., Gao, Q., Misawa, K., Fujiwara, M., Mori, K., Hajnal, J.V., Rueckert, D.: Discriminative dictionary learning for abdominal multi-organ segmentation. Medical Image Analysis 23(1), 92–104 (2015)
12. Wang, H., Yushkevich, P.A.: Multi-atlas segmentation without registration: a supervoxel-based approach, pp. 535–542 (2013)
13. Wolz, R., Chu, C., Misawa, K., Fujiwara, M., Mori, K., Rueckert, D.: Automated abdominal multi-organ segmentation with subject-specific atlas generation. IEEE Transactions on Medical Imaging 32(9), 1723–1730 (2013)
14. Zikic, D., Glocker, B., Criminisi, A.: Encoding atlases by randomized classification forests for efficient multi-atlas label propagation. Medical image analysis, July 2014
15. Zitova, B., Flusser, J.: Image registration methods: a survey. Image and vision computing 21(11), 977–1000 (2003)

Non-rigid Free-Form 2D-3D Registration Using Statistical Deformation Model

Guoyan Zheng$^{(\boxtimes)}$ and Weimin Yu

Institute for Surgical Technology and Biomechanics, University of Bern,
3014 Bern, Switzerland
Guoyan.Zheng@ieee.org

Abstract. This paper presents a non-rigid free-from 2D-3D registration approach using statistical deformation model (SDM). In our approach the SDM is first constructed from a set of training data using a non-rigid registration algorithm based on b-spline free-form deformation to encode *a priori* information about the underlying anatomy. A novel intensity-based non-rigid 2D-3D registration algorithm is then presented to iteratively fit the 3D b-spline-based SDM to the 2D X-ray images of an unseen subject, which requires a computationally expensive inversion of the instantiated deformation in each iteration. In this paper, we propose to solve this challenge with a fast B-spline pseudo-inversion algorithm that is implemented on graphics processing unit (GPU). Experiments conducted on C-arm and X-ray images of cadaveric femurs demonstrate the efficacy of the present approach.

1 Introduction

Recently, intensity-based non-rigid 2D-3D registration has drawn more and more attentions [1–7]. The reported techniques can be split into two main categories: those based on statistical shape and appearance models [1–4] and those based on one template image that is either derived from CT scan(s) [7] or from visual hull computation [5]. Methods in the former categories, in comparison with methods in the latter categories, are usually more efficient due to the less number of parameters to optimize. They are also more robust due to the statistical constraints applied by the shape and appearance models. In methods of both categories, the registration is conducted by iteratively comparing the reference 2D X-ray images with the floating simulation images called digitally reconstructed radiographs (DRR), which are obtained by ray casting a 3D volume data.

The contribution of this paper is a non-rigid free-from 2D-3D registration approach for personalized reconstruction of the proximal femur from a limited number (e.g., 2) of 2D X-ray images. Unlike existing approaches, where statistical shape and appearance models [1–4] are used, our approach uses b-spline-based statistical deformation model (SDM) introduced in [8]. The SDM is learned from a set of known deformations of proximal femur images to a given common template space. This SDM accounts for the mean and variability of the

© Springer International Publishing Switzerland 2015
L. Zhou et al. (Eds.): MLMI 2015, LNCS 9352, pp. 102–109, 2015.
DOI: 10.1007/978-3-319-24888-2_13

known deformations and thus encodes *a priori* information about the underlying anatomy [8–11]. It has the further advantages of constraining the 2D-3D registration procedure to produce only statistically likely types of warps and of reducing the number of parameters to optimize [12]. The iterative registration of the 3D b-spline-based SDM to the 2D X-ray images requires a computationally expensive inversion of the instantiated deformation in each iteration. In this paper, we propose to solve this challenge with a fast B-spline pseudo-inversion algorithm that is implemented on graphics processing unit (GPU).

The rest of the paper is arranged as follows. Section 2 presents the materials and methods. Experimental results are presented in Section 3, followed by discussions and conclusions in Section 4.

2   Materials and Methods

Our non-rigid free-from 2D-3D registration approach consists of two processes: the training process, where the SDM will be constructed from a set of training images, and the reconstruction process, where given X-ray images of an unseen subject, we will derive a patient-specific volume by non-rigidly matching the SDM to the input images. Note that the training process needs to be performed only once in order to be able to statistically register X-ray images of any unseen subject. Below details about each process will be given.

2.1   Training Process

Following the idea introduced in [8], we construct the SDM from CT data of 40 left cadaveric proximal femurs based on a two-stage procedure. More specifically, in the first stage, we randomly chose one of the proximal femur from this given training population as the reference volume $\mathbf{V}_0^{1st}$. All other volumes $\{\mathbf{V}_i^{1st}, i = 1, ..., 39\}$ were aligned to this reference volume with similarity registrations. We then applied the b-spline-based free-from deformation (FFD) algorithm [14] as implemented in the registration toolbox 'elastix' [13] to establish correspondences between the reference volume and each one of the 39 floating volumes. Each time, the output from the b-spline-based FFD algorithm is a local displacement expressed as the 3D tensor product of the 1D cubic B-splines [14]:

$$T_i^{FFD}(\mathbf{x}) = \sum_{r=0}^3 \sum_{s=0}^3 \sum_{t=0}^3 B_r(u)B_s(v)B_t(w)\mathbf{c}_{l+r,m+s,n+t} \qquad (1)$$

where $\mathbf{c}$ denotes the B-splines coefficients for a number of control points that form a regular lattice size of $(L+3) \times (M+3) \times (N+3)$; l, m, n are the indexes of the control points satisfying $-1 \leqslant l \leqslant (L+1), -1 \leqslant m \leqslant (M+1), -1 \leqslant n \leqslant (N+1)$, and $0 \leqslant u, v, w < 1$ corresponds to the relative positions of $\mathbf{x}$ in lattice coordinates.

By concatenating $(L+3) \times (M+3) \times (N+3)$ 3D control points for each local displacement, we have 39 FFDs described as control point vectors $\mathbf{C}_1^{1st}, ..., \mathbf{C}_{39}^{1st}$, where $\mathbf{C}_i^{1st} = vec(\mathbf{c}_1, ..., \mathbf{c}_{(L+3) \times (M+3) \times (N+3)})$. Here we use the operator, *vec*, to

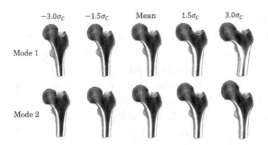

Fig. 1. The mean and the first two modes of variations of the SDM.

represent control point vectorization, and the operator, vec^{-1}, as the inverse of vectorization. Similarly, we can create 39 non-rigidly deformed floating volumes $\{\mathbf{I}_i^{1st}, i = 1, ..., 39\}$, where $\mathbf{I}_i^{1st}$ is a concatenation of gray values in the ith warped floating volume. From these data, we computed the average control point vector $\bar{\mathbf{C}}^{1st} = (39^{-1}) \cdot \sum_{i=1}^{39} \mathbf{C}_i^{1st}$ and the average intensity distribution $\bar{\mathbf{I}} = (40^{-1}) \cdot \sum_{i=0}^{39} \mathbf{I}_i^{1st}$, with $\mathbf{I}_0^{1st}$ standing for gray values of the reference data.

The purpose of the second stage is to remove the possible bias introduced by the reference volume selection. To achieve this goal, we applied the FFD generated from the average control point vector $\bar{\mathbf{C}}^{1st}$ to the reference volume $\mathbf{V}_0^{1st}$ to create a new volume $\mathbf{s}_0$ and assigned the average intensity distribution $\bar{\mathbf{I}}$ to this newly created volume. The new volume $\mathbf{s}_0$ was named as the atlas. It was used as the new reference volume in the second stage and all other 40 proximal femur volumes were regarded as the floating volumes. The b-spline-based FFD algorithm was used again to establish the correspondences between the atlas and the other 40 floating volumes. We thus obtained a set of 40 new control point vectors $\{\mathbf{C}_i; i = 1, ..., 40\}$. We could then construct the SDM as:

$$\begin{aligned}
\mathbf{S}_C &= ((m-1)^{-1}) \cdot \sum_{i=1}^{m} (\mathbf{C}_i - \bar{\mathbf{C}})(\mathbf{C}_i - \bar{\mathbf{C}})^T \\
\bar{\mathbf{C}} &= (m^{-1}) \cdot \sum_{i=1}^{m} \mathbf{C}_i \\
\mathbf{P}_C &= (\mathbf{p}_C^1, \mathbf{p}_C^2, ...); \mathbf{S}_C \cdot \mathbf{p}_C^i = (\sigma_C^i)^2 \cdot \mathbf{p}_C^i \\
\mathbf{C} &= \bar{\mathbf{C}} + \sum_{k=1}^{M_C} \alpha_C^k \sigma_C^k \mathbf{p}_C^k
\end{aligned} \tag{2}$$

where $m = 40$ is the number of training samples; $\bar{\mathbf{C}}$ and $\mathbf{S}_C$ are the average and the covariance matrix of the control point vectors, respectively; $\{(\sigma_C^i)^2\}$ and $\{\mathbf{p}_C^i\}$ are the descendingly ordered eigen values and associated eigen vectors, respectively; $\{\alpha_C^i\}$ are the model parameters; M_C is the cut-off points.

Fig. 1 shows the mean and the first two modes of variations of the SDM. Each instance of the SDM was generated by evaluating $\mathbf{I}_s = \bar{\mathbf{I}}(T^{FFD}(\mathbf{C}) \circ \mathbf{s}_0)$, where $T^{FFD}(\mathbf{C}) = \sum_{r=0}^{3} \sum_{s=0}^{3} \sum_{t=0}^{3} B_r(u)B_s(v)B_t(w)vec^{-1}(\mathbf{C})$ is the FFD generated from the instantiated control point vector $\mathbf{C} = \bar{\mathbf{C}} + \alpha_C \sigma_C^i \mathbf{p}_C^i$, with $\alpha_C \in \{-3.0, -1.5, 0, 1.5, 3.0\}$ and $i \in \{1, 2\}$ corresponding to the first two modes.

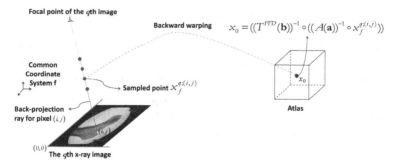

Fig. 2. A schematic illustration of the backward wapring.

2.2   Reconstruction Process

For an unseen proximal femur, we assume that we have a set of $Q \geq 2$ X-ray images and that all images are calibrated and co-registered to a common coordinate system called $\mathbf{f}$. Given an initial estimation of the registration parameters, our algorithm iteratively generates an 3D image and update the parameter estimation by minimizing the dissimilarity between the input 2D X-ray images and the associated DRRs that are created from the instantiated 3D image.

3D Image Instantiation and Alignment. The 3D image instantiation and alignment process is parametrized by two sets of parameters, i.e., the set of shape parameters $\mathbf{b} = (\alpha_C^1, \alpha_C^2, ..., \alpha_C^{Mc})^T$ determining a forward FFD from the atlas $\mathbf{s_0}$ to an instantiated 3D image $\mathbf{s}$ and the set of parameters $\mathbf{a} = (\Lambda, \beta, \gamma, \theta, t_x, t_y, t_z)^T$ determining a similarity transformation from the space of the instantiated image $\mathbf{s}$ to the common coordinate system $\mathbf{f}$, where Λ is the scaling parameter; β, γ, θ are rotational parameters and t_x, t_y, t_z are translational parameters. An instantiated 3D image that is aligned to the common coordinate system $\mathbf{f}$ is defined by following equation:

$$\bar{\mathbf{I}}(x_f(\mathbf{a}, \mathbf{b})) = \bar{\mathbf{I}}(\mathbf{A}(\mathbf{a}) \circ T^{FFD}(\mathbf{b}) \circ x_0) \tag{3}$$

where $\mathbf{A}(\mathbf{a})$ is the similarity transformation and $T^{FFD}(\mathbf{b})$ is the forward FFD.

Eq. (3) describes a forward warping. It is known that implementing this forward warping may result in holes in the aligned 3D image and a backward warping as follows should be used instead (see Fig. 2 for an illustration).

$$\bar{\mathbf{I}}(x_f^{q;(i,j)}) = \bar{\mathbf{I}}(x_0) = \bar{\mathbf{I}}((T^{FFD}(\mathbf{b}))^{-1} \circ ((A(\mathbf{a}))^{-1} \circ x_f^{q;(i,j)})) \tag{4}$$

where $x_f^{q;(i,j)}$ is a sampled discrete point (see Fig. 2) along the back-projection ray of a pixel (i, j) in the qth input X-ray images.

It is straightforward to compute the inverse of the similarity transformation $\mathbf{A}(\mathbf{a})$. However, it is computationally expensive to compute the inverse of the forward FFD $T^{FFD}(\mathbf{b})$. In this paper, instead of computing the inverse of the forward FFD, we propose to compute a pseudo-inverse of the instantiated B-spline transformation using the B-spline pseudo-inverse algorithm introduced in

[15]. The computed pseudo-inverse B-splines coefficients then allow us to compute a backward FFD in order to warp the atlas to the instantiated volume **s**. For details about this algorithm, we refer to [15]. To speed up the 3D B-spline pseudo-inverse computation, we have implemented the algorithm on GPU with the Compute Unified Device Architecture (CUDA) programming environment.

Registration Criterion. We chose to use the robust dissimilarity measure introduced in [16] to compare the floating DRRs to the associated reference X-ray images. This robust dissimilarity measure is defined as:

$$E(\mathbf{a},\mathbf{b}) = \sum_{q=1}^{Q} [\lambda \sum_{i,j}^{I,J} D_{q;(i,j)}^2(\mathbf{a},\mathbf{b})+ \tag{5}$$
$$(1-\lambda) \sum_{i,j}^{I,J} \frac{1}{card(N_{i,j}^r)} \sum_{(i',j')\in N_{i,j}^r} (D_{q;(i,j)}(\mathbf{a},\mathbf{b}) - D_{q;(i',j')}(\mathbf{a},\mathbf{b}))^2]$$

where $I \times J$ is the size of each X-ray image; $D_q = \{D_{q;(i,j)}\}$ is the qth observed difference image; $N = \{N_{i,j}^r\}$ are the rth order neighborhood systems and $card(N_{i,j}^r)$ is the number of pixels in $N_{i,j}^r$. We refer interesting readers to [16] for the details about how the difference images are computed and about the details of above equation.

Optimization Strategy. Considering the least-squares form of Eq. (5), we decided to use Levenberg-Marquardt optimizer to minimize $E(\mathbf{a},\mathbf{b})$. More specifically, the following two stages are executed until convergence.

- Similarity registration stage: The shape parameters are fixed to the current estimation $\mathbf{b}_t$ and the Levenberg-Marquardt optimizer is used to iteratively minimize the image dissimilarity energy $E(\mathbf{a},\mathbf{b}_t)$ in order to obtain a new estimation of the similarity transformation parameters $\mathbf{a}_{t+1}$.
- Non-rigid registration stage: The similarity transformation parameters are fixed to $\mathbf{a}_{t+1}$ and the Levenberg-Marquardt optimizer is used again to iteratively estimate the new shape deformation parameters $\mathbf{b}_{t+1}$. At each iteration, following two steps are performed.
  - Step 1: Following the Levenberg-Marquardt optimizer, compute the gradient and the regularized Hessian of Eq. (5) with respect to the shape parameters, and then calculate an additive update $\Delta\mathbf{b}_t$ of the shape parameters to get a new estimation $\mathbf{b}_{t+1} = \mathbf{b}_t + \Delta\mathbf{b}_t$.
  - Step 2: Based on $\mathbf{b}_{t+1}$, we first instantiate the control point vector $\mathbf{C} = \bar{\mathbf{C}} + \sum_{k=1}^{M_C} \alpha_C^k \sigma_C^k \mathbf{p}_C^k$. We then compute its pseudo-inverse. Based on the computed pseudo-inverse B-splines coefficients, we can compute a backward FFD, which will be used to warp the atlas to the instantiated image **s** to generate DRRs for the next iteration.

3   Experiments and Results

The atlas has a resolution of $192 \times 128 \times 192$ voxels with a voxel size of $0.664 \times 0.664 \times 1.0mm^3$. The control point lattice has a size of $25 \times 18 \times 35$ points with a

Table 1. Pseudo-inverse validation results where R_x, R_y, and R_z are correlation coefficients of the two backward FFDs along x, y, and z axis, respectively.

Quantity		#1	#2	#3	#4	#5	#6	#7	#8	#9	#10	Average
R_x		0.993	0.997	0.998	0.994	0.991	0.997	0.995	0.997	0.998	0.997	0.996
R_y		0.996	0.997	0.997	0.996	0.996	0.997	0.997	0.997	0.997	0.996	0.997
R_z		0.998	0.995	0.993	0.998	0.998	0.995	0.993	0.995	0.993	0.994	0.995
$Mean\_M$ (mm)		0.049	0.086	0.081	0.095	0.104	0.097	0.097	0.094	0.084	0.096	0.088
$Median\_M$ (mm)		0.014	0.024	0.023	0.023	0.025	0.027	0.027	0.023	0.021	0.027	0.023
Computing	elastix	202	200	199	201	204	205	205	204	202	203	202.5
Time (s)	Ours	1.33	1.22	1.02	1.06	1.01	1.09	1.05	1.03	1.09	0.98	1.09

grid spacing of $6.0 \times 6.0 \times 6.0 mm^3$. For all the registration experiments, the cutoff point M_C was empirically chosen to be 9. Shape parameters **b** were initialized to zeros and pose parameters **a** were initialized with anatomical landmark based registration. Implemented on a laptop with 2.5 GHz Intel Core i5 processor and Nvidia GeForce GT 750M graphics card, it took about 5-7 minutes to register the SDM to 2 X-ray images with a resolution of 768×576 pixels.

Pseudo-Inverse Validation Experiment. Due to the facts that no direct validation was conducted in [15] to validate the accuracy of the 2D bspline pseudo-inverse algorithm and that we have implemented a GPU-based 3D version of the 2D pseudo-inverse algorithm introduced in [15], we designed this experiment to validate the accuracy of our 3D pseudo-inverse algorithm by comparing the backward FFD calculated from the results of our pseudo-inverse algorithm with the one computed by 'elastix' [13] via non-rigid registration. Please note that in 'elastix' a smaller grid spacing than the forward FFD is chosen for the inverse transform which prevents a direct comparison of the inverted B-splines coefficients generated by these two different methods. This experiment was conducted on the registration outputs of the first 10 proximal femurs in the second stage of the SDM construction. Correlation along each axis of the two backward FFDs, the mean and median magnitudes ($Mean\_M$ and $Median\_M$) of the difference vectors at all voxels, and the computing time are presented in Table 1, which demonstrates that our b-spline pseudo-inverse algorithm is accurate and fast.

Experiment on C-arm Images of 10 Cadaveric Femurs. In this experiment, 10 cadaveric femurs (none of them was used in the SDM construction) were used. For each femur, we acquired two calibrated C-arm images around the proximal region. The reconstruction accuracies were evaluated by randomly digitizing dozens points from the surface of each femur and then computing the distances from those digitized points to the associated surface model which was segmented from the reconstructed volume. Mean and median reconstruction errors for each femur are presented in Table 2. The mean reconstruction errors range from 1.0 mm to 1.6mm and an average accuracy of 1.3 mm was found.

Experiment on X-Ray Images of 6 Cadaveric Femurs. In this experiment, X-ray images of another 6 cadaveric femurs (again, none of them was used in the SDM construction) were used, where 3 of them were part of complete hips.

Table 2. Results of experiment on C-arm images of 10 cadaveric femurs.

Quantity	#1	#2	#3	#4	#5	#6	#7	#8	#9	#10	Average
Mean (mm)	1.5	1.0	1.1	1.0	1.4	1.6	1.4	1.3	1.1	1.1	1.3
Median (mm)	1.2	0.7	0.8	0.8	1.1	1.4	1.2	1.1	0.9	0.9	1.0

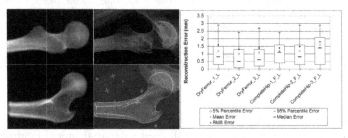

Fig. 3. Results of applying the present approach to X-ray images of 6 cadaveric femurs. Left column shows DRRs of a reconstructed volume, middle column shows X-ray images (for visualization purpose, only regions around the proximal femur are shown) super-imposed with edges extracted from the DRRs, and right image shows the errors of reconstructing all 6 cadaveric femurs.

For each femur, the ground truth surface models were either obtained with a CT-scan reconstruction method (for 3 complete hips) or with a hand-held laser-scan reconstruction method (for others). The surface models segmented from the reconstructed volumes were then compared to the associated ground truth models to evaluate the reconstruction accuracies. A reconstruction example as well as the errors of reconstructing volumes of all 6 femurs is shown in Fig. 3. An average mean reconstruction accuracy of 1.2 mm was found.

4   Discussions and Conclusions

We presented a non-rigid free-from 2D-3D registration approach using statistical deformation model. The iterative registration of the SDM to the input X-ray images required a computationally expensive inversion of the instantiated deformation in each iteration. In this paper, we solved this challenge with a fast B-spline pseudo-inversion algorithm that was implemented on GPU. Results from comprehensive experiments conducted on both simulated and real X-ray images of cadaveric femurs demonstrated the efficacy of the present approach.

In comparison to the state of the art, our approach has several advantages. For example, the shape model presented in [3] was constructed on the dense deformation fields while we constructed our SDM on sparse B-splines control point vectors, which required much less storage space. Furthermore, Using the pseudo-inverse B-splines coefficients to compute the backward FFD can be viewed as a smoothing alternative in which explicit regularization is achieved through B-splines approximation. Thus, no additional regularization is needed.

Acknowledgments. This work was partially supported by the Japanese-Swiss Science and Technology Cooperation Program. We thank Dr P. Zysset for providing training CT data.

References

1. Sadowsky, O., Chintalapani, G., Taylor, R.H.: Deformable 2D-3D registration of the pelvis with a limited field of view, using shape statistics. In: Ayache, N., Ourselin, S., Maeder, A. (eds.) MICCAI 2007, Part II. LNCS, vol. 4792, pp. 519–526. Springer, Heidelberg (2007)
2. Ahmad, O., Ramamurthi, K., et al.: Volumetric DXA (VXA) - A new method to extract 3D information from multiple in vivo DXA images. J. Bone Miner. Res. **25**, 2468–2475 (2010)
3. Zheng, G.: Personalized x-ray reconstruction of the proximal femur via intensity-based non-rigid 2D-3D registration. In: Fichtinger, G., Martel, A., Peters, T. (eds.) MICCAI 2011, Part II. LNCS, vol. 6892, pp. 598–606. Springer, Heidelberg (2011)
4. Whitmarsh, T., Humbert, L., et al.: Reconstructing the 3D shape and bone mineral density distribution of the proximal femur from dual-energy X-ray absorptiometry. IEEE T. Med. Imaging **30**, 2101–2114 (2011)
5. Lucas, B.C., Otake, Y., Armand, M., Taylor, R.H.: An active contour method for bone cement reconstruction from C-arm X-ray images. IEEE T. Med. Imaging **31**, 860–869 (2012)
6. Markelj, P., Tomazevic, D., et al.: A review of 3D/2D registration methods for image-guided interventions. Med. Image Anal. **16**, 642–661 (2012)
7. Yu, W., Zheng, G.: Personalized x-ray reconstruction of the proximal femur via a new control point-based 2D–3D registration and residual complexity minimization. In: VCBM 2014, pp. 155–162 (2014)
8. Rueckert, D., Frangi, A.F., Schnabel, J.A.: Automatic construction of 3D statistical deformation models using non-rigid registration. In: Niessen, W.J., Viergever, M.A. (eds.) MICCAI 2001. LNCS, vol. 2208, pp. 77–84. Springer, Heidelberg (2001)
9. Loeckx, D., et al.: Temporal subtraction of thorax CR images using a statistical deformation model. IEEE T. Med. Imaging **22**, 1490–1504 (2003)
10. Barratt, D.C., et al.: Instantiation and registration of statistical shape models of the femur and pelvis using 3D ultrasound imaging. Med. Image Anal. **12**, 358–374 (2008)
11. Onofrey J., Papademetris X., Staib L.: Low-Dimensional Non-rigid Image Registration Using Statistical Deformation Models from Semi-Supervised Training Data. IEEE T. Med. Imaging (2015) (in press)
12. Pszczolkowski, S., Pizarro, L., Guerrero, R., Rueckert, D.: Nonrigid free-form registration using landmark-based statistical deformation models. In: Proc. SPIE, Medical Imaging, vol. 8314 (2012). doi:10.1117/12.911441
13. Klein, S., Staring, M., et al.: Elastix: a toolox for intensity-based medical image registration. IEEE T. Med. Imaging **29**, 196–205 (2010)
14. Rueckert, D., Sonoda, L.I., et al.: Nonrigid registration using free-form deformations: Application to breast MR images. IEEE T. Med. Imaging **18**, 712–721 (1999)
15. Tristán, A., Arribas, J.I.: A fast B-spline pseudo-inversion algorithm for consistent image registration. In: Kropatsch, W.G., Kampel, M., Hanbury, A. (eds.) CAIP 2007. LNCS, vol. 4673, pp. 768–775. Springer, Heidelberg (2007)
16. Zheng, G.: Effective incorporating spatial information in a mutual information based 3D–2D registration of a CT volume to X-ray images. Comput. Med. Imag. Grap. **34**, 553–562 (2010)

Learning and Combining Image Similarities for Neonatal Brain Population Studies

Veronika A. Zimmer[1]([✉]), Ben Glocker[3], Paul Aljabar[4], Serena J. Counsell[4],
Mary A. Rutherford[4], A. David Edwards[4], Jo V. Hajnal[4],
Miguel Ángel González Ballester[1,2], Daniel Rueckert[3], and Gemma Piella[1]

[1] SIMBioSys Group, Universitat Pompeu Fabra, Barcelona, Spain
veronika.zimmer@upf.edu
[2] ICREA, Barcelona, Spain
[3] Biomedical Image Analysis Group, Imperial College London, London, UK
[4] Imaging Sciences & Biomedical Engineering, King's College London, London, UK

Abstract. The characterization of neurodevelopment is challenging due to the complex structural changes of the brain in early childhood. To analyze the changes in a population across time and to relate them with clinical information, manifold learning techniques can be applied. The neighborhood definition used for constructing manifold representations of the population is crucial for preserving the similarity structure in the embedding and highly application dependent. It has been shown that the combination of several notions of similarity and features can improve the new representation. However, how to combine and weight different similarites and features is non-trivial. In this work, we propose to learn the neighborhood structure and similarity measure used for manifold learning through Neighborhood Approximation Forests (NAFs). The recently proposed NAFs learn a neighborhood structure in a dataset based on a user-defined distance. A characterization of image similarity using NAFs enables us to construct manifold representations based on a previously defined criterion to improve predictions regarding structural and clinical information. In particular, NAFs can be used naturally to combine the affinities learned from multiple distances in a joint manifold towards a more meaningful representation and an improved characterization of the resulting embedding. We demonstrate the utility of NAFs in manifold learning on a population of preterm and in term neonates for classification regarding structural volume and clinical information.

1 Introduction

During early childhood, the brain undergoes complex structural changes, which makes it challenging to characterize normal and abnormal brain development. There is a need for identifying brain imaging biomarkers to improve the diagnostic and therapy. To analyze the changes and differences in a population and to relate them with clinical information, manifold learning techniques can be applied. Classical manifold learning techniques use the neighborhood of images,

© Springer International Publishing Switzerland 2015
L. Zhou et al. (Eds.): MLMI 2015, LNCS 9352, pp. 110–117, 2015.
DOI: 10.1007/978-3-319-24888-2_14

defined, e.g., by the L2-distance of intensities, to construct manifold representations of the population. The neighborhood definition is crucial for the quality of the resulting representation and highly application dependent. There has been much interest in identifying and combining additional information in the manifold learning step to improve the resulting embeddings. The manifold structure of brain images has been estimated in [1] based on pairwise non-rigid transformations, whereas in [2] similarities were derived from overlaps of their structural segmentations. In [3], shape and appearance information was combined in a joint embedding for an improved characterization of brain development and in [4] clinical information was incorporated into the embedding construction. However, in general it is not clear how to combine and weight multiple features.

For deriving manifold representations from imaging information, typically the whole image is used (e.g., the L2-distance between all the intensities). But it may not be known in advance which voxels or features are important for a given classification task and manifold learning does not provide insight into this question. The extraction of relevant features requires prior knowledge to the underlying data which might not be available for all applications.

Random forests, on the other hand, have shown to be a powerful approach to feature selection and classification. In [5], they were applied to manifold learning by deriving the pairwise similarity measures from random forest classifiers for different modalities. Additionally, the most important features for the classification problem could be extracted. Recently, the neighborhood approximation forests (NAFs) [6] have been proposed which learn the neighborhood structure in a dataset and the most discriminative features based on a user-defined distance.

In this work, we learn the neighborhood structure used for manifold learning through NAFs. The ability of NAFs to learn on arbitrary distances enables us to construct manifold representations for specific high-level information. NAFs generate affinities based on co-occurrence in leaf nodes and give a natural way to combine the affinities learned from multiple distances. We consider the problem of classification of the data samples regarding structural and clinical information. We train the NAFs on a population of preterm and in term neonatal MR images based on the differences in structural volume (cerebellum and left lateral ventricle volume) and clinical information (gestational age (GA) at scan, birth weight in kilograms (kg) and whether oxygen was supplied after birth). Using the obtained affinity matrices, we construct manifold representations and show their improved performance for classification regarding the learned information. In particular, we show that joint embeddings, obtained by combining affinity matrices from different NAFs, are able to encode simultaneously different information.

2   Methods

Neighborhood Approximation Forests. A NAF learns in a supervised manner a neighborhood structure of a given dataset induced by an arbitrary notion of similarity between images. In the training step, the algorithm uses features based on appearance to cluster the images according to the distance function.

For testing, the learned features are used to predict the closest neighbors in the training database of a test image. Given a population $\mathcal{I}$ of images, a subset $\mathbf{I} = \{I_p\}_{p=1}^{P} \in \mathcal{I}$ is used for training and each I_p is represented by a high-dimensional intensity-based feature vector $\mathbf{f}(I_p) \in \mathbb{R}^Q$. The population $\mathcal{I}$ is equipped with a user-defined distance function $\rho : \mathcal{I} \times \mathcal{I} \to \mathbb{R}$ which allows the definition of pairwise distances $\rho(I_m, I_n)$ between the training images.

Training Phase: In the training phase N individual trees are constructed. For each tree T, a random subset of features $\mathbf{f}_T \subset \mathbf{f}$ is selected with $\mathbf{f}_T \in \mathbb{R}^q$, $q < Q$. At each node of tree T, the algorithm divides the data samples present in the current node into two sets. This branching of the set of images $\mathbf{I}_s$ present in node s is based on a binary test: for $I_n \in \mathbf{I}_s$, $I_n \in \mathbf{I}_{s_R}$ if $\mathbf{f}_T^m(I_n) > \tau$ and $I_n \in \mathbf{I}_{s_L}$ if $\mathbf{f}_T^m(I_n) \leq \tau$. Here, $\tau \in \mathbb{R}$, s_R and s_L are the children nodes of s and $\mathbf{f}_T^m$ is the mth component of $\mathbf{f}_T$. For each node in each tree, t_s is optimized with respect to the parameters m and τ such that the data samples are clustered according to the distance function ρ in the most compact way.

Testing Phase: Given a test set $\hat{\mathbf{I}} = \{\hat{I}_r\}_{r=1}^{R} \in \mathcal{I}$, a test image $\hat{I}_r$ is passed down each tree in the forest. At a node, the binary test with the parameters learned in the training phase is applied. According to this test, the image is sent to the left or to the right child of the current node. This is repeated until the image arrives at a leaf node. If the leaf node contains the training image I_p, their affinity a_{pr} is increased by one. This procedure yields an affinity matrix $A = \{a_{pr}\}_{\substack{p=1,...,P \\ r=1...,R}}$ between the samples of the training and testing set.

Feature Selection: During the training phase of NAFs, the parameters m and τ of the binary test t_s in node s are optimized to obtain an optimal partitioning of the training data samples. The parameter m denotes the component of the feature vector $\mathbf{f}_T^m$ which is tested at the current node. There exist several ways of determining the importance of individual features for the growing of the decision trees. In [6], a feature is considered as important, if it is selected in the first three levels of the trees. A more sophisticated approach was used in [5], where the decrease in the Gini impurity criterion was measured for the individual features in each node. In this work, we adopt the former and simpler approach. The frequency of the selected features in the first three levels of the trees of the forest is recorded, and the values are normalized by the number of nodes in the tree level.

NAFs for Manifold Learning. The NAFs F_ρ are trained using the training set $\mathbf{I}$. For each distance function ρ, a pairwise affinity matrix $A_\rho \in \mathbb{R}^{P \times P} = \{a_\rho^{(ij)}\}_{i,j=1,...,P}$ is computed, where $a_\rho^{(ij)}$ reports, how often image $I_j \in \mathbf{I}$ and $I_i \in \mathbf{I}$ finish in the same node. The corresponding distance matrix D_ρ is constructed as $D_\rho = \{d_\rho^{(ij)}\}_{i,j=1,...,P}$ with $d_\rho^{(ij)} = 1 - a_\rho^{(ij)}/N$, where N is the number of trees in the forest. The matrix D_ρ can now be interpreted as pairwise distances of the image set $\mathbf{I}$ and can be used for constructing a manifold representation of the training set. We employ Isomap [7], a global approach, for learning the manifold which we found to give better embeddings than local approaches, such as Laplacian Eigenmaps. The combination of different affinity matrices A_{ρ_k}, $k = 1, \ldots, K$ learned with NAFs based on user-defined distances ρ_k, to create a joint embedding can be done by linear combination. That is, if the NAFs F_{ρ_k} contain the same number N of trees, the affinity matrices are additively combined by $A_{\rho_1, \ldots, \rho_K} = \frac{1}{K} \sum_{k=1}^{K} A_{\rho_k}$ and the components of the joint distance matrix $D_{\rho_1, \ldots, \rho_K}$ are $d_{\rho_1, \ldots, \rho_K}^{(ij)} = 1 - a_{\rho_1, \ldots, \rho_K}^{(ij)} / N$.

3   Data and Results

Data. We tested the proposed approach on a population of 343 neonatal brain T2 weighted MR images, both preterm and in term subjects, with an age range of $26.71 - 49.86$ GA at scan. For all subjects, automatic segmentation into 87 regions were available [8]. For a subset of 314 subjects, the weight at birth in kg is known and for a subset of 212 subjects it is known whether oxygen was supplied right after birth. In the experiments, we used this information to construct manifold representations of the populations.

All images were skull-stripped using BET [9], corrected for bias using N4 [10] and intensity normalized. To account for the size differences in the population, all subjects were affine aligned to an atlas template of 37 GA [11]. A non-rigid alignment was further applied with a large control point spacing to preserve detailed differences in the images. The aligned images in the atlas space were of size $117 \times 159 \times 126$ with an isotropic voxel size of $0.86 \, \text{mm}$. The images were smoothed using a Gaussian filter with physical size of $4.3 \, \text{mm}$ in each dimension.

NAF Construction. The feature vector for each image was composed of the intensities of randomly chosen voxels inside the brain mask of the atlas template. We chose a feature vector of length $Q = 100,000$. We trained NAFs for five different definitions of the distance function ρ: (i) F_{GA}, ρ is age difference; (ii) F_{BW}, ρ is difference in weight at birth; (iii) F_{LVV}, ρ is difference in left lateral ventricle volume; (iv) F_{CV}, ρ is difference in cerebellum volume. In addition, we trained a NAF on (v) F_{O2} using instead of a distance function the labels to train the trees. The parameters of the NAFs in the training phase were determinted empirically. We used 500 trees in each forest, in each tree $q = \text{round}(\sqrt{Q}) = 316$ features are evaluated, the maximum tree depth was 12 and the minimum sample size at a leaf was 5.

Manifold Learning and Regression. Isomap was applied to the affinity matrices obtained by the NAFs as described in Section 2. We kept the first 20 dimensions as new embedding coordinates. To evaluate the quality of the resulting embeddings, we predicted clinical and structural information for the test images and compared it to the real values. For each embedding, we predicted the following: (a) GA: GA at scan, (b) BW: birth weight in kg, (c) O2: O_2 supply after birth, (d) LVV: volume of the left ventricle, (e) CV: volume of the cerebellum. The prediction $\tilde{v}_i(I)$ of the real value $v_i(I)$, $i \in \{\text{GA}, \text{BW}, \text{O2}, \text{LVV}, \text{CV}\}$, for a test image I is obtained using the weighted mean: $\tilde{v}_i(I) = \dfrac{\sum_{I_n \in \mathbf{N}_\rho^k} \mathbf{w}(I, I_n) v_i(I_n)}{\sum_{I_n \in \mathbf{N}_\rho^k} \mathbf{w}(I, I_n)}$, where $\mathbf{N}_\rho^k$ is the set of k nearest neighbors of I in the training set and $\mathbf{w}(I, \cdot)$ are the affinities of I with respect to the training images.

Experiments and Results. We trained the forests F_{GA}, F_{LVV}, F_{CV}, F_{BW} and F_{O2} with two different configurations. For the first option, we trained the NAFs on the whole populations such that we get pairwise affinity matrices A_i and corresponding distance matrices D_i, $i \in \{GA, BW, O2, LVV, CV\}$, for the whole populations. Isomap was applied to each D_i in order to get a manifold representation of the dataset. For the evaluation of the performance in classification, we excluded the ground truth of the current test image in the regression step. For the second option, we performed leave-ten-out cross validations to estimate the performance of out-of-sample predictions. Multiple forests were constructed for each F_i, excluding ten samples each time, which were used for testing.

The regression results are shown in Table 1, where for each embedding the correlation between predicted and real value is presented. The columns correspond to the information we want to predict and the rows to the embeddings used for prediction. It can be seen that the quality of the predictions differ significantly between the different embeddings. All embeddings yield high correlation values for the prediction of the GA at scan. This is due to the fact, that the appearance of the images differ strongly between the age groups. Even the simple L2-distance between images is able to capture those differences. This is not the case for the predictions of the other clinical and structural information. All embeddings lead to poor correlation values for the prediction of the birth weight or the O2 supply, except for the embeddings based on F_{BW} and F_{O2}, respectively. This indicates that it is challenging to estimate neighborhoods which capture all the structural and functional changes in the brain. By constructing specified neighborhoods using various similarity definition, we are able to better classify and categorize the population according to previously defined criteria. When using leave-ten-out cross validation, the correlation values decrease in most of the cases. This expected effect was particularly marked for the embedding based on F_{O2}.

Table 1. Correlation between real and predicted values by the embedding based on normal L2-distance and NAFs as explained in Section 3.

	Whole population					Leave-ten-out				
	GA	BW	O$_2$	LVV	CV	GA	BW	O$_2$	LVV	CV
L2	0.93	0.51	-0.03	0.65	0.92	0.87	0.42	0.11	0.43	0.85
F_{GA}	**0.99**	0.44	0.09	0.43	0.94	**0.96**	0.42	0.02	0.52	0.92
F_{BW}	0.93	**0.96**	0.23	0.50	0.89	0.92	**0.73**	0.23	0.52	0.87
F_{O2}	0.91	0.49	**0.81**	0.56	0.86	0.87	0.48	**0.26**	0.61	0.79
F_{LVV}	0.93	0.30	0.12	**0.95**	0.92	0.92	0.34	-0.01	**0.89**	0.90
F_{CV}	0.96	0.55	0.16	0.49	**0.99**	0.95	0.50	-0.03	0.50	**0.94**

As an example, two embeddings, obtained with the simple L2-distance and with F_{BW}, are visualized through their first two embedding coordinates in Fig. 1.

The color coding is according to the weight at birth in kg. It can be clearly seen that the embedding based on the L2-distance is not able to separate the data samples according to birth weight, whereas the embedding based on F_{BW} provides a good separation.

L2-distance  F_{BW}

Fig. 1. Scatter plots of the first two embedding coordinates. Embeddings obtained with the L2-distance (left) and F_{BW} (right) as similarity measure. The color coding corresponds to the weight at birth in kg.

The embeddings based on NAFs are specialized embeddings, meaning that they are constructed to estimate the neighborhood according to one specific criteria. The downside of this approach can be seen, e.g., for the prediction of the left lateral ventricle volume. The embeddings based on the L2-distance, F_{GA}, F_{BW} and F_{O_2} obtain rather low correlation values in the range of $0.4 - 0.65$ for predicting the left lateral ventricle volume. However, the joint embedding, which combines the affinity matrices of the NAFs trained on the ventricle volume and the birth weight, as explained in Section 2, is able to predict both information more accurately. This is shown in Table 2, where the correlation of the real and predicted values are shown for three joint embeddings based on (i) $F_{BW,LVV}$: combination of F_{BW} and F_{LVV}, (ii) $F_{BW,CV}$: combination of F_{BW} and F_{CV} and (iii) $F_{LVV,CV}$: combination of F_{LVV} and F_{CV}.

Table 2. Correlation between real value of clinical and structural information and predicted values by the joint embedding as explained in Section 3.

	Whole population					Leave-ten-out				
	GA	BW	O$_2$	LVV	CV	GA	BW	O$_2$	LVV	CV
$F_{BW,LVV}$	0.95	**0.90**	0.14	**0.95**	0.92	0.95	**0.67**	0.05	**0.88**	0.91
$F_{BW,CV}$	0.97	**0.89**	0.05	0.55	**0.98**	0.97	**0.66**	0.13	0.55	**0.95**
$F_{LVV,CV}$	0.95	0.42	0.20	**0.96**	**0.93**	0.94	0.37	-0.10	**0.86**	**0.93**

Figure 2 plots the regression results using the joint embedding based on F_{BW-LVV} and the individual embeddings of F_{BW} and F_{LVV} for predicting the weight at birth and the left lateral ventricle volume. The differences are clearly seen. Neither F_{LVV} is able to predict the birth weight, nor F_{BW} to predict the volume of the left ventricle. The correlation between predicted and real values are poor and the root mean square error (RMS) is high. The joint embedding based on both NAFs, however, yields correlation values of 0.90 for the birth weight and 0.95 for the lateral ventricle volume and smaller RMS.

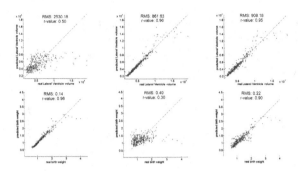

Fig. 2. Scatter plots for left lateral ventricle volume (top row) and birth weight prediction (bottom row) based on F_{BW} (left), F_{LVV} (middle) and joint $F_{BW,LVV}$ (right).

During training, NAF selects the most discriminative features according to the selected distance function. In Fig. 3, the features selected in the first three levels of the trees are shown for F_{LVV} and F_{GA}. As expected, the most discriminative features in forest F_{LVV} are in the left lateral ventricle. The most discriminative features in forest F_{GA} are found in the deep gray matter and part of the cortex. In this regions the appearance in MR differ strongly between younger (26-28 GA) and older neonates (37-42 GA).

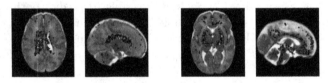

Fig. 3. Features selected in the first three levels of the trees for distance based on left ventricle volume (left: axial and sagittal) and GA at scan (right: axial and sagittal).

4   Conclusions

We have proposed a framework for manifold learning, where the pairwise similarities are learned and combined through NAFs. We used the resulting embeddings to perform classification regarding structural and clinical information. One key motivation of using NAFs is that they provide a natural way for the combination of similarities learned from multiple distances in the manifold learning step. In addition, the NAFs approximate neighborhoods based on arbitrary distances and select automatically the features which are most discriminative for the given distance function which make a priori feature extraction not necessary.

The method was applied to a population of preterm and in term neonatal MR images. We trained the NAFs on appearance features of the images based on differences in cerebellum and left lateral ventricle volume, GA at scan, birth weight and oxygen supply. The resulting embeddings were specific to the criterion their neighborhoods were trained on (structural volumes, birth weight, etc.)

and showed an accurate classification performance regarding this criterion while embeddings based on classical similarity measures fail. In particular, we showed how the combination of pairwise affinity matrices based on different NAFs can improve the overall performance of the joint embedding.

Encoding simultaneously different information (clinical and image-based) in the embeddings may help in studying abnormal brain development which is characterized by the change in multiple biomarkers.

Acknowledgments. The authors would like to thank E. Konukoglu for providing the implementation of the NAFs (publicly available at http://www.nmr.mgh.harvard. edu/~enderk/software.html).

V. A. Zimmer is supported by the grant FI-DGR 2013 (2013 FI_B00159) from the Generalitat de Catalunya. This research was partially funded by the Spanish Ministry of Economy and Competitiveness (TIN2012-35874).

References

1. Gerber, S., Tasdizen, T., Fletcher, P., Joshi, S., Whitaker, R.: Manifold modeling for brain population analysis. Med. Imag. Anal. **14**(5), 643–653 (2010)
2. Aljabar, P., Rueckert, D., Crum, W.: Automated morphological analysis of magnetic resonance brain imaging using spectral analysis. NeuroImage **43**(2), 225–235 (2008)
3. Aljabar, P., Wolz, R., Srinivasan, L., Counsell, S.J., Rutherford, M.A., Edwards, A.D., Hajnal, J.V., Rueckert, D.: A Combined Manifold Learning Analysis of Shape and Appearance to Characterize Neonatal Brain Development. IEEE Trans. Med. Imag. **30**(12), 2072–2086 (2011)
4. Wolz, R., Aljabar, P., Hajnal, J.V., Lötjönen, J., Rueckert, D.: Nonlinear dimensionality reduction combining MR imaging with nonimaging information. Med. Imag. Anal. **16**(4), 819–830 (2012)
5. Gray, K.R., Aljabar, P., Heckemann, R.A., Hammers, A. Rueckert, D., Alzheimer's Disease Neuroimaging Initiative: Random forest-based similarity measures for multi-modal classification of Alzheimer's disease. NeuroImage **65**, 167–175 (2013)
6. Konukoglu, E., Glocker, B., Zikic, D., Criminisi, A.: Neighborhood approximation using randomized forests. Med. Imag. Anal. **17**, 790–804 (2013)
7. Tenenbaum, J.B., de Silva, V., Langford, J.C.: A Global Geometric Framework for Nonlinear Dimensionality Reduction. Science **290**(5500), 2319–2323 (2000)
8. Makropoulos, A., Gousias, I.S., Ledig, C., Aljabar, P., Serag, A., Hajnal, J., Edwards, A.D., Counsell, S., Rueckert, D.: Automatic whole brain MRI segmentation of the developing neonatal brain. IEEE Trans. Med. Imag. **33**(9), 1818–1831 (2014)
9. Smith, S.M.: Fast robust automated brain extraction. Human Brain Mapping **17**(3), 143–155 (2002)
10. Tustison, N.J., Avants, B.B., Cook, P.A., Zheng, Y., Egan, A., Yushkevich, P.A., Gee, J.C.: N4ITK: Improved N3 Bias Correction. IEEE Trans. Med. Imag. **29**(6), 1310–1320 (2010)
11. Serag, A., Aljabar, P., Ball, G., Counsell, S.J., Boardman, J.P., Rutherford, M.A., Edwards, A.D., Hajnal, J.V., Rueckert, D.: Construction of a consistent high-definition spatio-temporal atlas of the developing brain using adaptive kernel regression. NeuroImage **59**(3), 2255–65 (2012)

Deep Learning, Sparse Coding, and SVM for Melanoma Recognition in Dermoscopy Images

Noel Codella[1]($\boxtimes$), Junjie Cai[1], Mani Abedini[2], Rahil Garnavi[2],
Alan Halpern[3], and John R. Smith[1]

[1] IBM T.J. Watson Research Center, Yorktown Heights, NY, USA
nccodell@us.ibm.com
[2] IBM Australia Research Labs, Melbourne, VIC, Australia
[3] Memorial Sloan-Kettering Cancer Center, New York, NY, USA

Abstract. This work presents an approach for melanoma recognition in dermoscopy images that combines deep learning, sparse coding, and support vector machine (SVM) learning algorithms. One of the beneficial aspects of the proposed approach is that unsupervised learning within the domain, and feature transfer from the domain of natural photographs, eliminates the need of annotated data in the target task to learn good features. The applied feature transfer also allows the system to draw analogies between observations in dermoscopic images and observations in the natural world, mimicking the process clinical experts themselves employ to describe patterns in skin lesions. To evaluate the methodology, performance is measured on a dataset obtained from the International Skin Imaging Collaboration, containing 2624 clinical cases of melanoma (334), atypical nevi (144), and benign lesions (2146). The approach is compared to the prior state-of-art method on this dataset. Two-fold cross-validation is performed 20 times for evaluation (40 total experiments), and two discrimination tasks are examined: 1) melanoma vs. all non-melanoma lesions, and 2) melanoma vs. atypical lesions only. The presented approach achieves an accuracy of 93.1% (94.9% sensitivity, and 92.8% specificity) for the first task, and 73.9% accuracy (73.8% sensitivity, and 74.3% specificity) for the second task. In comparison, prior state-of-art ensemble modeling approaches alone yield 91.2% accuracy (93.0% sensitivity, and 91.0% specificity) first the first task, and 71.5% accuracy (72.7% sensitivity, and 68.9% specificity) for the second. Differences in performance were statistically significant ($p < 0.05$), suggesting the proposed approach is an effective improvement over prior state-of-art.

Keywords: Melanoma recognition · Dermoscopy · Dermatology · Deep learning · Sparse coding

1 Introduction

The United States saw an estimated 76,100 new cases of melanoma in 2014, and 9,710 melanoma related deaths [1]. The incidence of melanoma has doubled

© Springer International Publishing Switzerland 2015
L. Zhou et al. (Eds.): MLMI 2015, LNCS 9352, pp. 118–126, 2015.
DOI: 10.1007/978-3-319-24888-2_15

in a generation, and is increasing at a faster rate than any other type of solid tumor [2]. Early diagnosis is critical to combating this disease: when diagnosed in initial stages, treatments achieve a 98% 5-year survival rate. Once disease reaches lymphatics, survival rate drops to 62%. As the disease metastasizes to other areas of the body, survival drops even further to 16%. While non-invasive diagnostic methods with high sensitivity are necessary to curb the mortality rate, high-specificity is also required to prevent unnecessary medical costs, disfiguring procedures, and patient anxiety. Recent literature demonstrates that among a sampling of 20,000 skin lesions surgically excised to rule out melanoma, less than 0.1% of these tested positive for the disease [3].

Unaided visual inspection by expert dermatologists has been shown to yield diagnostic accuracy of about 60% [4]. In order to improve performance, dermoscopic imaging was introduced. Dermoscopy is a technique of placing a high-resolution magnifying imaging device in contact with the skin. Lighting is controlled, and a liquid interface or polarization filter is applied to remove surface skin reflectance, exposing underlying layers of skin to inspection. Assuming adequate levels of expertise by the interpreter, dermoscopic imaging has been shown to improve recognition performance over unaided visual inspection by approximately 50%, resulting in absolute accuracies between 75%-84% [5].

In an effort to standardize diagnostic methodologies and curb inter and intra-observer variation of dermoscopic image interpretation, procedural assessment algorithms were developed for clinicians to follow [6]. These include the ABCD rule, the 7-point checklist, the Menzies method, the CASH method, pattern analysis, and the revised pattern analysis. Among these clinical evaluation algorithms, studies have shown that pattern analysis yields better diagnostic performance over other approaches [7]. Pattern analysis involves the identification of predefined visual patterns in the lesions [6,8]. Often the descriptive terms referring to visual patterns are nicknamed in accordance with analogous entities in the natural world the patterns most resemble: i.e. "honeycomb," "cobblestone," or "moth eaten border". This habit of analogous descriptions make intuitive sense, as the effectiveness of using analogies to describe and relate new knowledge to pre-existing knowledge has been well documented in education literature [9]. Studies also find that clinicians with the most experience in the field of dermoscopy tend to rely on that experience more-so than the results of any one particular analytic method [10].

Given melanoma recognition in the clinical setting has trended toward the use of pattern descriptions with analogies and expert experience, this work explores whether these same underlying principles could be used to improve the performance of automated approaches. Prior work toward automated melanoma recognition has followed classical computer vision approaches that extract hand-coded low-level visual features, combined with some form of classifier training [5,11–17]. Application of deep learning strategies, which have been successful for the task of recognition in natural photographs, have been limited by the relatively small size of the datasets. This work combines the use of deep convolutional networks trained in the domain of natural photographs, in addition to specialized features learned via an efficient sparse coding algorithm [18], to eliminate the need of large collections of annotated data to learn good features, and allowing the system to draw analogies. Improvements in performance are demonstrated compared to previous state-of-art work.

2   Related Work

Many years of work surround the topic of melanoma recognition from dermo-scopic imaging. Review articles covering a sampling of manuscripts in the most recent decade have been presented [5]. The diversity of approaches is fairly broad, but constricted within the space of classifical computer vision approaches, each work covering varying combinations of low-level visual feature extractions (color, edge, and texture descriptors, quantification of melanin based on color, etc), or machine learning techniques (kNN, SVM, etc.), and some also involving segmen-tation approaches [11–13]. A team from the Pedro Hispano Hospital of Portu-gal sought to evaluate the performance of several machine learning approaches [16,17], including global and local color, edge, and texture descriptors, training classifiers using an array of techniques, including SVM and KNN. The maximum accuracy achieved by algorithms studied was approximately 89%, on a limited dataset of 200 lesions containing 40 melanomas.

Aside from work to directly learn to recognize melanoma, there has also been work to learn to recognize specific skin lesion patterns that are indicative of melanoma, and are more easily visually verified by a clinician, such as "blue-white veil" [14,15]. While this line of modeling holds a great deal of promise to improve the accuracy of melanoma recognition, studies have again been limited by the availability of annotated data.

Recently, there has been activity to build large-scale public repository of dermoscopy data for the purposes of establishing a benchmark in the field of melanoma recognition, organized by the International Skin Imaging Collabora-tion (ISIC) [19]. Algorithms applied on this dataset used methods similar to other previous studies, involving a combination of low-level visual features, including color histogram, edge histogram, and a multiscale variant of color Local Binary Pattern (LBP), to achieve best performance [20]. In this work, data from the ISIC dermoscopy dataset is used for evaluation.

3   Methods

The following subsections describe the dataset used for performance evaluation, as well as the approaches for learning classifiers in this domain.

3.1   Dataset

The International Skin Imaging Collaboration (ISIC) dataset currently contains one of the largest collections of contact non-polarized dermoscopy images, com-plete with manual bounding boxes placed around the lesions for analysis. Exam-ples are shown in Fig. 1. The dataset presents those cases that are most difficult

Melanoma   Atypical   Benign

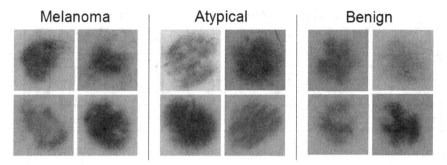

Fig. 1. Example images from the ISIC dermoscopy dataset, according to category.

for experts to distinguish, involving 334 images of melanoma and 144 images of atypical nevi, as well as 2146 clearly benign lesions (2624 total). Atypical nevi represent borderline cases: lesions that are not melanoma, but are visually similar to melanoma (as determined by expert analysis). Experiments of 2-fold cross-validation are performed 20 times (40 experiments total) for evaluation on this dataset. Two variants of the task are also performed: one task discriminating melanoma from both atypical and benign lesions (easier task), and one task discriminating melanoma from only atypical lesions (harder task).

3.2   Deep Learning Modeling Components

The presented deep learning approach uses two parallel paths: 1) transfer of convolutional neural network features learned from the domain of natural photographs, and 2) unsupervised feature learning, using sparse coding, within the domain of dermoscopy images. Classifiers are then subsequently trained for each using non-linear SVMs, and the models are then combined in late fusion (score averaging).

Convolutional Neural Network Features – The Caffe convolutional neural network (CNN) is a flexible and efficient deep learning architecture developed at Berkeley [21]. A pre-trained model from the Image Large Scale Visual Recognition Challenge (ILSVRC) 2012 is provided for download from the website. This pre-trained model includes 5 convolutional layers, 2 fully connected layers, and a final 1000 dimensional concept detector layer. In this work, the concept detector layer of this model (1000 dimensions, referred to as "FC8"), as well as the first fully connected layer (4096 dimensions, referred to as "FC6"), are used as visual descriptors for dermoscopy images.

Sparse Coding Features – Sparse coding is a class of unsupervised methods that seeks to learn a dictionary of sparse codes from which a given dataset can

☐ = "globule"-like patches   ☐ = "blue-whitish"-like patches

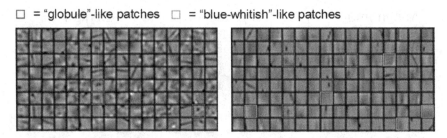

Fig. 2. Grayscale and RGB dictionary subsets learned from data. The method has identified common patterns that clinicians also search for, such as globules and blue-white structures.

be reconstructed. This is done by minimizing the following objective function:

$$\min_{D,\,\alpha} \quad \frac{1}{n} \sum_{i=1}^{n} \left(\frac{1}{2} \|x_i - D\alpha_i\|_2^2 + \lambda \|\alpha_i\|_1 \right) \qquad (1)$$

Where D is the learned dictionary, α_i is the sparse representation for data sample x_i, n is the number of samples, and λ is a regularization parameter. The SPAMS sparse coding dictionary learning algorithm [18] is an online optimization approach for this objective function, based on stochastic approximations. Because of its good efficiency, the SPAMS algorithm was employed to learn dictionaries on this dataset. Two dictionaries are constructed in color (RGB) and grayscale color spaces. Images are rescaled to 128x128 pixel dimensions before extraction of 8x8 patches, to learn dictionaries of 1024 elements. A λ value of 0.15, and 1000 iterations (recommended defaults in the SPAMS implementation) were used for minimization of the objective function. Representative dictionaries are depicted in Fig. 2.

Classifier Learning – To train melanoma classifiers from various deep features under study, a non-linear SVM using a histogram intersection kernel and sigmoid feature normalization was employed. SVM scores were mapped to probabilities using logistic regression on training data [22]. A probability of 50% is used as the binary classification threshold. Fusion is done by unweighted SVM score averaging (late fusion).

Table 1. Performance Results: Melanoma vs. Atypical and Benign

	Hand Coded	Caffe CNN			Sparse Coding			Fusions	
	Ensemble	4K FC6	1K FC8	Fusion	GRAY	RGB	Fusion	Deep	All
ACC	0.912	0.919	0.853	0.910	0.825	0.903	0.907	0.923	**0.931**
SEN	0.930	0.903	0.805	0.893	0.823	0.885	0.905	0.925	**0.949**
SPE	0.910	0.921	0.860	0.912	0.825	0.906	0.907	0.923	**0.928**

Table 2. Performance Results: Melanoma vs. Atypical

	Hand Coded	Caffe CNN			Sparse Coding			Fusions	
	Ensemble	**4K FC6**	**1K FC8**	**Fusion**	**GRAY**	**RGB**	**Fusion**	**Deep**	**All**
ACC	0.715	0.723	0.654	0.725	0.651	0.681	0.695	0.728	**0.739**
SEN	0.727	0.724	0.664	0.725	0.643	0.685	0.691	0.728	**0.738**
SPE	0.689	0.722	0.632	0.723	0.670	0.673	0.706	0.729	**0.743**

3.3 Classical Modeling Approach

Low-level visual features involved in prior reports to achieve top performance in the ISIC dermatology dataset [20], as well as the ImageCLEF 2013 medical modality recognition benchmark [23], were used in this study as a comparison baseline. These include color histogram, edge histogram, a multiscale variant of color LBP [23,24], Gist, color wavelets, thumbnail vector, and various image statistics [20,23]. The strength of this approach is that features are optimally combined through an ensemble fusion algorithm – no prior assumptions about the effectiveness of a feature are made; features are tested and chosen based on performance on the data. 80% of training data was used for model learning over features, and 20% of training data was used for optimizing the late fusion of the features, in accordance with prior literature [20]. SVM scores were mapped to probabilities using logistic regression on training data [22]. A probability of 50% is used as the threshold.

4 Results

Classifier performance, in terms of the accuracy (ACC), sensitivity (SEN), and specificity (SPE), as measured by 20 experiments of two-fold cross-validation, is shown in Tables 1 and 2. The first displays results of experiments distinguishing melanoma from all non-melanoma lesions in the dataset. The second displays results of experiments distinguishing melanoma vs. atypical lesions only, a more difficult task. Each set of experiments are broken into 4 groups using different modeling approaches: ensemble models of low-level features (Ensemble), models from transferred convolutional neural network features (Caffe CNN), models from unsupervised sparse coding features (Sparse Coding), and late fusions of the previous models (Fusions).

4.1 Ensembles of Low-Level Visual Features

The "Ensemble" columns of Tables 1 & 2 show the performance results of the ensemble modeling approach over low-level visual features, which has previously achieved top performance on both the ISIC melanoma recognition dataset, and ImageCLEF medical modality recognition dataset [20,23]. This experiment serves as our baseline, to understand what the current performance standards are from the prior literature. Clearly, the task of distinguishing melanoma from only atypical lesions is the most challenging of the two tasks, as classifier accuracy drops by more than 10%.

4.2 Convolutional Neural Networks

The performance of SVMs trained on features extracted with convolutional neural networks transferred from natural photographs is shown in columns "4K
FC6" (4096 dimensional fully connected FC6 layer of Caffe network), "1K FC8"
(1000 dimensional concept output layer of Caffe network), and "Fusion" (late
fusion of the two generated model outputs) under the "Caffe CNN" group. What
is clear from this experiment is that this approach alone is on par with ensembles of low-level features. This is an important finding – the network has been
optimized for natural photographs of real-world objects, which is a very different
application domain to dermoscopy imaging, yet is performing similarly as well.
Prior work has demonstrated transfer of deep networks between related domains
[25]. In this application, the only shared quality between domains is that both are
acquired from natural light, using similar image capture hardware. The content,
however, is different: dermoscopy images contain no perspective distortion, all
colors are restricted to those possible in skin tones, and sharp edges are scarce.
Nevertheless, the features remain effective for discrimination.

4.3 Sparse Coding

The performance of classifiers trained over sparse representations of the dataset
are shown in columns "GRAY" (grayscale), "RGB" (color), and "Fusion" (score
averaging) under the "Sparse Coding" group. Sparse coding is a feature type
that is similar to the first layer of a convolutional neural network, though the
learning process is unsupervised. The sparse codes represent patterns with which
the system can reconstruct the images with minimized error. Therefore, they are
specifically tuned to this task and dataset. What is clear from these experiments
is that color information is important to diagnosis. On average, these two features alone perform similarly well to an ensemble of several hand-coded low-level
visual features, demonstrating its ability to quickly and efficiently adapt to the
recognition task. The performance of the method was found to be robust to the
number of sparse codes: experiments were also done for 512 and 4096 dictionary elements. The first produced similar results, though the second produced
a significant performance drop, possibly due to overfitting (data not shown for
brevity).

4.4 Fusions

The performance of simple late fusions of models is shown in the "Fusions"
group of Tables 1 & 2. "Deep" represents the simple averaging of all Caffe and
sparse coding features. "All" represents this averaging across all model types,
ensembles of low-level features included, and achieved best accuracy in all tasks.
What is clear from this experiment is that the combination of networks trained
from natural photos, in addition to sparse codes trained directly within the
task domain, leads to performance gains. The further fusion with ensembles

of low-level features brings additional performance gains, as the low-level features represent complimentary information (non-convolutional-based statistics and pattern analyses). The performance improvements are similar in both discrimination tasks of melanoma vs. all non-melanoma lesions, and melanoma vs. atypical only.

5   Conclusion

Dermatologists describe lesions using terms corresponding to natural world entities or patterns that most resemble the skin structures exhibited (such as "honeycomb" or "moth-eaten border"), as well as using specialized terms and overall experience gained for the task. This work investigates an automated method that attempts to mimic this process using convolutional neural networks trained on images of natural photographs to create feature descriptors of lesions that relate them to patterns in the natural world, combined with sparse coding representations that are highly specialized to the task. The method is compared to ensemble approaches using only hand-coded low-level features, which have been the previous state-of-art in this field. Statistically significant performance gains are observed, suggesting the proposed approach may be useful for recognizing disease. Future work may focus on using the proposed modeling approach to identify specific clinical patterns that may be indicative of disease, in order to provide human verifiable evidence to support a disease diagnosis.

References

1. Cancer Facts & Figures 2014. American Cancer Society (2014)
2. Melanoma Research Gathers Momentum. The Lancet **385**(9985), 2323
3. Oliveria, S.A., Selvam, N., Mehregan, D., Marchetti, M.A., Divan, H.A., Dasgeb, B., Halpern, A.C.: Biopsies of Nevi in Children and Adolescents in the United States, 2009 Through 2013. JAMA Dermatology, December 2014
4. Kittler, H., Pehamberger, H., Wolff, K., Binder, M.: Diagnostic accuracy of dermoscopy. The Lancet Oncology **3**(3), 159–165 (2002)
5. Abder-Rahman, A.A., Deserno, T.M.: A systematic review of automated melanoma detection in dermatoscopic images and its ground truth data. In: Proc. SPIE, Medical Imaging 2012: Image Perception, Observer Performance, and Technology Assessment, vol. 8318 (2012)
6. Braun, R.P., Rabinovitz, H.S., Oliviero, M., Kopf, A.W., Saurat, J.H.: Dermoscopy of pigmented skin lesions. J. Am. Acad. Dermatol. **52**(1), 109–121 (2005)
7. Carli, P., Quercioli, E., Sestini, S., Stante, M., Ricci, L., Brunasso, G., De Giorgi, V.: Pattern analysis, not simplified algorithms, is the most reliable method for teaching dermoscopy for melanoma diagnosis to residents in dermatology. Br. J. Dermatol. **148**(5), 981–984 (2003)
8. Rezze, G.G., Soares de Sá, B.C., Neves, R.I.: Dermoscopy: the pattern analysis. An. Bras. Dermatol. **3**, 261–268 (2006)
9. Aubusson, P.J., Harrison A.G., Ritchie S.M.: Metaphor and Analogy in Science and Education. Springer Science & Technology Education Library, vol. 30 (2006)

10. Gachon, J., et al.: First Prospective Study of the Recognition Process of Melanoma in Dermatological Practice. Arch. Dermatol. **141**(4), 434–438 (2005)

11. Garnavi, R., Aldeen, M., Bailey, J.: Computer-aided diagnosis of melanoma using border and wavelet-based texture analysis. IEEE Trans. Inf. Technol. Biomed. **16**(6), 1239–1252 (2012)

12. Ganster, H., Pinz, A., Röhrer, R., Wildling, E., Binder, M., Kittler, H.: Automated Melanoma Recognition. IEEE Transactions on Medical Imaging **20**(3) (2001)

13. Colot, O., Devinoy, R., Sombo, A., de Brucq, D.: A colour image processing method for melanoma detection. In: Wells, W.M., Colchester, A.C.F., Delp, S.L. (eds.) MICCAI 1998. LNCS, vol. 1496, p. 562. Springer, Heidelberg (1998)

14. Madooei, A., Drew, M.S., Sadeghi, M., Stella Atkins, M.: Automatic Detection of Blue-White Veil by Discrete Colour Matching in Dermoscopy Images. Medical Image Computing and Computer-Assisted Intervention, 453–460 (2013)

15. Celebi, M.E., Iyatomi, H., Stoecker, W.V., Moss, R.H., Rabinovitz, H.S., Argenziano, G., Soyer, H.P.: Automatic detection of blue-white veil and related structures in dermoscopy images. Comput. Med. Imaging Graph. **32**(8), 670–677 (2008)

16. Mendonca, T., Ferreira, P.M., Marques, J.S., Marcal, A.R., Rozeira, J.: PH2 - a dermoscopic image database for research and benchmarking. In: Conf. Proc. IEEE Eng. Med. Biol. Soc., pp. 5437–5440 (2013)

17. Barata, C., Ruela, M., et al.: Two Systems for the Detection of Melanomas in Dermoscopy Images using Texture and Color Features. IEEE Systems Journal **99**, 1–15 (2013)

18. Mairal, J., Bach, F., Ponce, J.: Sparse Modeling for Image and Vision Processing. Foundations and Trends in Computer Graphics and Vision **8**(2/3), 85–283 (2014)

19. International Skin Imaging Collaboration Website. http://www.isdis.net/index.php/isic-project

20. Abedini, M., Codella, N.C.F., Connell, J.H., Garnavi, R., Merler, M., Pankanti, S., Smith, J.R., Syeda-Mahmood, T.: A generalized framework for medical image classification and recognition. IBM Journal of Research and Development **59**(2/3) (2015)

21. Jia, Y., Shelhamer, E, Donahue, J., Karayev, S., Long, J., Girshick, R., Guadarrama, S., Darrell, T.: Caffe: Convolutional Architecture for Fast Feature Embedding (2014). arXiv preprint arXiv:1408.5093

22. Kender, J.R.: Separability and refinement of hierarchical semantic video labels and their ground truth. In: 2008 IEEE International Conference on Multimedia and Expo, pp. 673–676, 23 June 2008

23. Codella, N., Connell, J., Pankanti, S., Merler, M., Smith, J.R.: Automated medical image modality recognition by fusion of visual and text information. In: Golland, P., Hata, N., Barillot, C., Hornegger, J., Howe, R. (eds.) MICCAI 2014, Part II. LNCS, vol. 8674, pp. 487–495. Springer, Heidelberg (2014)

24. Zhu, C., Bichot, C., Chen, L.: Multi-scale color local binary patterns for visual object classes recognition. In: 20th IAPR International Conference on Pattern Recognition (ICPR), pp. 3065–3068. IEEE Press, New York (2010)

25. Yosinski, J., Clune, J., Bengio, Y., Lipson, H.: How transferable are features in deep neural networks? In: Advances in Neural Information Processing Systems, vol. 27, pp. 3320–3328 (2014)

Predicting Standard-Dose PET Image from Low-Dose PET and Multimodal MR Images Using Mapping-Based Sparse Representation

Yan Wang[1,2], Pei Zhang[2], Le An[2], Guangkai Ma[2], Jiayin Kang[2], Xi Wu[3],
Jiliu Zhou[1], David S. Lalush[4,5], Weili Lin[6], and Dinggang Shen[2(✉)]

[1] College of Computer Science, Sichuan University, Chengdu, China
[2] IDEA Lab, Department of Radiology and BRIC,
University of North Carolina at Chapel Hill, Chapel Hill, NC, USA
dinggang_shen@med.unc.edu
[3] Department of Computer Science, Chengdu University of Information Technology,
Chengdu, China
[4] Joint Department of Biomedical Engineering,
University of North Carolina at Chapel Hill, Chapel Hill NC, USA
[5] North Carolina State University, Raleigh, NC, USA
[6] Department of Radiology and BRIC, University of North Carolina at Chapel Hill,
Chapel Hill, NC, USA

Abstract. Positron emission tomography (PET) has been widely used in clinical diagnosis of diseases or disorders. To reduce the risk of radiation exposure, we propose a mapping-based sparse representation (*m*-SR) framework for prediction of *standard-dose* PET image from its *low-dose* counterpart and corresponding multimodal magnetic resonance (MR) images. Compared with the conventional patch-based SR, our method uses a mapping strategy to ensure that the sparse coefficients estimated from the low-dose PET and multimodal MR images could be directly applied to the prediction of standard-dose PET images. An incremental refinement framework is also proposed to further improve the performance. Finally, a patch selection based dictionary construction method is used to speed up the prediction process. The proposed method has been validated on a real human brain dataset, showing that our method can work much better than the state-of-the-art method both qualitatively and quantitatively.

Keywords: Positron emission tomography (PET) · Sparse representation · Incremental refinement · Multimodal MR images

1 Introduction

Positron emission tomography (PET) is an emerging imaging technology that is able to reveal metabolic activities of a tissue (or an organ). Different from other imaging technologies (e.g., computed tomography (CT) and magnetic resonance imaging (MRI)) that capture anatomical changes in the tissue (or organ), PET scans can detect

© Springer International Publishing Switzerland 2015
L. Zhou et al. (Eds.): MLMI 2015, LNCS 9352, pp. 127–135, 2015.
DOI: 10.1007/978-3-319-24888-2_16

biochemical and physiological changes. As these changes often occur before anatomical changes, PET is widely used for proactive treatment and early disease detection, such as tumor and brain disorders [1, 2].

An injection of radioactive substance (tracer) with a sufficient high dose is often needed to generate the PET image with clinically acceptable quality. However, the use of a high-dose tracer inevitably leads to substantial radiation exposure, which may be detrimental to the subject's health, especially for children. On the other hand, it will degrade the quality of the PET image by reducing the dose since the image quality is proportional to the total injected dose and also the total acquisition time.

Although much effort has been put to tackle the above problem, most of the existing methods focus on the PET image itself [3, 4]. However, the emerging multimodality imaging systems such as PET/CT and PET/MRI suggest an alternative solution by using the information from other imaging modalities [5, 6] to help improve the quality of PET image. Specifically, as MRI offers high contrast among soft tissues and also complements the molecular information of PET [7], we explore the use of the low-dose PET (L-PET) image together with multimodal MR images (T1-weighted, fractional anisotropy (FA), Mean diffusivity (MD)) to predict the standard-dose (S-PET) image. Inspired by the success of patch-based sparse representation (SR) in super-resolution image reconstruction [8], we propose a similar method for S-PET image prediction.

However, due to huge difference in imaging mechanisms between MRI and PET, it is often unreliable to directly apply the sparse weights estimated from MR and L-PET images to S-PET images for prediction. In this paper, we propose a mapping-based SR (m-SR) framework to address this issue. Specifically, we first map the multimodal MR images and L-PET image of each training subject onto the corresponding S-PET image of the same subject by a graph-based linear mapping. We then use all mapped training MR images and L-PET images to build a dictionary, which can be used to represent the given testing MR and L-PET images (after a similar mapping) via SR. Finally, we can perform prediction by applying the obtained sparse coefficients to the training S-PET images associated with the mapped training MR and L-PET images. A novel refinement framework is proposed to further improve the prediction.

Below we briefly introduce the basic idea of the patch-based SR in Section 2, and then elaborate our method in Section 3. We show the experimental results in Section 4, and draw conclusions in Section 5.

2   Patch-Based Sparse Representation (SR)

For simplicity, we first introduce below the S-PET image prediction with the patch-based SR by using an L-PET image and a T1-weighted MR image. Suppose that we have N training subjects, each with an MR image, an L-PET image, and a corresponding S-PET image. All of these $3N$ images are used as the training set. Given a testing MR image and associated L-PET image, the goal is to predict an S-PET image, corresponding to the given L-PET image.

To predict the value of any voxel x in the unknown (testing) S-PET image, we first select a set of patches of the same size ($p \times p \times p$) from the training set to construct the coupled dictionaries: a coding dictionary (CD) and a reconstruction dictionary (RD). Specifically, we first define a neighborhood centered at voxel x with the size of $w \times w \times w$ in both training MR and L-PET images. We then generate the CD, D_x^{M-L}, by grouping all the patches within such neighborhood across all MR and L-PET images of training subjects. Each column in the CD is denoted as an atom, and there are total-ly $w \times w \times w \times N$ atoms in D_x^{M-L}. Furthermore, each atom contains $p \times p \times p \times 2$ intensity features, half of which are extracted from the training MR image and the other half are from the training L-PET image. Similarly, we can build the corresponding RD, D_x^S, containing $p \times p \times p$ dimensional column vectors extracted from the corresponding S-PET images of N training subjects.

Given the testing MR and L-PET images from a new testing subject, it is assumed that each patch in the testing images can be sparsely represented by a linear combination of the patches in D_x^{M-L}. Specifically, to predict the patch centered at x in the unknown S-PET image of the testing subject, a set of sparse coefficients, $\{\alpha_x\}$, is calculated by minimizing the following non-negative Elastic-Net problem [9]:

$$\min_{\alpha_x \geq 0} \left\| f^{M-L}(x) - D_x^{M-L}\alpha_x \right\|_2^2 + \lambda_1 \|\alpha_x\|_1 + \lambda_2 \|\alpha_x\|_2^2, \qquad (1)$$

where $f^{M-L}(x)$ is a feature vector containing the raw intensity values extracted at x from both the testing MR and L-PET images. There are three terms in (1). The first term measures how well the feature vector $f^{M-L}(x)$ can be represented by the CD. The second term enforces the sparsity on $\{\alpha_x\}$ via L_1 regularization, and the last term encourages similar patches to have similar coefficients. λ_1 and λ_2 are the two weights to balance these three terms.

Once we have $\{\alpha_x\}$, we can estimate the intensity values of the patch centered at x in the unknown S-PET for the testing subject, $f^S(x)$, as follows:

$$f^S(x) = D_x^S \alpha_x. \qquad (2)$$

Then, the intensity value at voxel x of the unknown S-PET of the testing subject can be obtained by taking the center value of vector $f^S(x)$.

3   Proposed Method

3.1   Mapping Based SR

Graph-Based Mapping Procedure. The underlying assumption of the patch-based SR is that the embedding geometric relationship of patches in the training S-PET images is very similar to the relationship of patches in the training multimodal MR and L-PET images. However, this assumption may not be true, due to the noise in acquisition and transmission, as well as the huge difference in imaging mechanisms between PET and MRI. To solve this problem, we propose to transform the training multimodal MR and L-PET patches to their respective S-PET patch by using a graph-based distribution mapping method. Note that a graph here represents the distribution of feature vectors of training patches, and consists of a set of nodes and edges (linking similar patches). Each node in the graph represents a training patch, and each edge describes the geometric relationship between a pair of training patches. Specifically, we use graphs g^M/g^L to describe the distributions of feature vectors of patches from the training MR and L-PET images, respectively, and use graph g^S for describing patches from the training S-PET images. The mapping procedure aims to make the transformed graphs $g^{M\prime}/g^{L\prime}$ match well with the graph g^S. This can be achieved by node-to-node matching, edge-to-edge matching, or even high-order matching between g^M/g^L and g^S. Specifically, the mapping procedure for graph of L-PET, g^L, is given below as an example:

$$\min_{H^L} \Sigma_i \left\| A_i^S - H^L * A_i^L \right\|_2^2 + \beta_1 \Sigma_i \Sigma_j \left\| (A_i^S - A_j^S) - H^L * (A_i^L - A_j^L) \right\|_2^2 +$$
$$\beta_2 \Sigma_i \Sigma_j \Sigma_k \cdots + \cdots, \tag{3}$$

where A_i^S is an S-PET image patch, A_i^L is its corresponding L-PET image patch, and H^L is a mapping matrix to transform A_i^L. The first term represents the node-to-node matching between the graphs g^S and g^L, that is, the mapped L-PET image patch $H^L * A_i^L$ should be similar to A_i^S. The second term enforces that the relationship between the mapped patches $H^L * A_i^L$ and $H^L * A_j^L$ should be very similar to that between A_i^S and A_j^S. Note that the above procedure is to obtain the mapping matrix H^L between the L-PET and S-PET images. The mapping matrices H^{T1}, H^{FA}, H^{MD} between the single modal MR (T1, FA, MD) and S-PET images can be estimated in a similar way.

Fusion of multimodal MR images for Prediction of S-PET image. Once we obtain the mapping matrices H^{T1}, H^{FA} and H^{MD}, we can apply them to the multimodal MR images (T1, FA and MD), respectively, to obtain the mapped T1 (m-T1), mapped FA (m-FA), and mapped MD (m-MD) images, and then perform SR. Note that we have to balance the contribution of each channel of multimodal MR images before any SR. Otherwise, the errors for representing multimodal MR images will dominate over the L-PET image. To determine the weights for each channel, we use the following equation:

$$\min_{\mathbf{w}} \Sigma_i \left\| I_i^S - (w_1 I_i^{T1} + w_2 I_i^{FA} + w_3 I_i^{MD}) \right\|_2^2 \quad \text{s.t.} \ \Sigma_{j=1}^3 w_j = 1, \tag{4}$$

where I_i^S is the S-PET image of subject i, I_i^{T1}, I_i^{FA}, and I_i^{MD} represent the mapped T1, mapped FA, and mapped MD images of subject i, respectively, and $\mathbf{w}=[w_1, w_2, w_3]$ is the weights associated with I_i^{T1}, I_i^{FA}, and I_i^{MD}. Then, we can obtain the multimodal MR fusion image of subject i by using

$$\tilde{I}_i^M = w_1 H^{T1} I_i^{T1} + w_2 H^{FA} I_i^{FA} + w_3 H^{MD} I_i^{MD}. \tag{5}$$

Similarly, the mapped L-PET (m-L-PET) image can be obtained after applying the mapping matrix H^L to L-PET images. Then, for each voxel x in the unknown S-PET image of the testing subject, it can be predicted via two procedures: the coding procedure and the reconstruction procedure. Finally, we will get the predicted S-PET image (S-PET)' by using voxel-wise prediction.

3.2   Incremental Refinement

Even if the distributions of the S-PET image patches and the multimodal MR/L-PET image patches could become more similar to each other after the above mapping strategy, discrepancies may still exist due to the nature of different sources of information, as well as the simple linearity of the mapping. To solve this problem, we propose an incremental refinement scheme to further improve the quality of the prediction. This scheme consists of a *training refinement stage* and a *testing refinement stage* as detailed below.

Training Refinement Stage: We construct multiple layers to iteratively refine the quality of prediction. Here, we use the set of training L-PET images $\mathbf{I}^L$ as the initial prediction $\mathbf{I}^{S(0)}$ and the set of training S-PET images $\mathbf{I}^S$ as the final prediction. For each layer, the prediction results of the previous layer are fed into m-SR to generate a new set of predictions. Specifically, at the b-th layer, the mapping matrices H^{T1}, H^{FA}, H^{MD} are learned to map the multimodal MR images to $\mathbf{I}^S$. Those matrices are then used to generate the set of MR fusion images $\tilde{\mathbf{I}}^M$ according to (5). Meanwhile, $H^{S(b)}$ is learned and used to map the prediction results of the previous layer $\mathbf{I}^{S(b-1)}$ to $\mathbf{I}^S$, thus obtaining the new mapped images $\tilde{\mathbf{I}}^{S(b)}$. For each sample $\tilde{I}_i^{S(b)} \in \tilde{\mathbf{I}}^{S(b)}$, a leave-one-out strategy is then utilized to construct the CD and RD in the SR (i.e., all other mapped samples, except for $\tilde{I}_i^M$, $\tilde{I}_i^{S(b)}$ and I_i^S, are utilized). The prediction $I_i^{S(b)}$ of the b-th layer is finally obtained via SR with the new dictionaries.

Testing Refinement Stage: Suppose that we have a new L-PET image I_t^L, together with its corresponding multimodal MR images I_t^{T1}, I_t^{FA}, I_t^{MD} from a testing subject, where t denotes for testing subject. We use the following scheme to obtain the final prediction. Take the b-th layer for example. The mapping matrices H^{T1}, H^{FA}, H^{MD} and $H^{S(b)}$ learned for that layer in the training stage are applied, respectively, to the MR images and the previously predicted S-PET $I_t^{S(b-1)}$ of the testing subject, leading to the mapped MR images and the mapped prediction $\tilde{I}_t^{S(b)}$. After applying the fusion strategy, we obtain the MR fusion image of the testing subject $(\tilde{I}_t^M)$. Then, based on all the mapped samples $(\tilde{\mathbf{I}}^M, \tilde{\mathbf{I}}^{S(b)})$ learned from the same layer in the training stage and also the S-PET samples $(\mathbf{I}^S)$, the CD and RD can be built, respectively. Finally, the prediction $I_t^{S(b)}$ can be obtained via SR and used as the input to the next layer. By going through all the layers, we can obtain the final estimation of the S-PET for the testing subject.

3.3   Patch Selection Based Dictionary Construction

To efficiently construct a dictionary, we propose a patch selection based dictionary construction method. Given an image patch to be encoded, we select the most relevant patches from all the patches within the search window across the training set to construct the dictionary. Similarity between patches is used as a criterion for patch selection. Here, we measure the similarity by computing the intensity difference between patches. By using patch selection, we can *not only* exclude those irrelevant patches *but also* guarantee the inclusion of those meaningful patches. All selected patches will be used as atoms to construct the dictionary. Since the given testing patch can now be better represented by the new dictionary, the whole S-PET image can be more accurately estimated, compared with that using a universal dictionary.

4   Experiments

We validated our method on a human brain dataset of 8 subjects. The noise in the L-PET and S-PET images is not correlated due to separate acquisition. Since the acquisition time of L-PET is a quarter of that of the S-PET, it can be assumed that the former dose is also a quarter of the latter dose. Meanwhile, a T1-weighted MPRAGE MRI sequence and a diffusion-weighted image (DTI) were also generated, and the resulting T1 and DTI images were further aligned to the PET image via affine transformation [10]. Finally, the FA and MD were computed from the resulting warped DTI image [11]. All images were obtained by a Siemens Biograph mMR system. Iterative reconstruction was employed with the ordered subsets expectation maximization (OSEM) algorithm [12]. Each image has a size of 256×256×256, and a resolution of 2.09×2.09×2.03 mm³.

A leave-one-out cross-validation (LOOCV) strategy was used for evaluation. We used the first term and the second term of (3) for mapping. We set the following parameters for the patch-based SR in all experiments throughout this paper: patch size 5×5×5, neighborhood/search window size 15×15×15, the number of atoms in dictionary after patch selection $R = 800$, $\beta_1 = 0.8$, $\lambda_1 = 0.1$, and $\lambda_2 = 0.01$. Specifically, we use normalized mean square error (NMSE) and peak signal-to-noise ratio (PSNR) for quantitative evaluation.

4.1   Comparison of *m*-SR and Classic SR

We first compare our method (without the refinement strategy) with the classic SR. An example of the prediction results by the two methods is shown in Fig. 1.

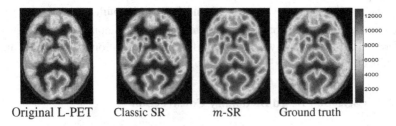

Original L-PET   Classic SR   *m*-SR   Ground truth

Fig. 1. An example of the prediction results by the classic SR and *m*-SR.

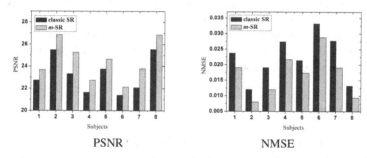

Fig. 2. The performance of the classic SR and m-SR in terms of PSNR and NMSE.

Figure 1 clearly shows that the prediction by our method significantly improves the details over the original L-PET image, and is much better than the one given by the classic SR. This can be further validated by the quantitative results given in Fig. 2.

4.2   Efficacy of the Incremental Refinement Strategy

Now we evaluate the performance of the incremental refinement procedure on the m-SR. The number of layers for the refinement was set to 3. We used both the multi-modal MR and L-PET images in the experiments. Figure 3 shows an example of the prediction result at each layer.

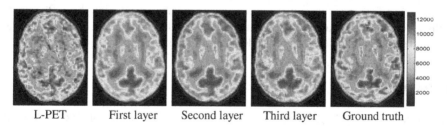

L-PET   First layer   Second layer   Third layer   Ground truth

Fig. 3. An example showing the influence of the incremental refinement strategy.

We can see that the prediction quality is gradually improved with the increase of layers. The detailed quantitative results on all testing subjects are given in Fig. 4.

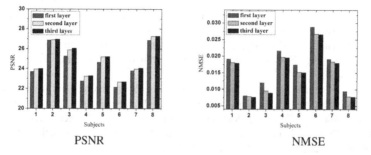

Fig. 4. Influence of the incremental refinement strategy on the m-SR.

Figure 4 shows that the performance improves gradually with the increase of the number of layers, indicating that the incremental refinement procedure can further improve image quality of the predicted S-PET image. However, the number of layers is proportional to the computational time. Thus, the number of layers should not be excessive in order to retain the computational efficiency.

5   Conclusion

We have presented a novel sparse representation method for predicting the S-PET image by using the multimodal MR and L-PET images with two new strategies: a mapping strategy and an incremental refinement scheme. The first strategy aims to reduce the patch distribution differences between MR/L-PET and S-PET images, while the second strategy is used to gradually improve the quality of the prediction. Experimental results show that our method can predict high-quality PET images, suggesting its great potential in clinical diagnosis by reducing the radiation exposure to the patients.

To the best of our knowledge, this is the first work that can well predict the S-PET image by using multimodal MR and L-PET images. In the proposed method, the training samples need to be tripled, i.e., any training subject should have the full set of multimodal MR images, L-PET, and S-PET. This excludes subjects with unavailable MR images or L-PET images (which often occurs in the dataset) for training our model. Therefore, our future work will focus on robustly predicting the S-PET image with different set of available image modalities. In addition, we also plan to rigorously evaluate our method on a larger scale dataset in the future.

References

1. Chen, W.: Clinical applications of PET in brain tumors. Journal of Nuclear Medicine 48(9), 1468–1481 (2007)
2. Quigley, H., Colloby, S.J., O'Brien, J.T.: PET imaging of brain amyloid in dementia: a review. International Journal of Geriatric Psychiatry 26(10), 991–999 (2011)
3. Bai, W., Brady, M.: Motion correction and attenuation correction for respiratory gated PET images. IEEE Transactions on Medical Imaging 30, 351–365 (2011)
4. Gigengack, F., Ruthotto, L., Burger, M., Wolters, C.H., Jiang, X., Schafers, K.P.: Motion correction in dual gated cardiac PET using mass-preserving image registration. IEEE Transactions on Medical Imaging 31(3), 698–712 (2012)
5. Liu, Y., Ghesani, N.V., Zuckier, L.S.: Physiology and pathophysiology of incidental findings detected on FDG-PET scintigraphy. Seminars in Nuclear Medicine 40(4), 294–315 (2010)
6. Lumbreras, B., Donat, L., Hernandez-Aguado, I.: Incidental findings in imaging diagnostic tests: a systematic review. The British Journal of Radiology 83(988), 276–289 (2014)
7. Boss, A., Bisdas, S., Kolb, A., Hofmann, M., Ernemann, U., Claussen, C.D., Stegger, L.: Hybrid PET/MRI of intracranial masses: initial experiences and comparison to PET/CT. Journal of Nuclear Medicine 51(8), 1198–1205 (2010)

8. Yang, J., Wright, J., Huang, T.S., Ma, Y.: Image super-resolution via sparse representation. IEEE Transactions on Image Processing **19**(11), 2861–2873 (2010)
9. Zou, H., Hastie, T.: Regularization and variable selection via the elastic net. Journal of the Royal Statistical Society: Series B (Statistical Methodology) **67**(2), 301–320 (2005)
10. Smith, S.M., Jenkinson, M., Woolrich, M.W., Beckmann, C.F., Behrens, T.E., Johansen-Berg, H., Matthews, P.M.: Advances in functional and structural MR image analysis and implementation as FSL. NeuroImage **23**(S1), S208–S219 (2004)
11. Tournier, J.D., Mori, S., Leemans, A.: Diffusion tensor imaging and beyond. Magnetic Resonance in Medicine **65**(6), 1532–1556 (2011)
12. Hudson, H.M., Larkin, R.S.: Accelerated image reconstruction using ordered subsets of projection data. IEEE Transactions on Medical Imaging **13**(4), 601–609 (1994)

Boosting Convolutional Filters with Entropy Sampling for Optic Cup and Disc Image Segmentation from Fundus Images

Julian G. Zilly[1], Joachim M. Buhmann[2], and Dwarikanath Mahapatra[2]([⊠])

[1] Department of Mechanical Engineering, ETH Zurich, Zurich, Switzerland
[2] Department of Computer Science, ETH Zurich, Zurich, Switzerland
mahapatd@vision.ee.ethz.ch

Abstract. We propose a novel convolutional neural network (CNN) based method for optic cup and disc segmentation. To reduce computational complexity, an entropy based sampling technique is introduced that gives superior results over uniform sampling. Filters are learned over several layers with the output of previous layers serving as the input to the next layer. A softmax logistic regression classifier is subsequently trained on the output of all learned filters. In several error metrics, the proposed algorithm outperforms existing methods on the public DRISHTI-GS data set.

1 Introduction

Glaucoma is one of the leading causes of irreversible vision loss in the world. Due to the aging world population, the WHO estimates that the number of people affected by glaucoma disease may increase to almost 80 million by 2020 [13]. Glaucoma progression is characterized by increase of optic cup area in color fundus images. Our work aims to develop a learning based algorithm using convolutional neural networks (CNN) to segment the optic disc (OD) and optic cup (OC) from retinal fundus images.

There exist numerous approaches for automatic optic cup and disc segmentation such as morphological features [1] and active contours [10]. Their performance depends upon contour initialization and ability to identify weak edges. Machine learning (ML) methods [4] have gained importance as they provide a powerful tool for feature classification. Success of ML methods depends on carefully hand designed features. However, hand crafted features limit their applicability to different datasets. This work proposes to learn the most discriminative features for OC and OD segmentation in the form of convolutional filters.

Mayraz and Hinton [12] proposed a hierarchical learning procedure based on a probabilistic learning framework called the product of experts [3], where the probability of an image is described by the normalized product of learned individual distributions. Another approach that also employs a hierarchical network and was evaluated on medical images is used in [11], where a CNN is learned from multiple scales by optimizing a 2-norm orthogonal matching pursuit problem.

© Springer International Publishing Switzerland 2015
L. Zhou et al. (Eds.): MLMI 2015, LNCS 9352, pp. 136–143, 2015.
DOI: 10.1007/978-3-319-24888-2_17

Ciresan et al. [5] used a Deep Neural Network (DNN) to segment neuronal structures in electron microscopy (EM) images and significantly outperform state of the art. Turaga et al. [17] segment neuronal structures in EM images by learning an affinity graph using a CNN. Our work proposes a novel CNN architecture for OC and OD segmentation without the need to define hand crafted features. This improves the algorithm's generalization ability. The primary contributions of this paper are: 1) a novel sampling strategy is introduced to identify landmarks that provide high information content to train our CNN architecture; and 2) a boosting framework is introduced to learn convolutional filters in our CNN architecture.

2   Method

Preprocessing: Each image is cropped with the optic disc or cup relatively central to the image and some background pixels around the OD and OC. This allows the algorithm to capture the essential characteristics of the image while focusing on the OC and OD. All images are downsampled by a factor of 4 to reduce computation complexity. The RGB images are converted to L*a*b color space. The intensity mean is subtracted from all pixel values and divided by the standard deviation. The intensities are then normalized to $[0, 1]$. Figures 1 (a),(b) show an example original image and the normalized image after preprocessing.

Entropy Sampling: Entropy maps are calculated for each color channel using entropy filtering [8] and highly informative points selected to reduce the computational. They are used to training our CNN architecture. Figure 1 (c) shows the entropy filtered output of the original image. The informative points have higher value in the image.

2.1   Boosting Convolutional Filters

Figure 1 (d) illustrates our method's architecture. Convolutional networks are composed of individual convolutional filters which can be regarded as classifiers in an ensemble. In that sense, the question may be posed how one could learn such filters in a principled manner. Different principled methods exist to arrive at an ensemble classifier of which the most popular are Boosting [7] and Bagging [2]. Kiros et al. [11] proposed to learn a generative convolutional network with two layers through bagging and solving an optimization problem for each filter using orthogonal matching pursuit. The key requirement is successive filters need to be orthogonal to previously learned filters. In contrast, in this work we propose a more direct way of exploring different filters through boosting to learn a discriminative convolutional network.

As a first step, 3×3 patches around each sampled point are extracted. To ensure that the filters do not need to learn superfluous patterns, such as similar patterns with different magnitude, all patches are subjected to *Local Contrast Normalization* as done in [11]. To this end, each patch is reshaped into a vector

x_{patch} and divided by the l_2-norm of the patch. The mean of the patch vector is then subtracted.

Using the extracted patch data, the following optimization problem is solved for each filter individually

$$\underset{w}{\text{minimize}} \sum_{i=1}^{N} v_i \cdot |y_i - x_i w| \tag{1}$$

where $y_i \in Y = \{-1, +1\}$ is the label of a given training point i, $x_i \in X_{patch}$ represents the corresponding patch around point i. w is the convolutional filter in vector form that is to be learned, and v_i are the positive weights on an individual data point. The CVX optimization environment [9] was used. The architecture specifications can be summarized as:

1. Filters of size $3 \times 3 \times n_{maps}$ are trained, where n_{maps} corresponds to the number of channels of each input image, e.g. three for a regular RGB image.
2. 500 points are sampled to learn convolutional filters for each scale.
3. Filters are learned for five scales in the first layer and four scales in the second layer. This gives the local algorithm (3×3 filters) a more global understanding.
4. Two layers of convolutional filters are implemented. For the optic disc, five filters per scale are learned in the first layer and one filter per scale in the second layer. For the optic cup, six filters per scale are learned in the first layer and one filter per scale in the second layer. This makes for a total of 29 filters for the optic disc and 34 filters learned for the optic cup segmentation. Since optic cup segmentation is more challenging, more filters lead to better segmentation

Exploration of different filters is done through reweighting of data points based on *Gentle AdaBoost* [6] as it generalizes better by avoiding overfitting. The following reweighting is performed:

Initialize the weights as $v_i = \frac{1}{m}$, for $i = 1, \ldots, m$. For $n = 1, \ldots N$:

1. Estimate the "weak" hypothesis $h_n(x)$, i.e. learn filter w and bias b in the optimization problem 1.
2. Update weights

$$v_i \leftarrow \frac{v_i \cdot exp(-y_i h_n(\mathbf{x_i}))}{Z_n} \tag{2}$$

with Z_n chosen so that $\sum_{i=1}^{m} v_i = 1$.

α is always set to 1 and is determined by the error ϵ of the individual classifier, where a highly accurate classifier yields a high α factor and an inaccurate classifier yields low α factor as can be inferred from the equation defining α in this paragraph. The output of the convolution of each filter is passed through a *tanh* saturation function. As previously done for preprocessing, the mean of the image is subtracted and all values are divided by the standard deviation. Again, values are rescaled to lie in the range $[0, 1]$. These convoluted images are then passed through a max-pooling operation [15] to introduce further robustness into the system. In a second layer, the stacked output maps of the filters learned in the first layer are used as input. This second layer can be regarded as an extended ensemble classifier. The ensemble classifier is extended in the sense that not only values of one point for multiple individual classifiers are treated but the patch around these points as well. This reads as

$$H_{conv}(x) = \sum_{i=1}^{K} \sum_{p \in patch} w_{i,p} h_i(p) \tag{3}$$

where $H_{conv}(x)$ is a convolutional filter of the second layer (or any further layers), p denotes the positions of points in the patch around point x, $w_{i,p}$ are the learned weights for the convolutional filter in layer two and $h_i(p)$ describes the processed output of convolutional filter i of the previous layer. The processed output of the convolution of filters with the input images provide a good impression of which characteristics of the image a filter is focusing on. Figure 1 e) shows the output of the first filter in the first layer, while Figure 1 f) shows the output of the first filter in the second layer, i.e. an extended ensemble filter. Figure 2 (a) shows a subset of the learned filters for OC and OD.

2.2   Classification

A classifier is trained on the extracted features of all sampled points, which are the output of each convolutional filter, the color values at these points and a "centricity" score. To extract the output of each convolutional filter, filters at smaller scales are upsampled to the original image size. For each image, 5000 points are sampled for which the L*a*b colors as well as the output of each convolutional filter at these points are extracted. Additionally, a "centricity number" of the sampled points is extracted which is meant to be a value measuring the "radius" from the center of the optic disc. The centricity is calculated by finding the weighted centroid c of the maximum intensity region of the L-color in L*a*b color space and calculating the outward radius from this point for a given sampled point as

$$C = \frac{(p_x - c_x)^2}{l_x} + \frac{(p_y - c_y)^2}{l_y} \tag{4}$$

where l_x, l_y is the width and height of a the given image, p is the position of the sampled point and c denotes the centroid's position. These are the features on which subsequently a softmax logistic regression classifier is trained as in [11]. The resulting probability map is shown in Figure 1 g).

Postprocessing: After classification, an unsupervised graph cut algorithm [14] is applied to the probability map in the previous subsection to smooth the results as demonstrated on the sample image in Figure 1 h). A convex hull transform is applied to the graph cut output. Given the oval shape of both the optic disc

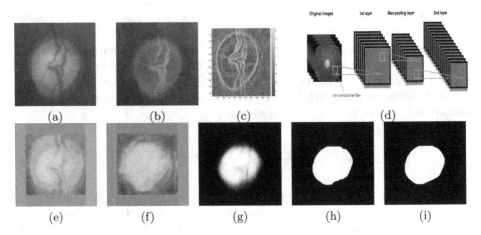

Fig. 1. (a)Example original image; (b) image after preprocessing and normalization of (a); (c) entropy filtered output; (d) illustration of CNN architecture; (e) output of the first filter in the first layer; (f) output of the first filter in the second layer; (g) probability map from logistic regression classifier; (h) graph cut segmentation; (i) final output after convex hull fitting.

and cup it is apriori known that a convex shape is to be detected. Taking the convex hull of the graph cut output unites previously disjoint regions that all belong to the optic disc or cup. The improved segmentation is demonstrated in Figure 1 i).

3   Experimental Results

Our proposed method for optic disc and cup segmentation was validated on the DRISHTI-GS dataset [16] which consists of 50 patient images obtained using 30 degree FOV at a resolution of 2896 × 1944. We use a 5 fold cross validation scheme with 40 training images and 10 test images in each fold. The ground truth disc and cup segmentation masks were obtained by a majority voting of manual markings by 4 ophthalmologists. Quantitative evaluation is based on F-score ($F = 2\ P \times R/(P + R)$) to measure the extent of region overlap and absolute pointwise localization error B in pixels (measured in the radial direction); P is precision and R is recall. Additionally we report the overlap measure $S = Area(M \cap A)/Area(M \cup A)$. M is the manual segmentation while A is the algorithm segmentation. Our whole pipeline was implemented in MATLAB on a 2.66 GHz quad core CPU running Windows 7.

3.1   Segmentation Performance

Table 1 summarizes the segmentation performance of different methods. Our proposed method, CNN, outperforms all the competing methods as is evident from the higher F and S values, and lower B values. The difference is also

Table 1. Segmentation performance for OC and OD segmentation using different methods.

	Optic Disc					Optic Cup				
	CNN	[4]	[18]	[10]	[16]	CNN	[4]	[18]	[10]	[16]
F	94.7	93.0	92.2	90.8	95.0	83.0	80.8	78.4	78.9	80.7
S	89.5	87.3	86.8	85.0	85.2	86.4	82.1	80.1	82.5	84.2
B	9.1	9.4	9.9	12.1	11.7	16.5	19.3	20.6	17.2	16.2

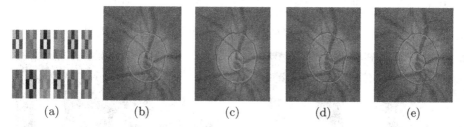

| (a) | (b) | (c) | (d) | (e) |

Fig. 2. (a) Subset learned filter for OD (top row) and OC (bottom row). Segmentation results for different methods: (b) our proposed CNN model; (c) integrated disc and cup segmentation method of [18]; (d) superpixel segmentation method of [4] and ; (e) [10]

statistically significant since $p < 0.01$ (from Student-t tests) for all methods compared to CNN. Segmenting the optic cup is more challenging than the disc due to absence of distinguishing depth information. While pallor is one factor, it is not always reliable due to similar intensity profiles of neighboring regions. CNN obtains high segmentation accuracy than hand crafted features by learning image priors for the cup region.

Since [4] is a superpixel based approach, pixels from different classes may be grouped in one superpixel which affects its performance. [10] uses a modified Chan-Vese model, which finds it challenging to segment the optic disc using only intensity information. [1] uses only morphological features which is good enough for disc segmentation, but does not perform as well for cup segmentation. However CNN outperforms all these methods. Figure 2 shows the comparative results of FoE and the combined disc and cup segmentation methods of [4],[18] and [10].

For optic disc segmentation all the methods perform almost at the same level since OD is much easy to segment. However CNN's advantages are prominent for cup segmentation. CNN outperforms the state-of-the-art approaches tested by Sivaswamy et al. [16] which achieve a maximal F-score of 0.80 on the training set. On the other hand CNN achieves a F-score of 0.83 with a smaller standard deviation than the other methods. CNN also has lower boundary localization error than other competing methods. We also show the best and worst case results for optic disc (Figure 3) and optic cup (Figure 4).

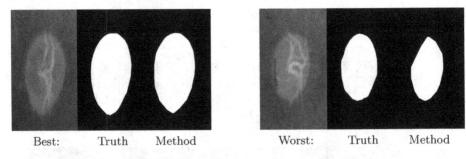

Best: Truth   Method   Worst: Truth   Method

Fig. 3. Results of best/worst case segmentation for optic disc, respectively

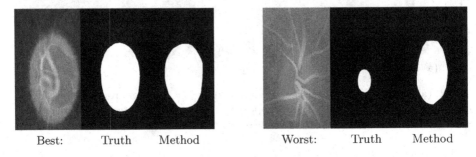

Best: Truth   Method   Worst: Truth   Method

Fig. 4. Results of best/worst case segmentation for optic cup, respectively

4   Discussion and Conclusion

This paper introduced a novel entropy sampling method within a CNN architecture. Building upon this technique, an original framework for learning convolutional filters in a principled manner using boosting was described. The boosted network of convolutional filters was shown to outperform existing methods on the DRISHTI-GS data set. Entropy sampling competently finds more relevant points than uniform sampling. Boosting convolutional filters is able to learn very discriminative convolutional filters even for small data sets. Our proposed CNN architecture, helped by entropy sampling, focuses to learn discriminative features from more relevant points.

References

1. Aquino, A., Gegundez-Arias, M.: Marin., D.: Detecting the optic disc boundary in digital fundus images using morphological edge detection and feature extraction techniques. IEEE Trans. Med. Imag. **20**(11), 1860–1869 (2010)
2. Breiman, L.: Bagging predictors. Machine Learning, 123–140 (1996)
3. Brown, A., Hinton, G.: Products of hidden markov models. Technical report GCNU TR 2000–008, Gatsby Computational Neuroscience Unit, University College London, November 2000

4. Cheng, J., Liu, J., et al.: Superpixel classification based optic disc and optic cup segmentation for glaucoma screening. IEEE Trans. Med. Imag. **32**(6), 1019–1032 (2013)
5. Ciresan, D., Giusti, A., Gambardella, L.M., Schmidhuber, J.: Deep neural networks segment neuronal membranes in electron microscopy images. In: Pereira, F., Burges, C., Bottou, L., Weinberger, K. (eds.) Advances in Neural Information Processing Systems, vol. 25, pp. 2843–2851. Curran Associates, Inc. (2012). http://papers.nips.cc/paper/4741-deep-neural-networks-segment-neuronal-membranes-in-electron-microscopy-images.pdf
6. Doğan, H., Akay, O.: Using adaboost classifiers in a hierarchical framework for classifying surface images of marble slabs. Expert Syst. Appl. **37**(12), 8814–8821 (2010). http://dx.doi.org/10.1016/j.eswa.2010.06.019
7. Freund, Y., Schapire, R.E.: A short introduction to boosting (1999)
8. Gonzalez, R.C., Woods, R.E., Eddins, S.L.: Digital Image Processing Using MATLAB. Prentice-Hall Inc., Upper Saddle River (2003)
9. Grant, M., Boyd, S.: CVX: Matlab software for disciplined convex programming, version 2.1., March 2014. http://cvxr.com/cvx
10. Joshi, G., Sivaswamy, J., Krishnadas, S.: Optic disk and cup segmentation from monocular color retinal images for glaucoma assessment. IEEE Trans. Med. Imag. **30**(6), 1192–1205 (2011)
11. Kiros, R., Popuri, K., Cobzas, D., Jagersand, M.: Stacked multiscale feature learning for domain independent medical image segmentation. In: Wu, G., Zhang, D., Zhou, L. (eds.) MLMI 2014. LNCS, vol. 8679, pp. 25–32. Springer, Heidelberg (2014). http://dx.doi.org/10.1007/978-3-319-10581-9_4
12. Mayraz, G., Hinton, G.: Recognizing handwritten digits using hierarchical products of experts. IEEE Transactions on Pattern Analysis and Machine Intelligence **24**(2), 189–197 (2002)
13. Organization, W.H.: Vision 2020. the right to sight. global initiative for the elimination of avoidable blindness. WHO Press (2006)
14. Salah, M., Mitiche, A., Ayed, I.: Multiregion image segmentation by parametric kernel graph cuts. IEEE Transactions on Image Processing **20**(2), 545–557 (2011)
15. Scherer, D., Müller, A., Behnke, S.: Evaluation of pooling operations in convolutional architectures for object recognition. In: Diamantaras, K., Duch, W., Iliadis, L.S. (eds.) ICANN 2010, Part III. LNCS, vol. 6354, pp. 92–101. Springer, Heidelberg (2010). http://dl.acm.org/citation.cfm?id=1886436.1886447
16. Sivaswamy, J., Krishnadas, S., Datt Joshi, G., Jain, M., Syed Tabish, A.: Drishti-GS: retinal image dataset for optic nerve head(ONH) segmentation. In: 2014 IEEE 11th International Symposium on Biomedical Imaging (ISBI), pp. 53–56, April 2014
17. Turaga, S.C., Murray, J.F., Jain, V., Roth, F., Helmstaedter, M., Briggman, K., Denk, W., Seung, H.S.: Convolutional networks can learn to generate affinity graphs for image segmentation. Neural Computation 22(2), 511–538, May 17, 2015 2009. http://dx.doi.org/10.1162/neco.2009.10-08-881
18. Wong, D., et al.: Level set based automatic cup to disc ratio determination using retinal fundus images in argali. In: Proc. IEEE EMBC, pp. 2266–2269 (2008)

Brain Fiber Clustering Using Non-negative Kernelized Matching Pursuit

Kuldeep Kumar[1]([✉]), Christian Desrosiers[1], and Kaleem Siddiqi[2]

[1] Software and IT Engineering, École de Technologie Supérieure, Montreal, Canada
kkumar@livia.etsmtl.ca
[2] Centre for Intelligent Machines, McGill University, Montreal, Canada

Abstract. We present a kernel dictionary learning method to cluster fiber tracts obtained from diffusion Magnetic Resonance Imaging (dMRI) data. This method extends the kernelized Orthogonal Matching Pursuit (kOMP) model by adding non-negativity constraints to the dictionary and sparse weights, and uses an efficient technique based on non-negative tri-factorization to compute these parameters. Unlike existing fiber clustering approaches, the proposed method allows fibers to be assigned to more than one cluster and does not need to compute an explicit embedding of the fibers. We evaluate the performance of our method on labeled and multi-subject data, using several fiber distance measures, and compare it with state of the art fiber clustering approaches. Our experiments show that the method is more accurate than the ones we compare against, while being robust to the choice of distance measure and number of clusters.

1 Introduction

To simplify the visualization and analysis of white matter fiber tracts obtained from diffusion Magnetic Resonance Imaging (dMRI) data, it is often necessary to group them into larger clusters, or *bundles*. The methods proposed for this task can either represent fibers explicitly, with a fixed set of features, or use a distance measure. Methods using explicit features, such as B-splines or the distribution parameters (i.e., mean and covariance) of fiber points [1], are often unable to capture qualitative fiber bundle shape and can be sensitive to fiber length and endpoint location. The second category of methods avoid computing explicit features by using specialized distance measures, such as the Hausdorff, endpoints, and mean of closest points (MCP) distances [4,10]. Fiber clustering approaches can also be divided based on the technique employed to group fibers, which include spectral embedding [1,5], hierarchical clustering [4], Gaussian [15] or Dirichlet [14] processes, and k-means [5].

While most of these methods assume a crisp membership of fibers to bundles, as shown in Figure 1, such a separation of fibers into hard clusters is often arbitrary. In practice, fiber bundles may overlap and intersect each other, making their extraction and analysis difficult. Moreover, when used to label the fibers of a new subject, the clusters learned using crisp methods may give poor results,

L. Zhou et al. (Eds.): MLMI 2015, LNCS 9352, pp. 144–152, 2015.
DOI: 10.1007/978-3-319-24888-2_18

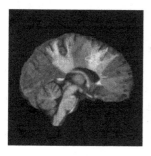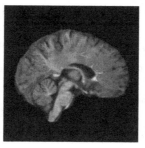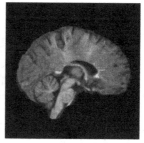

Fig. 1. Clustering of Corpus Callosum by our method: hard clustering (**left**); membership of each fiber to two bundles (**center** and **right**). Dark green represents a zero membership and bright red a maximum membership to the bundles.

due to the variability across individual brains [12]. Recently, clustering methods based on dictionary learning [13] and non-negative matrix factorization [6] have shown clear advantages over traditional approaches, by representing more accurately the soft membership of objects to clusters. In the case of fiber clustering, such methods could be more robust to overlapping bundles and less sensitive to the parameter controlling the target number of bundles. Since these methods provide additional information on the membership of fibers to bundles, they could also facilitate the visualization and analysis of clustering results. Lastly, if the dictionary is used as an atlas to label new fiber data, soft memberships would be more robust to inter-subject variability.

The present article is, to our knowledge, the first to use dictionary learning and sparse coding for fiber clustering. Our specific contributions include:

1. A kernelized dictionary learning approach for the soft clustering of fibers that provides a simple way to control the degree to which fibers may be assigned to more than one cluster. Unlike spectral methods, our approach does not enforce an explicit embedding of fibers;

2. A novel sparse coding method that extends the kernelized Orthogonal Matching Pursuit (kOMP) approach of [11] by imposing non-negativity constraints on the dictionary and sparse weights, and an efficient technique based on non-negative tri-factorization to compute these parameters. Non-negativity is an important theoretical consideration in the application of sparsity and dictionary learning to fiber clustering;

3. An extensive experimental evaluation, where several distance measures and clustering approaches are compared on labeled and multi-subject data.

In Section 2, we present our kernelized dictionary learning method and its link to other clustering techniques such as k-means. Section 3 then evaluates our method and analyzes the impact of its parameters. We conclude with a discussion of our main contributions as well as potential extensions of our work.

2 Kernelized Dictionary Learning for Clustering

2.1 Dictionary Learning Using Kernelized k-means

We start by defining the fiber clustering task considered in this work. Let $X \in \mathbb{R}^{d \times n}$ be the data matrix of n fibers, where each column contains the feature vector $x_i \in \mathbb{R}^d$ of a fiber tract i. The *hard* clustering problem can be defined as finding a matrix $D \in \mathbb{R}^{d \times m}$ of m bundle prototypes (i.e., *cluster centers*), as well as a fiber-to-bundle assignment matrix $W \in \{0,1\}^{m \times n}$, that optimize the following problem:

$$\underset{\substack{D \in \mathbb{R}^{d \times m} \\ W \in \{0,1\}^{m \times n}}}{\arg\min} \quad \frac{1}{2} \|X - DW\|_F^2 \quad \text{subject to: } \|w_i\|_1 = 1, \ i = 1, \ldots, n. \quad (1)$$

Here, L_1-norm constraints are added on the columns w_i of W so that each tract is assigned to exactly one bundle. Note that this model can be considered as a special case of dictionary learning, where D is the dictionary and W is constrained to be binary and have a single non-zero element per column.

The model described above encodes fibers using a fixed set of features, such as 3D points. Since fibers can have very different lengths and endpoints, this can lead to a poor description of the bundles. This problem can be avoided by using a kernelized formulation, where each fiber tract is projected to a q-dimensional space using a mapping function $\phi : \mathbb{R}^d \rightarrow \mathbb{R}^q$, such that $\phi(x)^\top \phi(x') = k(x, x')$ is a kernel function. Let $\Phi \in \mathbb{R}^{q \times n}$ be the matrix of mapped features and define as $K = \Phi^\top \Phi$ the kernel matrix. The *kernelized* clustering problem can be expressed as:

$$\underset{\substack{D \in \mathbb{R}^{q \times m} \\ W \in \{0,1\}^{m \times n}}}{\arg\min} \quad \frac{1}{2} \|\Phi - DW\|_F^2 \quad \text{subject to: } \|w_i\|_1 = 1, \ i = 1, \ldots, n. \quad (2)$$

Because the dictionary prototypes are defined in the kernel space, D cannot be computed explicitly. To overcome this problem, we follow the strategy proposed in [11], and define the dictionary as $D = \Phi A$, where $A \in \mathbb{R}_+^{n \times m}$ is a non-negative matrix representing a convex combination of the columns in Φ.

This kernelized model can be solved using an iterative approach, which optimizes A and W alternatively, until convergence. Given a fixed A, W can be updated by assigning each fiber i to the prototype j whose features in the kernel space are the closest:

$$w_{ji} = \begin{cases} 1 : \text{if } j = \arg\min_{j'} \ \frac{1}{2}[A^\top K A]_{j'j'} - [A^\top k_i]_{j'}, \\ 0 : \text{otherwise.} \end{cases} \quad (3)$$

where k_i corresponds to the i-th column of K. Moreover, recomputing A for a given W corresponds to solving the following linear regression:

$$A = W^\top (WW^\top)^{-1}. \quad (4)$$

This optimization process is known as *kernelized k-means* [5].

Algorithm 1. Non-negative kernelized orthogonal matching pursuit

---

Input: The dictionary matrix $A \in \mathbb{R}_+^{n \times m}$ and kernel matrix $K \in \mathbb{R}^{n \times n}$;
Input: The fiber index i and sparsity level $S_{\max}$;
Output: The set of non-zero weights I_s and corresponding weight values w_s;

Initialize set of selected atoms and weights: $I_0 = \emptyset$, $w_0 = \emptyset$;

for $s = 1, \ldots, S_{\max}$ **do**

$\quad \tau_j = \left[A^\top (k_i - K A_{[I_s]} w_s) \right]_j / \left[A^\top K A \right]_{jj}, \quad j = 1, \ldots, m;$

$\quad j_{\max} = \arg\max_{j \notin I_{s-1}} \tau_j, \quad I_s = I_{s-1} \cup j_{\max};$

$\quad w_s = \arg\min_{w \in \mathbb{R}_+^s} w^\top A_{[I_s]}^\top K A_{[I_s]} w - 2 k_i^\top A_{[I_s]} w;$

return $\{I_s, w_s\}$;

Note: $A_{[I_s]}$ contains the columns of A whose index is in I_s ;

2.2   Non-negative Kernelized Sparse Clustering

Because they map each fiber to a single bundle, hard clustering approaches like (kernelized) k-means can be sensitive to poorly separated bundles and fibers which do not fit in any bundle (outliers). This section describes a new clustering model that allows one to control the hardness or softness of the clustering. In this model, the hard assignment constraints are replaced with non-negativity and L_0-norm constraints on the columns of W. Imposing non-negativity is necessary because the values of W represent the membership level of fibers to bundles. Moreover, since the L_0-norm counts the number of non-zero elements, fiber tracts can be expressed as a combination of a small number of prototypes, instead of a single one. When updating the fiber-to-bundle assignments, the columns w_i of W can be optimized independently, by solving the following sub-problem:

$$\arg\min_{w_i \in \mathbb{R}_+^m} \frac{1}{2} \|\phi(x_i) - \Phi A w_i\|_2^2 \quad \text{subject to: } \|w_i\|_0 \leq S_{\max}. \tag{5}$$

Parameter $S_{\max}$ defines the maximum number of non-zero elements in w_i (i.e., the sparsity level), and is provided by the user as input to the clustering method.

To compute non-negative weights w_i, we modify the kernelized Orthogonal Matching Pursuit (kOMP) approach of [11], as shown in Algorithm 1. Unlike kOMP, the most *positively* correlated atom is selected at each iteration, and the sparse weights w_s are obtained by solving a non-negative regression problem. Note that, since the size of w_s is bounded by $S_{\max}$, computing w_s is fast.

In the case of a soft clustering (i.e., when $S_{\max} \geq 2$), updating A using Equation (4) can lead to negative values in the matrix. As a result, the bundle prototypes may lie outside the convex hull of their respective fibers. To overcome this problem, we adapt a strategy proposed for non-negative tri-factorization [6] to our kernelized model. In this strategy, A is recomputed by applying the following update scheme, until convergence:

$$A_{ij} \leftarrow A_{ij}\frac{\left(KW^{\top}\right)_{ij}}{\left(KAWW^{\top}\right)_{ij}}, \quad i = 1,\ldots,n, \quad j = 1,\ldots,m. \tag{6}$$

In terms of computational complexity, the bottleneck of the method lies in computing the kernel matrix. For large datasets, we could reduce this computational complexity by approximating the kernel matrix with the Nyström method [12].

3   Experiments

Data: Two datasets were used in our experiments. The first dataset, provided by the Sherbrooke Connectivity Imaging Laboratory (SCIL), contains labeled fiber tracts generated from the dMRI data of a 25 year old healthy volunteer [7]. To evaluate the clustering methods, we used 10 of the most prominent bundles (i.e., left/right cingulum, corticospinal tract, superior cerebellar penduncle, inferior longitudinal fasciculus, and inferior fronto-occipital fasciculus) for a total of 4449 fibers. Figure 4 (**left**) shows the right sagittal and inferior axial views of the ground truth set. To evaluate the performance of our method on multiple subjects, we also used the data of 12 healthy volunteers (6 males and 6 females, 19 to 35 years of age) from the freely available MIDAS dataset [2]. For fiber tracking, we used the tensor deflection method [9] with the following parameters: minimum fractional anisotropy of 0.1, minimum fiber length of 100 mm, threshold for fiber deviation angle of 70 degrees. A mean number of 9124 fiber tracts was generated for the 12 subjects.

Experimental Methodology: We tested three distance measures used in the literature for the fiber clustering problem: 1) the Hausdorff distance (Haus) [4] which measures the maximum distance between any point on a fiber and its closest point on the other fiber, 2) the mean of closest points distance (MCP) [4,12] which computes the mean distance between any point on a fiber and its closest point on the other fiber, and 3) the endpoints distance (EP) [10] which measures the mean distance between the endpoints of a fiber and their respective closest endpoints on the other fiber.

Fiber distances were converted into similarities using a radial basis function (RBF) kernel: $k_{ij} = \exp\left(-\gamma \cdot dist(\text{fiber}_i, \text{fiber}_j)^2\right)$. Parameter γ was adjusted separately for each distance measure, using the distribution of values in the corresponding distance matrix. Since the tested distance measures are not all metrics, we applied spectrum shift to make kernels positive semi-definite: $K' = K + |\lambda_{\min}|I$, where $\lambda_{\min}$ is the minimum eigenvalue of K. This technique only modifies the self similarities and is well adapted to clustering [3]. Following the convergence rate shown in Figure 3 (**right**), we set the maximum number of iterations to 30. We initialized W using the output of a spectral clustering method [12], which applies the k-means algorithm on the 10 first eigenvectors of the normalized Laplacian matrix of K. Finally, to compare our method with

Table 1. Clustering accuracy of our KSC method ($S_{\max} = 3$), kernelized k-means (KKM), spectral clustering (Spect), and hierarchical clustering (HSL), using the Hausdorff, MCP and EP distances, on the SCIL dataset. For KSC, KKM and Spect, the mean accuracy over 10 initializations is reported. The best results for a distance and accuracy metric are shown in boldface type. Bilateral clustering results for KSC ($S_{\max} = 3$) and KKM are also provided.

Distance	Method	RI mean (std)	ARI mean (std)	NARI mean (std)	SI mean (std)
Haus	KSC	**0.924 (0.013)**	**0.658 (0.068)**	**0.634 (0.030)**	**0.425 (0.022)**
	KKM	0.904 (0.020)	0.589 (0.082)	0.573 (0.068)	0.365 (0.054)
	Spect	0.884 (0.018)	0.517 (0.041)	0.538 (0.054)	0.317 (0.069)
	HSL	0.891 (0.000)	0.640 (0.000)	0.609 (0.000)	0.221 (0.000)
	QB	0.851 (0.000)	0.468 (0.000)	0.485 (0.000)	0.143 (0.000)
	KSC+Bilat	0.931 (0.018)	0.710 (0.072)	0.698 (0.125)	0.439 (0.042)
	KKM+Bilat	0.909 (0.025)	0.635 (0.077)	0.628 (0.086)	0.374 (0.064)
MCP	KSC	**0.948 (0.012)**	**0.780 (0.051)**	**0.716 (0.047)**	**0.543 (0.032)**
	KKM	0.947 (0.011)	0.777 (0.049)	**0.716 (0.046)**	0.541 (0.028)
	Spect	0.942 (0.014)	0.752 (0.058)	0.701 (0.047)	0.515 (0.059)
	HSL	0.915 (0.000)	0.704 (0.000)	0.612 (0.000)	0.474 (0.000)
	QB	0.943 (0.000)	**0.780 (0.000)**	0.696 (0.000)	0.486 (0.000)
	KSC+Bilat	0.949 (0.010)	0.793 (0.036)	0.782 (0.078)	0.543 (0.065)
	KKM+Bilat	0.947 (0.025)	0.791 (0.077)	0.768 (0.086)	0.540 (0.081)
EP	KSC	**0.919 (0.005)**	**0.634 (0.026)**	**0.641 (0.006)**	**0.422 (0.020)**
	KKM	0.915 (0.013)	0.621 (0.052)	0.634 (0.034)	0.410 (0.032)
	Spect	0.911 (0.014)	0.603 (0.053)	0.616 (0.040)	0.408 (0.031)
	HSL	0.842 (0.000)	0.539 (0.000)	0.445 (0.000)	0.197 (0.000)
	QB	0.885 (0.000)	0.534 (0.000)	0.550 (0.000)	0.129 (0.000)
	KSC+Bilat	0.939 (0.010)	0.735 (0.037)	0.766 (0.076)	0.428 (0.052)
	KKM+Bilat	0.929 (0.020)	0.703 (0.058)	0.702 (0.111)	0.397 (0.058)

hard clustering approaches, we mapped each fiber i to the bundle j for which w_{ji} is maximum.

We compared our kernelized sparse clustering (KSC) approach to four other methods: kernelized k-means (KKM) using the same K and initial clustering, the spectral clustering (Spect) approach described above, single linkage hierarchical clustering (HSL) [10], and QuickBundles (QB) [8]. The performance of these methods was evaluated using four clustering metrics: Rand index (RI), adjusted Rand index (ARI), normalized adjusted Rand index (NARI) and silhouette (SI) [10]. Unlike other measures, the SI measure does not use the ground truth. Following [12], we also performed bilateral clustering by reflecting fibers across the midsagittal plane, and grouping together fibers of both hemispheres that correspond symmetrically. Since our clustering method does not depend upon bilateral matching, most of the results are presented without this extension.

Comparison of Methods and Distance Measures: Table 1 gives the accuracy obtained by KSC ($S_{\max} = 3$) and the four other tested methods on the SCIL dataset, for the same number of clusters as the ground truth ($m = 10$). Since the output of spectral clustering depends on the initialization of its k-means clustering step, for Spect, KSC and KKM, we report the mean performance and standard deviation obtained using 10 different random seeds. We see that our KSC method improves the initial solution provided by spectral clustering

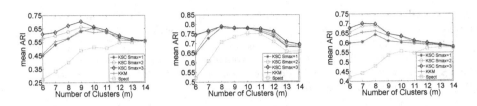

Fig. 2. Mean ARI obtained on the SCIL dataset by KSC ($S_{max} = 1, 2, 3$), KKM and Spect, using Haus (**left**), MCP (**center**), EP (**right**); for varying m.

($\geq 4\%$ mean ARI improvement) and, in most cases, gives a higher accuracy than the other clustering methods. We also observe that KSC is more robust to the choice of distance measure and, as reported in [10], that MCP is consistently better than other distance measures.

Table 1 also shows bilateral clustering results for KSC and KKM. We see that adding bilateral symmetry improves the performance of both methods, although KSC still outperforms KKM when using this property. While not reported in the table, we also tested our KSC method without the non-negativity constraints. Results have shown that imposing non-negativity can improve the mean ARI by 5% (for KSC+MCP, $m = 10$).

Impact of the Parameters: Figure 2 shows the mean ARI (over 10 runs) obtained on the SCIL dataset by our KSC approach, using $S_{max} = 1, 2, 3$, for an increasing number of clusters (i.e., dictionary size m). For comparison, the performance of KKM and Spect is also shown. When the Spectral Clustering initialization is near optimal (i.e., when m is near the true number of clusters and using MCP), both methods find similar solutions. However, when the initial spectral clustering is poor (e.g., Haus and EP distance or small number of clusters) the improvement obtained by KSC is more significant than KKM. Hence, KSC ($S_{max} \geq 2$) is more robust than hard clustering approaches (i.e., Spect, KKM or KSC $S_{max} = 1$) to the number of clusters and distance measures. We also observe that KKM is slightly better than KSC ($S_{max} = 1$), even though both methods limit the membership of fibers to a single bundle. This could be due to the fact that KKM minimizes the distance between fibers and their bundle prototype, while the matching pursuit algorithm of KSC is based on correlation.

Figure 3 (left) shows the mean SI (averaged over all clusters) obtained by KSC ($S_{max} = 3$), KKM and Spect with MCP, on 12 subjects of the MIDAS dataset. We see that our soft clustering method outperforms the hard clustering approaches, especially for a small number of clusters. In Figure 3 (center), the results obtained for $m = 35$ are detailed for each subject. Error bars in the plot show the mean and variance of SI values obtained over 10 different initializations. As can be seen, our method shows a greater accuracy and less variance across subjects.

Qualitative Evaluation: Figure 4 compares the ground truth clustering of the SCIL dataset with the outputs of KSC ($S_{max} = 3$) using the Haus, MCP

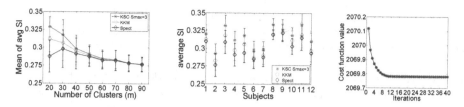

Fig. 3. Mean of average SI computed over 12 MIDAS subjects, using MCP and increasing values of m (**left**). Per-subject average SI and variance for $m = 35$ (**center**). Convergence plot (**right**)

and EP distances. Except for the superior cerebellar peduncle bundle (cyan and green colors in the ground truth), the bundles obtained by KSC+MCP and KSC+Haus are similar to those of the ground truth clustering. Also, we observe that the differences between KSC+MCP and KSC+Haus occur mostly in the right inferior fronto-occipital fasciculus and inferior longitudinal fasciculus bundles (yellow and purple colors in the ground truth). Possibly due to the large variance of endpoint distances in individual bundles, the clustering results obtained by KSC+EP are less accurate.

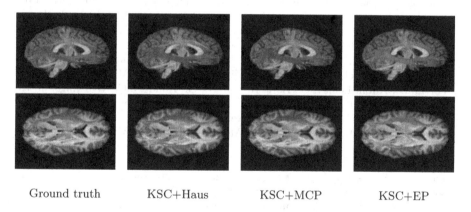

| Ground truth | KSC+Haus | KSC+MCP | KSC+EP |

Fig. 4. Right sagittal (**top**) and inferior axial (**bottom**) views of the ground truth, and bundles obtained by KSC ($S_{max} = 3$) using the Haus, MCP and EP.

4   Conclusion

We proposed a new method based on kernelized dictionary learning to cluster white matter fibers into significant bundles. This method allows fibers to be assigned to more than one cluster and does not enforce an explicit fiber embedding. We also presented an extension of the kOMP model that imposes nonnegativity constraints on the dictionary and sparse weights, and proposed an efficient technique to compute these parameters. We evaluated the performance of our method using various distance measures and compared it with state of the art clustering approaches. The results show our soft clustering method to be more accurate than these approaches, while being robust to the choice of distance measure and number of clusters. In future work, we will use the learned dictionary as an atlas to label new fibers, and enhance our current method by incorporating anatomical prior information. We will also make it scalable to large multi-subject datasets by approximating the kernel matrix with the Nyström method.

References

1. Brun, A., Knutsson, H., Park, H.-J., Shenton, M.E., Westin, C.-F.: Clustering fiber traces using normalized cuts. In: Barillot, C., Haynor, D.R., Hellier, P. (eds.) MICCAI 2004. LNCS, vol. 3216, pp. 368–375. Springer, Heidelberg (2004)
2. Bullitt, E., Zeng, D., Gerig, G., Aylward, S., Joshi, S., Smith, J.K., Lin, W., Ewend, M.G.: Vessel tortuosity and brain tumor malignancy: a blinded study. Academic Radiology 12(10), 1232–1240 (2005)
3. Chen, Y., Gupta, M.R., Recht, B.: Learning kernels from indefinite similarities. In: ICML 2009, pp. 145–152. ACM (2009)
4. Corouge, I., Gouttard, S., Gerig, G.: Towards a shape model of white matter fiber bundles using diffusion tensor MRI. In: ISBI 2004, pp. 344–347. IEEE (2004)
5. Dhillon, I.S., Guan, Y., Kulis, B.: Kernel k-means: spectral clustering and normalized cuts. In: SIGKDD 2004, pp. 551–556. ACM (2004)
6. Ding, C., Li, T., Peng, W., Park, H.: Orthogonal nonnegative matrix trifactorizations for clustering. In: Proceedings of the 12th ACM SIGKDD (2006)
7. Fortin, D., Aubin-Lemay, C., Boré, A., Girard, G., Houde, J.C., Whittingstall, K., Descoteaux, M.: Tractography in the study of the human brain: a neurosurgical perspective. The Canadian Journal of Neurological Sciences 39(6), 747–756 (2012)
8. Garyfallidis, E., Brett, M., Correia, M.M., Williams, G.B., Nimmo-Smith, I.: Quickbundles, a method for tractography simplification. Frontiers in Neuroscience 6 (2012)
9. Lazar, M., Weinstein, D.M., et al.: White matter tractography using diffusion tensor deflection. Human Brain Mapping 18(4), 306–321 (2003)
10. Moberts, B., Vilanova, A., van Wijk, J.J.: Evaluation of fiber clustering methods for diffusion tensor imaging. In: VIS 2005, pp. 65–72. IEEE (2005)
11. Nguyen, H., Patel, V.M., Nasrabadi, N.M., Chellappa, R.: Kernel dictionary learning. In: ICASSP 2012, pp. 2021–2024. IEEE (2012)
12. O'Donnell, L.J., Westin, C.F.: Automatic tractography segmentation using a high-dimensional white matter atlas. IEEE Trans. Med. Imag., 1562–1575 (2007)
13. Sprechmann, P., Sapiro, G.: Dictionary learning and sparse coding for unsupervised clustering. In: 2010 IEEE International Conference on Acoustics Speech and Signal Processing (ICASSP). IEEE (2010)
14. Wang, X., Grimson, W.E.L., Westin, C.F.: Tractography segmentation using a hierarchical dirichlet processes mixture model. NeuroImage 54(1), 290–302 (2011)
15. Wassermann, D., Bloy, L., Kanterakis, E., Verma, R., Deriche, R.: Unsupervised white matter fiber clustering and tract probability map generation: Applications of a Gaussian process framework for white matter fibers. NeuroImage 51(1) (2010)

Automatic Detection of Good/Bad Colonies of iPS Cells Using Local Features

Atsuki Masuda[1], Bisser Raytchev[1(✉)], Takio Kurita[1], Toru Imamura[2,3],
Masashi Suzuki[3], Toru Tamaki[1], and Kazufumi Kaneda[1]

[1] Department of Information Engineering, Hiroshima University, Hiroshima, Japan
bisser@hiroshima-u.ac.jp
[2] School of Bioscience and Biotechnology, Tokyo University of Technology,
Tokyo, Japan
[3] Biotechnology Research Institute for Drug Discovery, AIST, Tokyo, Japan

Abstract. In this paper we propose a method able to automatically detect good/bad colonies of iPS cells using local patches based on densely extracted SIFT features. Different options for local patch classification based on a kernelized novelty detector, a 2-class SVM and a local Bag-of-Features approach are considered. Experimental results on 33 images of iPS cell colonies have shown that excellent accuracy can be achieved by the proposed approach.

1 Introduction

Ever since their discovery in 2006, induced pluripotent stem (iPS) cells [4] have attracted a lot of attention and hope, due to their inherent potential to revolutionize medical therapy by personalizing regenerative medicine and creating novel human disease models for research and therapeutic testing (see e.g. [2] for a review of iPS cell technology, which also discusses potential clinical applications). Like embryonic stem (ES) cells, iPS cells have the ability to *differentiate* into any other cell type in the body, like neurons, heart, liver cells, etc. Still iPS cells offer distinct advantages over ES cells. As iPS cells can be derived from adult somatic tissues, they do not invoke the same ethical issues like ES cells, which can only be derived from embryos. Also, in a clinical setting iPS cells do not engender immune rejection since they are autologous cells unique to each patient. This also makes it possible to model disease in vitro on a patient-by-patient basis.

In order to fulfill their promise in regenerative medicine and drug discovery, a steady supply of iPS cells obtained through harvesting of individual cell colonies is needed. However, cultivating iPS cell colonies is a sensitive process, and even if care is taken abnormalities can appear, which need to be detected. It is therefore important to automate the process of detecting such abnormalities and one plausible way is to use machine learning techniques on images of the cultivated cell colonies. Some first steps in this direction have already been taken. In [7] an in-house developed image analysis software is used to detect cell colonies, and

© Springer International Publishing Switzerland 2015
L. Zhou et al. (Eds.): MLMI 2015, LNCS 9352, pp. 153–160, 2015.
DOI: 10.1007/978-3-319-24888-2_19

then colonies are classified as iPS or non-iPS based on morphological rules represented in a decision tree. This method needs a huge amount of data (more than 2000 colonies being used) to learn the rules and average accuracy of 80.3% is achieved. Joutsijoki et al. [3] use intensity histograms calculated over the whole image of a colony as features and SVMs with linear kernel function as a classifier, obtaining 54% accuracy on 80 colony images.

While the above methods try to learn the characteristics on a global colony-level, in this paper we propose to extract local invariant feature patches densely on a grid over each iPS colony image, and learn either a novelty detector or a classifier to discriminate *locally* between *undifferentiated* cells which would form Good colonies, and *differentiated* cells which would appear predominantly in Bad colonies. The advantage of the proposed local approach is that a huge amount of training samples can be obtained even from very few colony images, which otherwise would have been insufficient to learn the specific characteristics of differentiated vs. undifferentiated cells. Additionally a visualization on a pixel level is possible with the proposed approach, which would provide feedback about accuracy on a cell level, rather than for the whole image.

In the next section we describe the proposed approach in more detail, starting with the local feature extraction and then considering several alternative ways to classify the cells on a local level. In section 3, experimental results are reported on 33 images of Bad and Good colonies, showing that excellent accuracy can be achieved by the proposed method. Finally, section 4 concludes the paper.

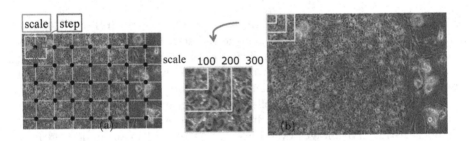

Fig. 1. (a) Illustration of the *scale* and *step* parameters used to control the size and sampling density of the local feature patches; (b) Scale (in pixels) related to cell and image size.

2   Methods

2.1   Extracting Local Features from iPS Cell Colony Images

As shown in Fig. 1a, we extract SIFT features [5] densely on a grid over each iPS colony image. SIFT features have been shown to achieve state-of-the-art performance on many object recognition tasks, and we expect that they would be able to successfully represent iPS cells on a local level. Two important parameters are *scale*, which determines the size of the local patches representing the features, and *step*, which determines the density of the sampling over the images. These parameters are illustrated in Fig. 1b and suitable values discussed in the Experiments section.

2.2 Cell Colony Classification with a Kernelized Novelty Detector

As undifferentiated cells look more or less similar to each other (round and compact), while differentiated cells can take quite different forms and texture, it seems most natural to formulate the colony classification problem in terms of novelty (abnormality) detection. In this subsection we describe the Novelty Detector [6] used to discriminate between Good and Bad colonies of iPS cells. We assume that sufficient training data is available so that the distribution of local feature patches corresponding to typical *Good* (undifferentiated) cells can be modeled in some (possibly transformed) feature space. In such a feature space, a hypersphere with minimal radius R and center $\mathbf{a}$ is sought, which contains most of the training data, so that anomalous data points (differentiated cells in this case) would lie outside the boundary of the hypersphere. If the local patches extracted from the training images are represented as vectors $\mathbf{x}_i$ $(i = 1, ..., m)$, the task is to minimize the radius of the hypersphere

$$\min \quad R^2 + \frac{1}{m\nu} \sum_i \xi_i \quad \text{subj. to} \quad (\mathbf{x}_i - \mathbf{a})^T (\mathbf{x}_i - \mathbf{a}) \le R^2 + \xi_i \qquad (1)$$

where the nonnegative slack variables ξ_i are used to account for outliers outside the sphere, and ν controls the trade-off between the two terms in the cost function. Using Lagrange multipliers the primal formulation of the optimization problem can be formulated as

$$L(R, \mathbf{a}, \alpha_i, \mathbf{x}_i) = R^2 + \frac{1}{m\nu} \sum_{i=1}^{m} \xi_i - \sum_{i=1}^{m} \gamma_i \xi_i$$

$$- \sum_{i=1}^{m} \alpha_i \left(R^2 + \xi_i - (\mathbf{x}_i \cdot \mathbf{x}_i - 2\mathbf{a} \cdot \mathbf{x}_i + \mathbf{a} \cdot \mathbf{a}) \right) \qquad (2)$$

with α_i and γ_i non-negative. Applying the kernel trick (RBF kernels being used in the experiments), we need to maximize

$$W(\alpha) = \sum_{i=1}^{m} \alpha_i K(\mathbf{x}_i, \mathbf{x}_i) - \sum_{i=1}^{m} \alpha_i \alpha_j K(\mathbf{x}_i, \mathbf{x}_j) \qquad (3)$$

with respect to α_i and subject to $\sum_{i=1}^{m} \alpha_i = 1$ and $0 \le \alpha_i \le 1/m\nu$. Then a test patch $\mathbf{z}$ is abnormal if the decision function $\phi(\mathbf{z})$ is negative:

$$\phi(\mathbf{z}) = R^2 - K(\mathbf{z}, \mathbf{z}) + 2 \sum_{i=1}^{m} \alpha_i K(\mathbf{z}, \mathbf{x}_i) - \sum_{i,j=1}^{m} \alpha_i \alpha_j K(\mathbf{x}_i, \mathbf{x}_j) < 0. \qquad (4)$$

2.3   Cell Colony Classification with 2-Class Support Vector Machine

Although the novelty detector approach described in the previous subsection seems most natural for the task at hand, when only a small training dataset is available this might be insufficient to learn all the variability inherent in the shapes and texture of the undifferentiated cells, i.e. it might be advantageous to learn the characteristics of both Good and Bad colonies, i.e. to use a 2-class classifier. Here we use a Support Vector Machine SVM [1] to utilize its well-known ability to generalize well to knew (unseen) data. SVMs learn a maximum margin hyperplane in transformed (through the kernel trick) features space to separate the 2 classes. Details are ommited for lack of space, but see [1].

2.4   Cell Colony Classification with the Bag-of-Features Approach

Although in this paper we take a purely local approach to information representation, it might be instructive to consider whether combining information across larger areas in the colonies might be advantageous. For this we adapt the popular Bag-of-Features (BoF) framework. All local feature patches extracted from all training images are clustered into k clusters, whose centers represent the *visual words*. Then a window of size larger than the scale of the features is slid sequentially over the colony image, and the content in each window is represented as a histogram of similarities to the visual words. The histograms are used as features in a SVM which classifies each window separately.

3   Experimental Results

For the experiments reported in this paper we have used a dataset containing 33 images of iPS cell colonies obtained under phase-contrast microscopy, which were taken at the Biotechnology Research Institute for Drug Discovery, AIST. Each image was labeled by an expert into 2 categories: in the *Good colonies* most cells appear to be undifferentiated (compact, round), while in the *Bad colonies* many (but *not all*) cells appear to be differentiated (spread, flattened). In total there were 27 images of Good and 6 images of Bad colonies. Some representative images are shown in Fig. 2. The size of the images is 4272×2848 pixels, and a typical undifferentiated iPS cell is of size approximately 100×100 pixels.

We first evaluate *the novelty detection method* described in section 2.2. As explained in section 2.1 we extract SIFT features densely on a grid from all training images, where the sampling density is controlled by the parameter *step*, and the size of the descriptor patch by the parameter *scale*. The scale size is selected relatively to the cell size – a radius of 50–100 pixels set as a value for the *scale* parameter would roughly be able to cover a single cell. We change the number of training images between 10 and 23 to see how detection accuracy changes as more training images become available. Only images of Good colonies are used to train the novelty detector, and the remaining Good colonies images (which have not been used for training) plus all Bad colonies images were used for

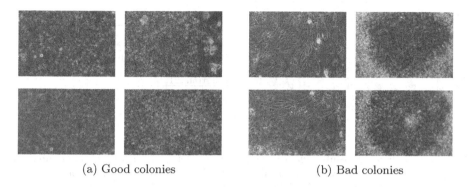

(a) Good colonies   (b) Bad colonies

Fig. 2. Examples of images of iPS colonies used in the experiments (see text for details)

test. The training images were selected randomly from all available Good images and this procedure was repeated 6 times to average the results. For the test, dense SIFT features were extracted from each test image in the same way (using the same scale and step parameters) as for the training images and classified as either Good or Bad depending on the output from the trained novelty detector. After this local patch classification the whole test image was classified by counting the number of patches classified as either Good or Bad and choosing the label corresponding to the higher number of votes.

Fig. 3 shows the results obtained for this experiment when the number of training images was changed from 10 to 15 to 21. Confusion matrices are shown on the right and average accuracy with standard deviation error bars on the left. The results indicate that when not enough training images are available (less than 21 here) the novelty detector is not able to detect reliably the bad colonies as novel events, but once sufficient information is supplied, very good result can be obtained (highest average accuracy was 95.85%). Additionally, a suitable value for the scale parameter seems to be crucial, and the results show that scale values corresponding roughly to the size of the individual cells (or a little larger) produce best results. The confusion matrices obtained for several different values of the scale parameter when using 21 training images are given in Fig. 4.

Next we show the results obtained when both Good and Bad colonies images were included in the training set and an SVM was used to learn and classify the local feature patches extracted from the images. Here again dense SIFT features were extracted and the scale and step parameters were varied in the same way as in the novelty detection experiment above. As we have more images from Good colonies in our dataset, to avoid unbalanced training we adopted the following experimental procedure. Since we have only 6 images with Bad colonies, we retain 1 such image for testing and use the other 5 for training, which procedure we repeat 6 times (i.e. leave-one-out on the Bad images). For each set of 5 Bad training images we randomly select 5 Good images for training and use the remaining 22 Good images for testing. As from the SVM we can obtain

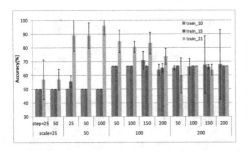

train_10	Good	Bad
Good	100.0%	0.0%
Bad	58.3%	41.7%

train_15	Good	Bad
Good	100.0%	0.0%
Bad	66.7%	33.3%

train_21	Good	Bad
Good	91.7%	8.3%
Bad	0.0%	100.0%

Fig. 3. Classification results when using a novelty detector with different number of training images. (Left) Average accuracy obtained for different values of the scale and step parameters; (Right) Confusion matrices obtained for the best parameter settings when respectively 10 (red bars), 15 (blue bars) and 21 (green bars) training images were used.

scale=50	Good	Bad
Good	91.7%	8.3%
Bad	0.0%	100.0%

scale=100	Good	Bad
Good	94.4%	5.6%
Bad	33.3%	66.7%

scale=200	Good	Bad
Good	100.0%	0.0%
Bad	52.8%	47.2%

Fig. 4. Confusion matrices obtained for different values of the *scale* parameter, when 21 Good training images were used to train a novelty detector. The value of the step parameter was fixed to 100 pixels.

the posterior probabilities for each local patch to belong to the Good colonies class (and for the areas where several neighboring patches overlap we average the posteriors from each contributing patch), we threshold the posteriors (for the experiments reported here we thresholded at the 0.5 probability level), then count the instances of Good and Bad predictions over the whole test image and report as its label the class corresponding to the majority of votes. The results from the above experimental procedure are shown in Fig. 5. On the left the average accuracy is given for different values of the scale and step parameters. Since the number of test images is different for the Good and Bad colonies, the reported accuracy is the mean of the accuracies for the Good and Bad colonies. More detailed results are given in the confusion matrices on the right for different values of the scale parameter. Here again we observe that the scale parameter is important, and consistently with the previous experiment best results are obtained when scale roughly corresponds to the cell size (50–100 pixels). Best accuracy of 99.25% was achieved for scale=50, step=50.

Although the classification results above provide an overall quantitative evaluation of the accuracy with which good and bad cell colonies can be detected, it might be more instructive to see how individual cells are classified. This is particularly easy to be done because of the local approach taken here. Fig. 6 shows representative examples of correctly classified colonies (top row for the novelty detector and bottom row for the 2-class SVM; left two columns for Good colonies and right two columns for Bad.) For the novelty detector Good patches are shown

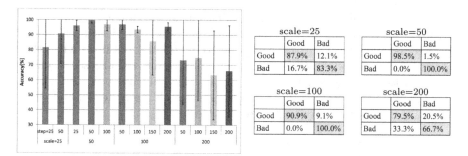

Fig. 5. Classification results when using a 2-class SVM. (Left) Average accuracy for different values of the scale and step parameters. Bars corresponding to the same values of the step parameter are shown in the same color; (Right) Confusion matrices for different values of the scale parameter (step fixed to 50 pixels).

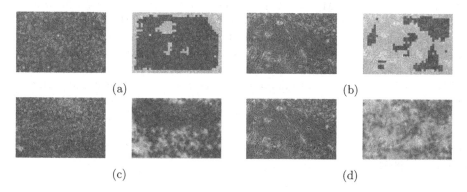

Fig. 6. Visualization of the detection/classification results at a patch level. (a), (b): using the novelty detector (scale=50, step=100 pixels, 21 Good training images) to detect (a) Good colony and (b) Bad colony images; (c), (d): using 2-class SVM (scale=step=50 pixels, using 5 Good and 5 Bad training images) to classify (c) Good colony and (d) Bad colony images.

in red, and Bad patches in white. For the SVM, posterior probabilities are visualized using different saturation levels of red – higher probability to belong to the Good class is shown in darker red, while the lower the probability, the more whitish the corresponding area becomes.

Finally, we performed experiments using the Bag-of-Features approach on the same dataset. Dense SIFT features were extracted from each image as in the previous two experiments, however now instead of classifying each feature (local patch) separately, the information from all patches inside a larger area (window) was represented in terms of a histogram of similarities to k visual words, obtained by clustering all features from the training images into k clusters (k-means clustering was used). The resulting histograms are fed to a 2-class SVM for learning and classification. The window is shifted left to right and top to bottom to cover the whole image, two neighboring windows having 50%

overlap. Results for different values of the scale, step and k parameters cannot be shown for lack of space but we observed that for any setting of these parameters BoF showed very low accuracy. Best accuracy of 68.6% was obtained when the sliding window was 600×600 pixels. The much worse results than those obtained for the purely local approaches from the previous 2 experiments indicate that, at least for the available dataset, the local approach should be preferred and that integration of information over larger areas is not helpful.

4   Conclusion

In this paper we have proposed a method to detect good and bad colonies of iPS cells by using local patches based on densely extracted SIFT features. We have shown that very good results can be obtained with either a kernelized novelty detector or a 2-class SVM, provided the local patches are extracted at a suitable scale. This should be determined relative to the size of the individual cells, i.e. at a similar or slightly larger scale. Combining information from multiple cells across larger areas using the Bag-of-Features framework did not produce good results, which seems to reinforce the proposed purely local approach. Still, validation of the obtained results on a much larger dataset is necessary, and we expect that for larger sets when the variation of differentiated cells could increase more significantly the novelty detector approach might gain the upper hand.

Acknowledgments. This work was supported in part by JSPS KAKENHI Grant Number 25330337.

References

1. Cristianini, N., Shawe-Taylor, J.: An Introduction to Support Vector Machines and Other Kernel-Base Learning Methods. Cambridge University Press (2000)
2. Ebben, J.D., Zorniak, M., Clark, P.A., Kuo, J.S.: Introduction to induced pluripotent stem cells: Advancing the potential for personalized medicine. World Neurosurg. **76**(3–4), 270–275 (2011)
3. Joutsijoki, H., et al.: Classification of ipsc colony images using hierarchical strategies with support vector machines. In: IEEE Symp. CIDM 2014, pp. 86–92 (2014)
4. Kazutoshi, T., Koji, T., Mari, O., Megumi, N., Tomoko, I., Kiichiro, T., Shinya, Y.: Induction of pluripotent stem cells from adult human fibroblasts by defined factors. Cell **131**(5), 861–871 (2007)
5. Lowe, D.G.: Distinctive image features from scale-invariant keypoints. International Journal Computer Vision **60**(2), 91–110 (2004)
6. Tax, D., Duin, R.: Data domain description by support vectors. In: Proceedings of ESANN 1999, pp. 251–256 (1999)
7. Watanabe, H., Tanabe, K., Kii, H., Ishikawa, M., Nakada, C., Uozumi, T., Kiyota, Y., Wada, Y., Tsuchiya, R.: Establishment of an algorithm for automated detection of ips/non-ips cells under a culture condition by noninvasive image analysis (2012)

Detecting Abnormal Cell Division Patterns in Early Stage Human Embryo Development

Aisha Khan[1(✉)], Stephen Gould[1], and Mathieu Salzmann[1,2,3]

[1] College of Engineering and Computer Science,
The Australian National University, Canberra, Australia
aisha.khan@anu.edu.au
[2] Computer Vision Research Group, NICTA, Canberra, Australia
[3] CVLab, EPFL, Lausanne, Switzerland

Abstract. Recently, it has been shown that early division patterns, such as cell division timing biomarkers, are crucial to predict human embryo viability. Precise and accurate measurement of these markers requires cell lineage analysis to identify normal and abnormal division patterns. However, current approaches to early-stage embryo analysis only focus on estimating the number of cells and their locations, thus failing to detect abnormal division patterns and potentially yielding incorrect timing biomarkers. In this work we propose an automated tool that can perform lineage tree analysis up to the 5-cell stage, which is sufficient to accurately compute all the known important biomarkers. To this end, we introduce a CRF-based cell localization framework. We demonstrate the benefits of our approach on a data set of 22 human embryos, resulting in correct identification of all abnormal division patterns in the data set.

1 Introduction

Predicting human embryo viability is one of the most relevant aspects of Assisted Reproductive Technology such as *in vitro* fertilization (IVF). Despite considerable research effort IVF have stagnant and unsatisfactory low success rate [2]. This is mainly due to little understanding of the basic biological aspects of early human embryo development, including factors that would aid in predicting successful development. In most cases embryologists assess embryo viability subjectively based on few visual observations, and critical events between observations may go unnoticed. Furthermore, embryo development is a complex process in which the exact timing and sequence of events are as essential as the successful completion of the events themselves. This requires continuous monitoring of each developing embryo and reliable embryo assessment biomarkers [2].

Recent advances in time-lapse microscopy has led to the study of the dynamics of developing embryos, and results in more reliable non-invasive embryo viability markers. A set of timing markers reported by Wong et al. [13] have been confirmed to be highly indicative of subsequent viability of the embryo [2]. These

We are grateful to Auxogyn, Inc. for their valuable support of this project.

L. Zhou et al. (Eds.): MLMI 2015, LNCS 9352, pp. 161–169, 2015.
DOI: 10.1007/978-3-319-24888-2_20

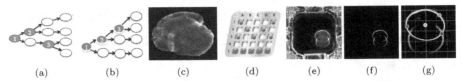

Fig. 1. Example of normal (a) and abnormal (b) division patterns. (c) Example of a 5-cell stage frame. (d) Petri Dish. (e) Raw image. (f) Hessian image. The Hessian image is used for proposing cell candidates by ellipse fitting (g).

markers are: (i) the duration of the first cleavage furrow from the beginning to the appearance of two cells; (ii) the duration of the 2-cell stage; and (iii) the time between the cleavage of each of the two cells to their respective daughter cells in the 4-cell stage. Recently, an additional timing parameter was proposed to complement the above-mentioned three parameters: (iv) the time to reach the 5-cell stage [9].

Current approaches [4,5,10,12,13] measure these timing parameters by performing cell detection and localization and ignore cell lineage. But cell lineage is vital for accurate measurement of the third timing parameter that requires identification of abnormal division patterns. Embryos can follow different courses of divisions after the first division (two cell stage). For the purpose of this study, a division pattern is considered normal when each of the cells at the 2-cell stage further divides to reach the 4-cell stage and is considered abnormal when only one of the two cells further divides to reach the 4-cell stage (see Fig. 1(a)–(b)). Two embryos classified to be at the same developmental stage (i.e., four cells) can be a product of completely different developmental processes. Since current approaches ignore lineage, they are unable to identify the cause of abnormal division patterns resulting in invalid timing measurements.

In this work, we introduce an approach that identifies abnormal division patterns in early stage human embryo development and allows accurate and precise measurements of timing parameters to be fully automated. Our approach allows embryologists to make use of detailed measurements that resolve cell ancestry. Manual characterization of the lineage requires biologist to maintain a rigorous observation regime and can also be prone to high inter-observer and intra-observer variability. This poses a huge hurdle for practical clinical implementation. By contrast, automated measurement of these tasks can alleviate this burden and may provide an objective, standardized embryo quality assessment free of human biases.

Our approach can be applied to any model that performs localization of individual cells. However, current models are limited to the 4-cell stage (e.g., [5,10]). Here, we therefore introduce a model that localizes cells beyond the 4-cell stage. We demonstrate the effectiveness of our model to detect and localize cells, and to trace their lineage in challenging microscopy images of developing human embryos. This allows us to identify abnormal cell division patterns and correctly assign timing parameters.

Related Work. Many authors have cited the complexities of monitoring human embryo development [4,5,10], which makes many of the standard detection, segmentation and tracking techniques not feasible (see Fig. 1(c) for an example of large overlap and poor visual features in the 5-cell stage). While some techniques have been proposed to detect cell divisions and perform cell tracking in microscopic images in general [3,7,8,11,14] and of embryos in particular [1,6], they typically require the cells to be stained, and thus cannot realistically be applied to human embryonic cells in an in vitro fertilization setting.

In the context of human embryonic cells, recent efforts have been made to automate the monitoring of early stage embryo development in an attempt to measure the timing parameters defined above. For example, Wang et al. [12] proposed a 3-level classification method to predict the embryo cell stage without explicit segmentation and tracking. However, our goal is to detect cell divisions by localizing and tracking cells to aid the biologists in the discovery and characterization of novel biological phenomena. Subsequently, a traditional particle filter based approach was proposed to detect cell divisions [13]. However, in the context of tracking multiple deforming objects, such as human embryos, traditional particle filters face problems due to the high dimensional search space. Similarly, Moussavi et al. [10] proposed a method to detect cell divisions by simultaneous segmentation and tracking cell boundaries in a conditional random field (CRF). However, the segmentation label space grows exponentially with number of cells and segments. Subsequently, a linear chain Markov model was proposed to detect and localize cells [5]. Their method uses cell spatial information along with a spatial continuity enforcement constraint, but suffers from label space exponential growth with the number of cells. The label space growth limits these models to the 4-cell stage. Moreover, these approaches detect cell divisions by tracking cell boundary between frames only, and no lineage tree analysis is performed. Importantly, all these methods are limited to the 4-cell stage, and measurement of timing parameters beyond four cells can only be performed manually.

While Khan et al. [4] recently proposed a method to identify the number of cells in an image up to five cells, their approach does neither localize the cells, nor track them. Furthermore, existing methods that construct lineage trees [1,3,6,7,11] have only been applied to stained cells with clear division patterns. As such, they are unable to handle the complexity of non-stained human embryos. In short, there exist no methods that can accurately measure the timing parameters of early-stage human embryo development and identify aberrant division patterns. In this work, we propose a CRF based model that identifies abnormal cell divisions by detecting and tracking individual cells. This allows accurate measurement of embryo viability markers and also provides biologists with detailed information about the developing embryo.

2   Methodology

Our goal is to monitor the patterns of cell division in microscopy images of evolving embryos. We achieve this by performing lineage tree analysis over the complete image sequence. Given cell location information for each of the cells within a frame our approach generates a complete ancestry by associating daughters to their mother in the previous frame. Importantly, our method can be applied to any system that outputs cell localization information.

Lineage Tree Construction. We propose to model the cell division ancestry as a lineage tree. To this end, and for the time being, let us assume that we are given the number of cells and their locations in a sequence of microscopy images. Our approach generates a lineage tree by associating each cell in a frame to its mother in the previous frame. If a cell is dividing, it is called a mother cell, and its two daughter cells share the same mother. Between consecutive frames, cell shape and location change in a confined manner. When a cell divides, its two daughters are almost half the size of their mother and, combined, present a similar shape to that of the mother. Using this fact, we associate cells between adjacent frames with highest intersection over union (IoU) between them. The IoU is computed by measuring the area of intersection of the two ellipses—one in each frame—divided by the area of their union.

Formally, let x^t and x^{t+1} denote the set of cells in the embryo at frames t and $t+1$, respectively. Then, an association between cells at frames t and $t+1$ is defined as

$$a^* = \operatorname*{argmin}_{a} \sum_{c \in x^{t+1}} \gamma(c, a(c)) \tag{1}$$

where $c \in x^{t+1}$ and $a(\cdot)$ is the association mapping from daughter to mother, where $a(c)$ returns the cell in x^t associated with cell c. To ensure a valid association, the following constraints are enforced; (i) each cell in frame $t + 1$ must have at most one mother; and (ii) each cell in frame t can either be assigned to a unique cell candidate in next frame or can divide and be associated with two or more cell candidates in the next time frame. The function γ measures the affinity of mapping c to $a(c)$ by computing the IoU between c and $a(c)$.

The lineage tree over the entire sequence can be obtained by finding a* between all consecutive frames. Since this only requires the locations of the cells, it can be applied to any existing cell localization method. However, existing methods are limited to the 4-cell stage, which is insufficient to obtain the last timing parameter (i.e., time to reach the 5-cell stage). Therefore, here, we introduce a new cell localization approach that can track the embryo beyond the 4-cell stage.

Cell Localization Model. Our model predicts the numbers and locations of the cells over time. We pose this problem in a CRF framework. We begin by preprocessing the images to produce a set of ellipses representing candidate cells within the image. The candidates define the label space for each time slice in our model. We infer the most likely number and location of cells for each frame with efficient exact inference.

Images of the developing embryos are captured by the $Eeva^{TM}$ System developed by Auxogyn, Inc. Embryos are placed in a petri dish inside the incubator where images are taken at 5-minute intervals over a three to five day period. Our method generates elliptical cell candidates for each frame using randomized sampling in conjunction with ellipse fitting [5]. This results in a small set of candidates (e.g., 100), which comprises the label space. Different frames have different label spaces as these are generated from evidence within each image (see Fig. 1 (d)–(g)).

We wish to annotate each frame in the image with the number and location of all cells within that frame. We formulate this by representing an embryo's state at time t by a set of variables. Let N_{max} be the maximum number of cells that can be predicted from the embryo's morphology (e.g., five). The variables are the number of cells $N^t \in \{1, 2, \ldots, N_{max}\}$, and cell location variables Y_m^t, one per cell, $m \in \{1, 2, \ldots, N_{max}\}$. Each location variable Y_m^t can take on a label from the label space $\mathbf{L}^t = \{c_1^t, \ldots, c_K^t, d^t\}$ corresponding to the K candidates, described above, and a special dummy label d^t, which allows us to account for frames containing less than N_{max} cells, and thus corresponding location variables should not be assigned a candidate. In a fully connected inter-slice graph we define four compatibility functions over the variables within one time slice: (i) a classifier probability on N^t (Φ_1); (ii) a unary potential over Y^t (Φ_2); (iii) a compatibility function between Y_m^t and N^t (Φ_3); and (iv) a similarity constraint on Y^t (Φ_4).

The function Φ_1 provides a prediction on N^t from the intensity images [4]. Briefly, a linear chain Markov model is applied on intensity images with learned unary and pairwise potentials to predict the number of cells directly in an image. The framework takes the feature vector of a frame as input, and returns a probability on the number of cells $p_N^t \in \mathbb{R}^{N_{max}}$. Then, the unary energy of the number of cells is equivalent to its negative log-probability.

Similarly, the function Φ_2 measures how much evidence there is for the candidate c^t in the image X^t. It is modeled as the output of a boosted decision tree classifier trained separately on a set of eight handcrafted and features extracted from the probability vector returned by Φ_1. The classifier takes the feature vectors of candidates c^t for frame t as input, and returns a probability of labels $\mathbf{L}^t$ for frame t. Then, we define Φ_2 as the negative log-probability of the boosted decision tree classifier.

The pairwise compatibility function Φ_3 between Y and N enforces that location variables $\{Y_i^t\}_{i=1,\ldots,N^t}$ get a label from $\mathbf{L}^t$ and the remaining location variables $\{Y_j^t\}_{j=N^t+1,\ldots,N_{max}}$ get the dummy label d^t while the other variables don't. The function is defined as

$$\Phi_3(Y_i^t, N^t) = \begin{cases} 0, & \text{if } (Y_i^t = d^t \wedge i > N^t) \vee (Y_i^t \neq d^t \wedge i \leq N^t) \\ \infty, & \text{otherwise.} \end{cases} \tag{2}$$

Function Φ_4 imposes a similarity constraint over Y^t such that no two location variables at time t represent the same part of the image. This is expressed as

$$\Phi_4(Y_i^t, Y_j^t, N^t) = \begin{cases} 0, & \text{if } \delta^t \leq \text{threshold}(N^t) \\ \infty, & \text{otherwise,} \end{cases} \tag{3}$$

where $\delta^t \in [0, 1]$ is a similarity measure between the candidates in label space $\mathbf{L}^t$ defined in terms of IoU. This also imposes mutual exclusion constraints over Y^t. Here threshold(N^t) is computed from training data by considering the IoU of all pairs of cell candidates (ellipses) close to the ground-truth (i.e., IoU w.r.t ground-truth ≥ 0.7) for each N^t separately. We set threshold(N^t) as the 90-th percentile IoU.

We then seek to model the evolution of the cells over time by adding an inter-slice compatibility function. More specifically, we introduce a pairwise potential that scores the compatibility of labels, Y^t and Y^{t+1}, for two consecutive frames. Since we wish to capture cell division events we use a simple model that enforces the number of cells not to decrease from time t to time $t+1$. It also penalizes the case where a transition is skipped from time t to time $t + 1$. This compatibility function is defined as

$$\psi_2^{t,t+1}(N^t, N^{t+1}) = \begin{cases} 0, & \text{if } (N^t = N^{t+1}) \vee (N^{t+1} = N^t + 1) \\ \infty, & \text{otherwise.} \end{cases} \tag{4}$$

We seek the most likely number of cells N^t and cell locations Y^t for each frame, and ultimately the most likely sequence. Formally, this corresponds to finding the variable configuration that minimizes the total CRF energy over all time frames, defined as

$$E(Y, N) = \sum_{t=1}^{T} \psi_1^t(Y_{\{1:\,N_{max}\}}^t, N^t) + \sum_{t=1}^{T-1} \psi_2^{t,t+1}(N^t, N^{t+1}), \tag{5}$$

where $\psi_1^t(Y^t, N^t)$ is the sum of intra-slice compatibility functions defined above. We achieve this by performing exact inference using a junction tree within the time slice and belief propagation between time slices. Exact belief updating is then performed by message passing over the junction tree.This allows us to perform exact inference over long sequences. However, belief propagation over junction tree is known to be computationally intensive in the general case. Its complexity may increase dramatically with the connectivity and state space cardinality of the nodes. Exact inference became computationally hard with a large label space (K>30) for $N_{max} = 5$. So in that case we applied max-product approximate inference within a time slice.

3 Experiments

We evaluated our approach on 22 developing embryos from eight different patients, consisting of a total of 9260 frames with 71 cell divisions. Ground truth for these sequences was generated by manually annotating each cell division, cell locations and cell lineage. Since our approach estimates the number of cells in each frame, their locations and the lineage tree, we report the following error metrics. Cell stage prediction: percentage of frames where the correct number of cells was predicted. Transition accuracy: number of frames between the ground-truth cell division and the predicted one. Localization: percentage of cells whose IoU with ground-truth is greater than 0.7. Lineage association: percentage of

Table 1. Cell stage prediction, cell transition (Trans.), localization (Loc.) and lineage resonstruction (Ling.) performance.

Experiments ($N_{max} = 5$)	Cell Stage Prediction (%)							Loc. (%)	Trans. Avg.	Ling. (%)	
	1-cell	2-cell	3-cell	4-cell	5-cell	Avg.	Overall			Ass.	Div.
Ours (MP)	100.0	99.6	95.5	91.7	88.2	95.0	95.5	74.2	4.0	74.0	81.7
Ours (JT)	100.0	99.6	95.5	91.8	88.2	95.0	95.6	82.6	4.0	80.8	86.0
Khan et al. [4]	100.0	99.6	95.5	88.7	88.2	94.4	94.6	—	6.4	—	—
($N_{max} = 4$)											
Ours (MP)	99.8	98.8	80.9	99.1	—	94.6	98.8	76.9	1.9	76.3	83.1
Ours (JT)	99.8	98.8	80.9	99.1	—	94.6	98.8	86.0	1.9	93.2	89.8
Khan et al. [5]	99.1	99.5	43.3	98.9	—	85.2	97.9	87.0	2.8	92.9	86.4
Khan et al. [4]	99.8	98.8	80.9	99.1	—	94.7	98.8	—	1.9	—	—

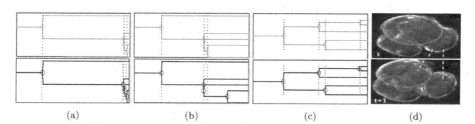

(a)   (b)   (c)   (d)

Fig. 2. Lineage tree examples. Green lines: Ground truth. Blue lines: Reconstructed lineage tree. The dotted red lines represents the ground-truth transitions. From left to right: Two examples of abnormal division patterns; an exampe of normal division pattern; an exmple of cell associations at the time of division.

correctly estimated mother-daughter relationships. Lineage division: percentage of correctly predicted divisions, i.e., correct association when a division occurs.

The results of these different metrics are reported in Table 1. The top half of the table contains results for the case where $N_{max} = 5$, which represents the scenario where all known biomarkers can be computed, and where only our cell localization approach is applicable. The bottom half of the table corresponds to $N_{max} = 4$, and thus our lineage tree estimation technique was applied either to our cell localization technique, or as a post-processing step to the method of [5].

As can be observed from the table, our approach yields accurate lineage tree estimates. In particular, for $N_{max} = 4$, it yields better results when applied with our cell localization method than with the one of Aisha et al. [5]. Fig. 2 illustrates an example of cell associations and localization for 3-4 cell division. Mother and daughters are marked in yellow. Importantly, our approach was able to identify all the abnormal cell division patterns, some of which are illustrated in Fig. 2, where only one of the cells in the 2-cell stage further divides to yield the four cell stage. In terms of cell stage prediction, both our inference strategies (MP and JT) yield very similar and accurate results. Note that, for $N_{max} = 4$, our approach yields much more accurate results than [5] for the 3-cell stage. Three cell periods tend to be very short and the hypotheses scoring function of [5] performs poorly here, which can be improved with more discriminating features. Importantly, this stage is crucial for the accuracy of the second and third timing biomarkers. For the cell transition accuracy, our approach also outperforms the results of [4] (for $N_{max} = 5$) and [5] (for $N_{max} = 4$). Finally, in terms of localization, our JT inference yields more accurate results than the MP one, and are similar to [5](for $N_{max} = 4$). The running time of inference with JT and MP is 5 hours and 1 hour per sequence, respectively, which is within the frame rate (300s).

4   Conclusion

We have presented an automated approach to identify abnormal division patterns in developing human embryos by performing lineage tree analysis. Our approach can be used in any model that can localize individual cells. Since existing models are either limited to the 4-cell stage or do not localize cells, we have also proposed a cell localization method that handles up to the 5-cell stage. Our results have shown that we can reliably identify abnormality in divisions and also detect and localize individual cells. Our approach therefore provides biologists with a tool to assist them in the embryo selection process, and, we believe, constitutes an important step towards understanding the human embryo development process. In the future we plan to automate the identification of other abnormalities in growing embryos, such as cell reabsorption and fragmentation.

References

1. Amat, F., Lemon, W., Mossing, D.P., McDole, K., Wan, Y., Branson, K., Myers, E.W., Keller, P.J.: Fast, accurate reconstruction of cell lineages from large-scale fluorescence microscopy data. Nature Methods (2014)
2. Chen, A.A., Tan, L., Suraj, V., Pera, R.R., Shen, S.: Biomarkers identified with TL imaging: discovery, validation, and practical app. Fertility and Sterility (2013)
3. El-Labban, A., Zisserman, A., Toyoda, Y., Bird, A.W., Hyman, A.: Discriminative semi-markov models for automated mitotic phase labelling. In: ISBI (2012)
4. Khan, A., Gould, S., Salzmann, M.: Automated monitoring of human embryonic cells up to the 5-cell stage in time-lapse microscopy images. In: ISBI (2015)
5. Khan, A., Gould, S., Salzmann, M.: A linear chain markov model for detection and localization of cells in early stage embryo development. In: WACV (2015)
6. Li, K., Miller, E., Chen, M., Kanade, T., Weiss, L., Campbell, P.: Computer vision tracking of stemness. In: ISBI (2008)
7. Liu, A.-A., Li, K., Kanade, T.: Mitosis sequence detection using hidden conditional random fields. In: ISBI (2010)
8. Lou, X., Hamprecht, F.: Structured learning for cell tracking. In: NIPS (2011)
9. Meseguer, M., Herrero, J., Tejera, A., Hilligse, K.M., Ramsing, N.B., Jose, R.: The use of morphokinetics as a predictor of embryo implantation. HR (2011)
10. Moussavi, F., Yu, W., Lorenzen, P., Oakley, J., Russakoff, D., Gould, S.: A unified graphical models framework for automated mitosis detection in human embryos. IEEE Trans. Med. Imaging 1551–1562 (2014)

11. Schiegg, M., Hanslovsky, P., Kausler, B.X., Hufnagel, L., Hamprecht, F.A.: Conservation tracking. In: ICCV (2013)
12. Wang, Y., Moussavi, F., Lorenzen, P.: Automated embryo stage classification in TLM video of early human embryo development. In: MICCAI (2013)
13. Wong, C., Loewke, K., Bossert, N., Behr, B., Jonge, C.D., Baer, T., Pera, R.R.: Non-invasive imaging of human embryos before embryonic genome activation predicts development to the blastocyst stage. Nature Bio. (2010)
14. Yang, F., Mackey, M.A., Ianzini, F., Gallardo, G., Sonka, M.: Cell segmentation, tracking, and mitosis detection using temporal context. In: Duncan, J.S., Gerig, G. (eds.) MICCAI 2005. LNCS, vol. 3749, pp. 302–309. Springer, Heidelberg (2005)

Identification of Infants at Risk for Autism Using Multi-parameter Hierarchical White Matter Connectomes

Yan Jin[✉], Chong-Yaw Wee, Feng Shi, Kim-Han Thung, Pew-Thian Yap,
and Dinggang Shen, for the Infant Brain Imaging Study (IBIS) Network

Department of Radiology and BRIC, School of Medicine, University of North
Carolina at Chapel Hill, Chapel Hill, NC 27599, USA
{yjinz,chongyaw_wee,fengshi,khthung,
ptyap,dinggang_shen}@med.unc.edu

Abstract. Autism spectrum disorder (ASD) is a variety of developmental disorders that cause life-long communication and social deficits. However, ASD could only be diagnosed at children as early as 2 years of age, while early signs may emerge within the first year. White matter (WM) connectivity abnormalities have been documented in the first year of lives of ASD subjects. We introduce a novel multi-kernel support vector machine (SVM) framework to identify infants at high-risk for ASD at 6 months old, by utilizing the diffusion parameters derived from a hierarchical set of WM connectomes. Experiments show that the proposed method achieves an accuracy of 76%, in comparison to 70% with the best single connectome. The complementary information extracted from hierarchical networks enhances the classification performance, with the top discriminative connections consistent with other studies. Our framework provides essential imaging connectomic markers and contributes to the evaluation of ASD risks as early as 6 months.

1 Introduction

Autism spectrum disorder (ASD) is a type of complex brain developmental disorders characterized by repetitive behaviors, both verbal and non-verbal communication difficulty, and social interaction obstacle. About 1% of the world population is affected by ASD. In the US, it is estimated that one in 68 children is affected by ASD. It is a life-long disease involving an annual healthcare cost of around $250 billion. Therefore, early diagnosis and medical intervention will significantly improve the life quality of subjects, and reduce the financial burden borne by the society. Unfortunately, so far, there is no single medical test for ASD diagnosis. Instead, it is based on the evaluations made by specially trained physicians and psychologists on specific behavioral tests, typically after the age of two [1]. On the other hand, studies have shown

This work was supported by the National Institute of Health grants EB006733, EB008374, EB009634, AG041721, MH100217, and AG042599. We thank the National Database for Autism Research (NDAR) for providing the data to this research.

© Springer International Publishing Switzerland 2015
L. Zhou et al. (Eds.): MLMI 2015, LNCS 9352, pp. 170–177, 2015.
DOI: 10.1007/978-3-319-24888-2_21

that a number of brain structural deficits may emerge in as early as the first year of life [2]. For example, white matter (WM) abnormalities have been observed over multiple locations such as corpus callosum [3] and the reduction of global network efficiency [4] was found in the brains of ASD infants between 7 months and 2 years of age. Nevertheless, few studies explored the ASD risk in infants before toddlerhood, especially in the first year of life.

Computer-aided diagnosis using features obtained from medical images have been successfully applied to identifying various clinical groups [5-8]. A number of studies attempted to classify autistic children, using features on regional structural MRI [9] and diffusion parameters of WM regions [10]. However, the subjects involved in these studies were over 7 years old, when ASD has progressed considerably. For early intervention, it is desirable to identify ASD at a much earlier stage, preferably even before the first trace of symptomatic behaviors. However, identifying ASD in infants is challenging and not well studied because of the difficulty of image acquisition from infants and also the lack of obvious symptoms at this stage.

In this paper, we propose a novel multi-channel machine-learning based classification framework to identify the six-month-old infants at high-risk for ASD. The major contributions of this study include: firstly, we develop a novel brain parcellation strategy to partition a publicly available atlas "infant AAL" [11] into anatomical meaningful regions of interest (ROIs) with adaptive sizes; secondly, unlike [10], we propose to use the features from a hierarchical set of whole-brain WM connectivity networks (i.e., connectomes), instead of conventional region-based features, to identify ASD infants; finally, we utilize an effective two-stage feature selection scheme and multi-kernel SVM classifier that can incorporate the complementary information from multi-channel sources to optimize the classification accuracy.

2   Multi-Parameter Hierarchical Connectome Classification

2.1   Overview

We employ in this study multi-parameter hierarchical WM connectivity networks as multi-source information for identification of infants who are at risk for ASD. The diagram of the complete workflow for our proposed method is shown in Fig. 1. To define the nodes in network, we start with the publicly available infant AAL atlas [9], and parcellate its 90 cerebral ROIs into 203 and 403 ROIs, respectively, for constructing more detailed brain networks (Section 2.2). Then, we define connections (edges) of the network using multiple diffusion properties, such as fractional anisotropy (FA), mean diffusivity (MD), and fiber length, over the fiber tracts connecting each pair of ROIs (nodes). Thus, three sets of hierarchical WM connectivity networks (nine in total) are constructed for each subject (Section 2.3). Finally, the relevant features selected from these networks using t-test and LASSO logistic regression are fed into a multi-kernel SVM classifier for patient identification (Section 2.4).

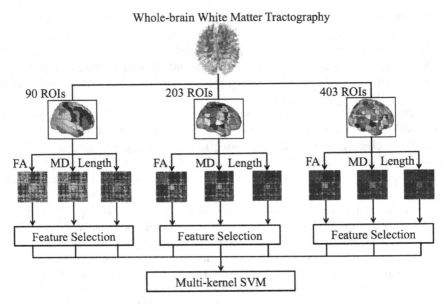

Fig. 1. The proposed classification framework based on multi-parameter hierarchical WM connectivity networks.

2.2   ROI Parcellation

The infant brain and the adult brain have large anatomical variances. Here, we used a 1-year-old infant AAL atlas that was adapted from the adult AAL atlas, which is a widely used single-subject high-resolution T1-weighted atlas [11]. The entire cerebrum was parcellated into 90 anatomically meaningful ROIs. However, to get more detailed connectivity information, it is necessary to divide the original ROIs into finer ROIs. We propose a novel strategy to parcellate the original ROIs into smaller sub-ROIs based on adaptive sizes. In our case, 203 and 403 ROIs were obtained when the size was chosen at around 20 mm and 16 mm, respectively. The detailed algorithm is described in Algorithm 1. Fig. 2 illustrates the 3D views of the three scales of infant AAL ROIs.

Algorithm 1. ROI Parcellation

Set the cube size a and load the original infant AAL ROIs.
Divide the entire volume (including the background) evenly into cubes of size a^3.
for ROI i=1:90 //compute the center of each new sub-ROI
   if any inside $V_{cube} > 0.3*a^3$, e.g., $V_{cube} > 0.3*a^3$, calculate the center of the cube.
   else Find a neighboring cube whose center is closest to its center and combine two regions.
     Recompute the new center of the combined region.
   end if
end for
for ROI i=1:90 //assign new ROIs
   Assign each inside voxel a new ROI index based on its shortest distance to an inside center.
end for

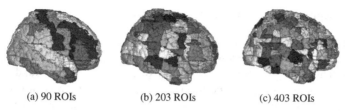

(a) 90 ROIs   (b) 203 ROIs   (c) 403 ROIs

Fig. 2. The 3D views of the three scales of infant AAL ROIs.

2.3   Hierarchical Connectomes

A connectome provides a comprehensive description of the complete structural connectivity of the entire brain. The features extracted from a connectome provide rich information for identifying ASD subjects due to its comprehensive characterization of the connections between brain regions. Furthermore, multi-scale connectomes may provide a range of complementary coarse-to-fine information for multi-level analysis of brain connections.

Two ROIs were considered anatomically connected if they were traversed by a common set of fibers. Connection strength between the two ROIs was computed as the average of FA, MD, and fiber length over the traversing fibers, respectively. Then, three connectivity networks (corresponding to FA, MD, and fiber length) can be constructed based on pair-wise connection strengths. By using all three different scales of the infant AAL atlas with 90, 203, and 403 ROIs, respectively, we constructed three sets of hierarchical connectivity networks (nine in total) for each subject. Fig. 3 illustrates a hierarchical set of FA connectomes from a pair of low-risk and high-risk subjects, respectively. Notice that the multi-scale networks of a low-risk subject contain stronger connections (i.e., more and thicker edges) than those of a high-risk subject.

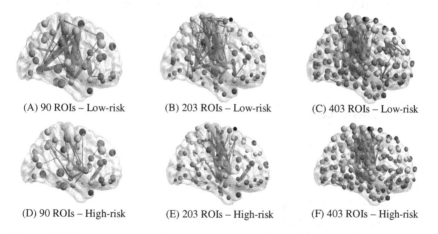

(A) 90 ROIs – Low-risk   (B) 203 ROIs – Low-risk   (C) 403 ROIs – Low-risk

(D) 90 ROIs – High-risk   (E) 203 ROIs – High-risk   (F) 403 ROIs – High-risk

Fig. 3. The 3D views of the hierarchical set of connectomes thresholded by mean FA = 0.4 from a pair of low-risk and high-risk subjects. Each sphere represents the center of an ROI and its size indicates the normalized volume of the ROI. The colors of the sub-ROIs in (B), (C), (E), and (F) correspond to those of the original ROIs in (A) and (D). The thickness of edges represents the mean value of FA averaged over the fibers connecting two respective ROIs.

2.4   Multi-Kernel Classification

We considered each element in each connectivity network as a feature. Thus, the number of features increased with the square of the number of ROIs, with tens of thousands of features for the finest scale. Many of them would be redundant or irrelevant for classification. Thus, we performed feature selection on each network separately to determine an optimal subset of features that were relevant. An initial subset of features was first selected using feature-wise t-tests performed between the high-risk group and the low-risk group. Features with p-values below an empirical threshold were further sieved using LASSO logistic regression.

Multi-kernel SVM has been proven to be more effective than single-kernel SVM [9] in utilizing the complementary information from multiple sources for improving classification accuracy. We applied it to the features selected from the nine networks, as described above. Let $\{(x_i^j, y_i), i = 1, ..., M, j = 1, ..., T\}$ be the set of training data, where $x_i^j \in \mathbb{R}^{n_j \times 1}$ represents the feature vector of the i-th subject for network j and $y_i \in 1$ (high-risk) or -1 (low-risk) is the label. M is the number of training subjects and T is the number of networks (i.e., $T = 9$ in our study). The primal formulation of multi-kernel SVM is given as

$$\min_{P_j, b, \xi_i} \frac{1}{2}\sum_{j=1}^{T} \beta_j \|P_j\|^2 + C\sum_{i=1}^{M} \xi_i \tag{1}$$
$$\text{s.t. } y_i\left(\sum_{j=1}^{T} \beta_j (P_j^T \phi_j(x_i^j) + b)\right) \geq 1 - \xi_i$$
$$\text{and } \xi_i > 0, \ \sum_{j=1}^{T} \beta_j = 1, \ \beta_j > 0$$

where β_j, P_j and ϕ_j denote the weight, the normal vector of the classification hyperplane, and the kernel-induced mapping function for the j-th network, respectively. b denotes the bias term, ξ_i denotes the slack variable (for misclassification), and C is a parameter that controls the degree of misclassification. Given a test subject x, the prediction of its label $\hat{y}$ will be $\hat{y} = sign(\sum_{j=1}^{T} \beta_j(P_j^T \phi_j(x) + b))$. We used an open-source software package SimpleMKL [12], which could decide the weight of each network simultaneously while solving the optimization problem.

3   Experiment Results

3.1   Subjects and Data Processing

The participants used in this study were chosen from the Infant Brain Imaging Study (IBIS, http://www.ibis-network.org), an ongoing study of brain and behavioral development in infants. The high-risk infants have at least one older sibling with ASD, while the low-risk infants have no first-degree relatives with ASD. Included in this study were 40 six-month-old high-risk infants (29 males/11 females) and also 40 low-risk infants (27 males/13 females).

The DWI images were acquired with a 2 mm isotropic spatial resolution, and consisted of one non-diffusion-weighted b_0 volume and 25 diffusion-weighted volumes with $b=1000$ s/mm^2. FA and MD images were then extracted from the data after diffusion tensor fitting. The infant AAL atlas was registered to the subjects' FA images. With the deformation fields generated, we warped all three sets of infant AAL ROIs (i.e., 90, 203, and 403 ROIs) to the DWI image space of each subject. Whole-brain tractography was performed using deterministic streamline tractography with peaks detected from the WM orientation distribution functions. Seed points were chosen as voxels with FA > 0.3. The maximum fiber turning angle was set to 45°, and tracking was stopped when FA < 0.15.

3.2   Experiment Setting

Three sets of hierarchical connectivity networks based on mean FA, mean MD, and mean fiber length were constructed as described in Section 2.3. The performance was evaluated using nested 5-fold cross validation with 10 randomized repetitions. In feature selection, for each network, an initial t-test was conducted to select the features with p-values < 0.001. Some features were further discarded using LASSO logistic regression. More specifically, the results of the binarized regression in the inner 5-fold cross validation within the training set were compared to the ground truth. The LASSO parameters with the best accuracy were used to select the features for the test fold. Finally, selected features from each network were fed into SimpleMKL for classification. Another inner 5-fold cross validation using the training set was performed to find the best parameter C in Eq. (1) and the test fold was classified with that C.

For performance evaluation, we used several metrics, i.e., accuracy (ACC), sensitivity (SEN), specificity (SPE), and the area under the receiver operating characteristic curve (AUC) for performance evaluation. Let TP, TN, FP, and FN denote, respectively, true positive, true negative, false positive, and false negative cases that the algorithm detects. The definitions of ACC, SEN, and SPE are: $ACC = \frac{TP+TN}{TP+TN+FP+FN}$, $SEN = \frac{TP}{TP+FN}$, and $SPE = \frac{TN}{TN+FP}$.

3.3   Classification Results

Fig. 4 shows the performance comparison between using a single network and multiple networks. In (A-C), the performance with the hierarchical set of networks (90, 203, and 403 ROIs) is compared to that of each single network, in terms of the parameter FA, MD, and fiber length, respectively. The accuracies of multi-network are ~73%, with a gain of ~5%, compared to the best single network. The AUCs are ~0.78 with a gain of ~13% against the best single network. Smaller standard deviations for most of the statistics, especially AUC, suggest a more stable performance by the hierarchical network framework. In (D), our proposed method, which includes all parameter networks, further outperforms each hierarchical network alone with an accuracy of 76% and an AUC of 0.80. To validate the significant improvements, we conducted the pair-wise t-tests based on ACC on the total 50 fold results. For both levels, i.e., the hierarchical networks vs. the single network with a single parameter and our proposed framework vs. those single-parameter hierarchical networks, $p < 0.05$. The results demonstrate that the complementary information provided by both multi-scale networks and multiple parameters indeed enhances the performance significantly.

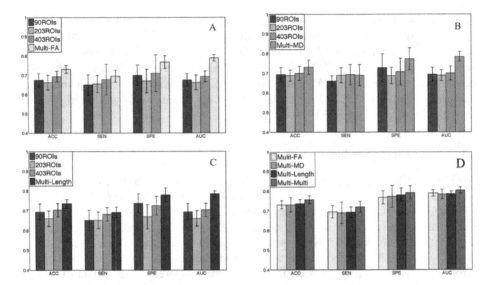

Fig. 4. Performance comparison for the 90-ROI (*blue*), 203-ROI (*cyan*), and 403-ROI (*green*) networks with (A) the hierarchical network framework (*yellow*) using FA; (B) the hierarchical network framework (*orange*) using MD; (C) the hierarchical network framework (*dark red*) using fiber length; and (D) the proposed hierarchical network framework using multiple diffusion statistics (*red*). The error bars denote the standard deviations obtained from 10 repetitions.

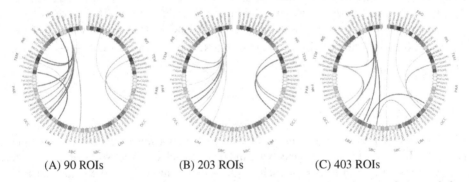

Fig. 5. Connectograms of the top 20 discriminative connections selected by our framework for (A) 90-ROI, (B) 203-ROI, and (C) 403-ROI networks, respectively. The intra- and inter-hemisphere connections are shown in red and black colors, respectively.

3.4   Most Discriminative Connections

We summed the counts of each connection selected by our proposed method for each level of connectome (90, 203, and 403 ROIs) over the 50 folds. The counts for FA, MD, and fiber length were combined at each level. The top 20 discriminative connections are reported using connectograms, a circular representation of connectomics, in Fig. 5. For the 203-ROI and 403-ROI networks, the original 90-ROI connections that contain those sub-ROI connections are shown. Thickness of each connection reflects its selection frequency, i.e., the thicker the line, the higher the selection frequency. Many connections are common to all three networks. However, the 403-ROI connectogram shows more diverse connections, even inter-hemisphere connections that are not shown in the coarser scales of connectomes. The connecting regions include frontal, parietal, temporal, occipital lobes, and a few subcortical regions, such as globus pallidus and putamen. Our findings are consistent with the previous studies [4]. Those top connections may serve as possible imaging markers for ASD diagnosis.

4   Conclusion

We propose a multi-channel classification framework that utilizes complementary information from a set of multi-parameter hierarchical WM connectivity networks to enhance the performance in identifying 6-month-old infants who are at high-risk for ASD. Our result of ACC/AUC of 76%/0.8 vs. 70%/0.7 for the best single network demonstrates the effectiveness of the propose method. Our method can be potentially applied to detecting other WM related diseases as well.

References

1. Prevalence of autism spectrum disorder among children aged 8 years, Centers for Disease Control and Prevention. Surveillance Summaries **63**(2), 1–21 (2014)
2. Ozonoff, S., et al.: A prospective study of the emergence of early behavioral signs of autism. J. Am. Acad. Child Adolesc. Psychiatry **49**(3), 256–266 (2010)
3. Wolf, J.J., et al.: Differences in white matter fiber tract development present from 6 to 24 months in infants with Autism. Am. J. Psychiatry **169**(6), 589–600 (2012)
4. Lewis, J.D., et al.: Network inefficiencies in autism spectrum disorder at 24 months. Transl. Psychiatry **4**, e388 (2014). doi:10.1038/tp.2014.24
5. Zhu, X., et al.: A novel matrix-similarity based loss function for joint regression and classification in AD diagnosis. Neuroimage **100**, 91–105 (2014)
6. Li, J., Jin, Y., Shi, Y., Dinov, I.D., Wang, D.J., Toga, A.W., Thompson, P.M.: Voxelwise spectral diffusional connectivity and its applications to alzheimer's disease and intelligence prediction. In: Mori, K., Sakuma, I., Sato, Y., Barillot, C., Navab, N. (eds.) MICCAI 2013, Part I. LNCS, vol. 8149, pp. 655–662. Springer, Heidelberg (2013)
7. Zhan, L., et al.: Comparison of nine tractography algorithms for detecting abnormal structural brain networks in Alzheimer's disease. Front Aging Neurosci **7**, 48 (2015). doi:10.3389/fnagi.2015.00048
8. Jin, Y., et al.: Automatic clustering of white matter fibers in brain diffusion MRI with an application to genetics. Neuroimage **100**, 75–90 (2014)
9. Wee, C.-Y., et al.: Diagnosis of autism spectrum disorders using regional and interregional morphological features. Hum. Brain Mapp. **35**(7), 3414–3430 (2014)
10. Ingalhalikar, M., et al.: Diffusion based abnormality markers of pathology: Toward learned diagnostic prediction of ASD. Neuroimage **57**(3), 918–927 (2012)
11. Shi, F., et al.: Infant brain atlases from neonates to 1- and 2-year-olds. PLos One **6**(4), e18746 (2011). doi:10.1371/journal.pone.0018746
12. Rakotomamonjy, A., et al.: SimpleMKL. J. Mach. Learn. Res. **9**, 2491–2521 (2008)

Group-Constrained Laplacian Eigenmaps: Longitudinal AD Biomarker Learning

R. Guerrero$^{(\boxtimes)}$, C. Ledig, A. Schmidt-Richberg, and D. Rueckert

Biomedical Image Analysis Group, Imperial College London, London, UK
reg09@imperial.ac.uk

Abstract. Longitudinal modeling of biomarkers to assess a subject's risk of developing Alzheimers disease (AD) or determine the current state in the disease trajectory has recently received increased attention.Here, a new method to estimate the time-to-conversion (TTC) of mild cognitive impaired (MCI) subjects to AD from a low-dimensional representation of the data is proposed. This is achieved via a combination of multi-level feature selection followed by a novel formulation of the Laplacian Eigenmaps manifold learning algorithm that allows the incorporation of group constraints.Feature selection is performed using Magnetic Resonance (MR) images that have been aligned at different detail levels to a template. The suggested group constraints are added to the construction of the neighborhood matrix which is used to calculate the graph Laplacian in the Laplacian Eigenmaps algorithm.The proposed formulation yields relevant improvements for the prediction of the TTC and for the three-way classification (control/MCI/AD) on the ADNI database.

1 Introduction

Nonlinear dimensionality reduction based on Laplacian Eigenmaps [1] or Isomap [2] is an essential technique in the exploration of high-dimensional medical imaging datasets. It is common for individual datasets to be not entirely independent from each other but to exhibit a certain degree of structure within them. For example, in a longitudinal studies multiple images of the same subject are acquired at several time points. These images will be highly correlated and thus similar to each other. Most classical nonlinear dimensionality techniques rely on finding similarities in the data to uncover the local manifold geometry. However, these approaches neglect potentially valuable grouping information. Treating images that are inherently correlated as independent could lead to a poor estimation of underlying manifold. It has been previously shown that exploiting a-priori knowledge of the underlying data grouping can lead to improved low-dimensional embeddings: In spatio-temporal Isomap [3] the original weights in the graph of local neighbors are empirically altered to emphasize similarity between temporally related points. In temporal Laplacian Eigenmaps (LE) [4] the temporal relationships are modeled as part of the objective function. However, these techniques focus on obtaining temporal consistency between within time series, rather than the overall geometrical shape of a population's manifold.

© Springer International Publishing Switzerland 2015
L. Zhou et al. (Eds.): MLMI 2015, LNCS 9352, pp. 178–185, 2015.
DOI: 10.1007/978-3-319-24888-2_22

Recently, the assessment and prediction of a subject's current and future risk of developing Alzheimers disease (AD), has received a substantial amount of attention. In [5] longitudinal patterns of brain atrophy are used to predict the conversion of mild cognitive impaired (MCI) patients to AD conversion. In [6] a discriminant analysis of longitudinal cortical thickness measurements are used to track changes in AD patients. In [7] LE have been explored to derive longitudinal features for AD from Magnetic Resonance (MR) images. Two approaches were explored: independent embedding of the baseline and follow-up scans, and embedding of the difference images. Given that the images were considered independent during embedding and only two time points per subject were used, the underlying trajectory of each subject might be poorly estimated.

In this work, a group-constraint graph Laplacian is introduced into the LE framework that allows the incorporation of a-priori knowledge of image grouping. Combined with multilevel feature selection a meaningful low-dimensional representation of the longitudinal data is derived. The proposed method is employed to calculate a low-dimensional embedding of T1-weighted MR images acquired from patients with memory complaints at multiple time points. It is shown that the incorporation of group-constraints allows the improved estimation of the time-to-conversion (TTC) of the subjects embedded in the manifold. The proposed approach also visualizes a subjects transition within the manifold across time as the disease progresses. The derived features show a natural ordering with regards to TTC and disease progress.

2   Manifold Learning MR Image Based Features

Manifold learning refers to a set of machine learning techniques that aim at finding a low-dimensional representation of high-dimensional data while preserving its intrinsic geometry. In the work presented here, feature selection, local binary patterns (LBP) and manifold learning are used to derive a low-dimensional representation of longitudinal MR image sets.

Deriving longitudinally meaningful biomarkers for AD based on manifold learning poses several challenges: Brain images reside in very high-dimensional space, although many dimensions (features or voxels) are not necessarily related to the disease being modeled. Relevant variable selection can be used to reduce the set of features. However, since images need to be aligned with each other for meaningful comparison, the question of which image alignment level is best needs to be addressed. Disease specific characteristics might manifest at different levels of image alignment, i.e. affinely aligned images of patients with AD might reveal discriminative information in the ventricles, while non-rigidly aligned images might reveal discriminative information of smaller structures such as the hippocampus. Additionally, due to the nature of MR images, changes in imaging protocols or acquisition parameters can produce images with distinct intensity characteristics that thus reside in distinct intensity spaces. This can be addressed by mapping all intensity features into a common space, e.g. by extracting LBP.

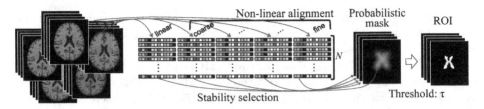

Fig. 1. Overview of the 4D relevant feature selection framework.

2.1 Multilevel Feature Selection

Feature selection reduces the amount of input features to those that are sensitive for a specific task. Elastic net [8] performs feature selection, encouraging the grouping of correlated features. In medical images, correlated features generally arise from neighboring regions, thus, feature selection can be viewed as ROI learning. Elastic net regression adds L_1 and L_2 regularization terms, each weighted by parameters $\lambda_1 > 0$ and $\lambda_2 > 0$, respectively, to ordinary least square regression. When $\lambda_2 \rightarrow \infty$, the optimization problem has for each predictor $\mathbf{x}_i$ a closed-form solution of the form that can be written as: $\hat{\beta}_i = (|\mathbf{1}^T\mathbf{x}_i| - \lambda_1/2)_+\mathrm{sign}(\mathbf{1}^T\mathbf{x}_i)$, where $(\cdot)_+$ is the positive part [8]. Stability selection [9] is used additionally to introduce robustness against sampling errors. A probabilistic mask that indicates the likelihood of a feature to be selected is then obtained. Thresholding the probabilities at τ yields a binary ROI [10]. In this work, independent features are MR image intensities, while the mini mental state examination (MMSE) score acts as the dependent variable. In order to address the uncertainty at which level of alignment the most relevant features can be found, each image is associated with R warped images. These correspond to alignments of the image to the template at R different alignment levels. A matrix $\mathbf{X}$ is built, where each column represents a spatial location in MNI space at a certain level of alignment to MNI space. Each row $\mathbf{x}_n$ in matrix $\mathbf{X}$ represents a subject at a specific time point $n \in N$ and is formed by concatenating R vectorized images at multiple levels $\mathbf{x}_n = [\mathrm{x}_{n1}, ..., \mathrm{x}_{nr}, ..., \mathrm{x}_{nR}]$. Elastic net regression then selects a subset of D features from $\mathbf{X}$, that correspond to column indices of $\mathbf{X}$. Finally, this yields a 4D mask, where the first three dimensions are spatial coordinates in MNI space and the fourth is the alignment level of the image to the template. Fig. 1 illustrates the described framework.

2.2 Local Binary Patterns

MR images acquired with different acquisition protocols have different intensity appearance. Thus, their intensities cannot be easily combined within a single framework without first mapping the image intensities into a common space. Many intensity normalization approaches (such as histogram matching) work very well for images absent of pathologies. In the case of pathology the basic assumption of these techniques does not necessarily hold (the mean, variance or quantiles can be shifted) and intensity normalization can potentially reduce disease related signal changes. In this work LBPs [11] around the 26-connected neighborhood of each selected voxel (according to Sec. 2.1) were extracted and encoded as binary vectors. This transforms the MR intensity features to an augmented binary space in $\mathbb{R}^{26D}$. In this space images that originally had distinct intensity characteristics can be combined, assuming that the original acquisition protocols are reasonably similar (e.g. both are T1-weighted).

2.3   Laplacian Eigenmaps

After feature selection, the high-dimensional feature space $\mathbf{V} = \{\mathbf{v}_1, \mathbf{v}_2, ..., \mathbf{v}_N\}$ $\in \mathbb{R}^{N \times D}$ is given by N vectors of length $\boldsymbol{D} = 26D$ that represent LBP extracted around the most relevant voxels from a set of R images at different levels of alignment. Here $\mathbf{v}_i = \{v_1, v_2, ..., v_D\}$ are LBPs extracted around the D most relevant voxels from the ith subject's set of R images. The aim is to learn the underlying low-dimensional manifold in $\mathbb{R}^d$ ($d \ll \boldsymbol{D}$) that best represents the population $\mathbf{V}$. LE [1] transforms data points to a low-dimensional space while preserving the local geometric properties of the manifold. The local geometry is determined by converting pairwise sum of squared differences (SSD) to a similarity matrix $\mathbf{W}$ using a Gaussian heat kernel. From $\mathbf{W}$, the k-neighborhoods of data points are used to construct a sparse neighborhood matrix $\mathbf{W}^*$. LE can be formulated as generalized eigenproblem $\mathbf{L}\nu = \mu\mathbf{M}\nu$, where $\mathbf{L} = \mathbf{M} - \mathbf{W}^*$ is the graph Laplacian and $\mathbf{M}$ is a degree matrix. Here ν and μ are the eigenvectors and eigenvalues, where the d eigenvectors corresponding to the smallest (non-zero) eigenvalues represent the new coordinate system.

Group-Constrained Graph Laplacian: The graph Laplacian $\mathbf{L}$ in LE acts as a design matrix that can be modified and adjusted, via changing the similarity matrix $\mathbf{W}$ to incorporate prior knowledge. In [1] $\mathbf{W}$ is sparsified using the data points' k-neighborhoods to form $\mathbf{W}^*$, which subsequently is used to calculate $\mathbf{L}$. In this work our interest lies in the modeling of longitudinal image data, specifically the modelling of several image instances of a subject acquired at different time points. Since the standard formulation does not allow the incorporation of grouping information an additional grouping feature $\mathbf{g}$ is introduced. Data points that belong to the same entity or group are associated with $\mathbf{g}$, e.g. g_i is categorical and all instances in the same category belong to the same group. In order to avoid nearest neighbors being biased towards any group g_i, a constraint is added so that at most one member per group $g_i \in \mathbf{g}$, for $i = 1, 2, ..., N$, is admitted into the neighborhood (within group connections are not permitted). This allows only a single time point per subject to form part of the local neighborhood, so that the space where the manifold resides is sampled as evenly as possible. Henceforth this modified sparse neighborhood matrix is referred to as $\mathbf{W}^{**}$. Fig. 2 (left) illustrates the differences between the sparse unconstrained neighborhood matrix $\mathbf{W}^*$ as obtained in [1] and the proposed group-constrained $\mathbf{W}^{**}$. The neighborhoods shown in Fig. 2 are made to be symmetric (undirected graph), and as such each point might have a different amount of neighbors.

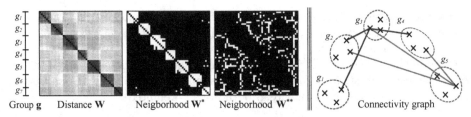

Fig. 2. Left: L_2 pairwise distance matrix **W**, sparse unconstrained (symmetric) neighborhood **W*** and the proposed group-constrained sparse (symmetric) neighborhood **W****, for 7 subjects with 5-9 time points each. Right: Schematic illustration of a spatial connectivity graph, where dotted and solid lines show the original LE (**W***) and the proposed (**W****) neighborhoods, respectively.

Fig. 2 (right) gives an illustrative example of a connectivity graph. It is easy to see that the local neighborhood of instances in a group would be poorly defined using only similarity or distance (dotted circles). However, by adding the proposed group constrains to the local neighborhood definition (solid lines) the underlying geometry of the data is better sampled.

3   Experiments and Results

Data used in this work was obtained from the Alzheimer's Disease Neuroimaging Initiative (ADNI) database. To date, ADNI (ADNI-1, -GO and -2) has recruited over 1500 adults, aged between 55 and 90 years, to participate in the study. Participants consist of cognitive normal (CN), significant memory concerns (SMC), MCI or early MCI (eMCI), and early AD subjects. In this work, a subset of subjects has been considered for which T1-weighted MR images and MMSE scores on at least five time points (over 8 years) were available. This resulted in 204 subjects and 1524 MR images: 790 MCI, 414 CN and 320 AD, with no SMC or eMCI subjects fulfilling the criteria. Of particular interest were 84 subjects with 610 images (302 MCI and 308 AD): These subjects were initially diagnosed as MCI and converted to AD during the study. Images were brain extracted using pyramidal intra-cranial masking [13]. Two types of registrations were used in the feature selection: Affine registration was used for longitudinal alignment of baseline and follow-up images, which encode pathological changes such as atrophy as intensity differences between the images. Cross-sectional registrations between baseline images and the MNI152 template were performed using non-rigid free-form-deformations [12] with different control point spacings (affine, 20mm, 10mm, 5mm and 2.5mm), which aim to eliminate inter-subject variability. The focus of the multilevel feature selection is thus to choose the optimal level of deformation that best compensates for inter-subject variability. A separate set of 292 subjects from ADNI-1 was used for multilevel feature selection to learn a probabilistic 4D relevance mask. The mask was thresholded at $\tau = 0.1$ yielding: 660, 922, 856, 580 and 190 voxels corresponding to the used deformation levels.

Table 1. Correlation coefficient between TTC or MMSE score, and first (D1) or second dimension (D2) of MLc, ML and PCA.

Features	TTC-D1	TTC-D2	MMSE-D1	MMSE-D2
MLc	**0.624**	**0.586**	**-0.548**	**-0.544**
ML	0.324	0.160	-0.318	-0.069
PCA	-0.459	0.073	0.441	-0.013

LBPs were extracted from the ROI of unseen images and used to learn a low-dimensional representation using: Principal component analysis (PCA) in order to demonstrate the nonlinear nature of the manifold, LE with an unconstrained neighborhood matrix (ML) and the proposed group-constrained LE (MLc). Parameters for LE were empirically set to: $k = 25$ nearest neighbors for the neighborhood graph (similar results obtained for $15 \leq k \leq 35$) and $\sigma = 1$ for the heat kernel. Fig. 3 shows the first two dimensions of the learned manifolds using MLc, ML and PCA. Marker color indicates time to/from conversion in months. It can be observed that there is a more coherent ordering (with respect to TTC) of the data with the proposed MLc embedding. The trajectory of an exemplar subject is shown by arrows. Feature ordering was empirically tested in the first two dimensions independently. Tab. 1 summarizes the results of calculating the correlation coefficient (CC) between the first or second dimension of the low-dimensional embeddings (MLc, ML and PCA) and TTC or MMSE. It can be seen that in every case the MLc embedding has higher absolute CC, which can be interpreted as a more coherent ordering of features.

The local neighborhood of images was used to estimate a subject's "state" along the disease "progression" trajectory. TTC was defined as the half way time point between the last MCI diagnosis and the first AD. Considering that the time between scans was on average 8.4 (range: [6; 48]) months, there is a minimum expected absolute error of 2.1 months. The performance of the low-dimensional coordinate systems (MLc, ML, PCA) and the full set of features (FULL), as defined in Sec. 2.1 and 2.2, were evaluated leave one out experiment. TTC was calculated using differently sized neighborhoods by finding the average time in the defined neighborhood. The lowest absolute mean error, $\sim$13 months, was obtained with the proposed method (MLc) using neighborhoods of between 30-75 instances. This compares to an absolute mean error $\sim$17 for ML, $\sim$16 for PCA and $\sim$15 months for FULL. ML performs poorly in the experiments due to the fact that local manifold geometry is not well estimated by the definition of neighborhoods that contain several points of the same subject. All methods converged to $\sim$18 months when the neighborhoods included most data points.

The discriminative power of the first two dimensions was compared in a classification experiment using linear discriminant analysis (LDA). Images were randomly split into train and test sets, where special care was taken not to include subjects that have at least one time point in the train set as part of the testing data. Average results from 1000 leave 10% out cross-validation runs are shown in Tab. 2. There seems to be little difference between the discriminative power of features in the binary classification, however MLc performs better than

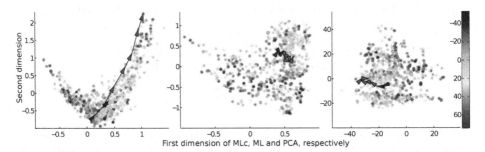

Fig. 3. 2D low-dimensional representations. Data points colored with respect to TTC in months (best seen in color). Arrows (blue MCI and red AD) indicate a subject's "flow" across time.

Table 2. Classification accuracy (sensitivity/specificity) results of a 1000 run leave 10% out cross-validation. Statistical significance (p<0.01) between methods are indicated with ⋄, * and † for MLc-ML, MLc-PCA and ML-PCA, respectively.

Features	AD - CN	AD - MCI$^{\diamond * \dagger}$	MCI - CN$^{\diamond *}$	AD - MCI - CN$^{\diamond * \dagger}$
MLc	89.0(90.5/87.8)	**80.7(85.5/68.9)**	68.7(67.3/71.5)	**61.3**
ML	89.1(87.4/90.6)	67.3(62.4/79.6)	**69.5(67.0/74.6)**	51.9
PCA	**89.1(89.3/88.9)**	71.6(67.8/81.3)	69.5(66.0/76.5)	55.1

PCA or ML in three-way classification. If MCI is considered a transitional stage between CN and AD, the three-way classification experiments suggests that MLc orders features more efficiently (see Fig. 3). Accuracy of the three-way classification was considered as the sum of diagonal elements of the confusion matrix divided by the total number of samples across all runs. Due to the high dimensionality of FULL, LDA could not be used to classify these features, further highlighting the importance of a compact representation.

4   Discussion and Future Work

Adding more dimensions to ML or PCA generally improves their performance, with PCA always outperforming ML in the TTC estimation experiment. However, neither of these approaches performs as good as MLc regardless of how many dimensions are included. Results also indicate that a more compact representation of the proposed MLc features over ML or PCA is obtained, while displaying an improved ability in the temporal ordering of the features, without compromising in discriminative power. Additionally, the proposed method is able to estimate the intrinsic nonlinear geometry of the data without any bias towards the amount of samples per subject. The derived biomarkers contain several confounding aspects, e.g. MR imaging artifacts of apparent anatomical fluctuations that affect the appearance of the MR images. Disease "progress" obtained directly from these biomarkers might be poorly estimated. Due to the unknown nature of the measurement's confounding aspects, fitting a general model to these measurements could be used as an outlier removal. These models could be used to project the movement of a subject in the manifold and along the disease trajectory. Another interesting aspect that can be addressed is the use of more than one type of biomarker, i.e. cognitive, volumetric, CSF measurements, etc. Specifically, models could be generated for several biomarkers and combined to give an aggregate estimate of the disease progress.

References

1. Belkin, M., Niyogi, P.: Laplacian eigenmaps and spectral techniques for embedding and clustering. Advances in Neural Information Processing Systems **14**, 585–591 (2002)
2. Tenenbaum, J.B., Silva, V., Langford, J.C.: A global geometric framework for nonlinear dimensionality reduction. Science **290**(5500), 2319–2323 (2000)
3. Jenkins, O.C., Matarić, M.J.: A spatio-temporal extension to Isomap nonlinear dimension reduction. In: International Conference on Machine Learning, pp. 441–448 (2004)
4. Lewandowski, M., Martinez-del-Rincon, J., Makris, D., Nebel, J.: Temporal extension of laplacian eigenmaps for unsupervised dimensionality reduction of time series. In: International Conference on Pattern Recognition, pp. 161–164 (2010)
5. Misra, C., Fan, Y., Davatzikos, C.: Baseline and longitudinal patterns of brain atrophy in MCI patients, and their use in prediction of short-term conversion to AD: results from ADNI. NeuroImage **44**(4), 141522 (2009)
6. Li, Y., Wang, Y., Wu, G., Shi, F., Zhou, L., Lin, W., Shen, D.: Discriminant analysis of longitudinal cortical thickness changes in Alzheimers disease using dynamic and network features. Neurobiology of Aging **33**(2), 427.e1530 (2012)
7. Wolz, R., Aljabar, P., Hajnal, J.V., Rueckert, D.: Manifold learning for biomarker discovery in MR imaging. In: Wang, F., Yan, P., Suzuki, K., Shen, D. (eds.) MLMI 2010. LNCS, vol. 6357, pp. 116–123. Springer, Heidelberg (2010)
8. Zou, H., Hastie, T.: Regularization and variable selection via the elastic net. Journal of the Royal Statistical Society, Series B **67**, 301–320 (2005)
9. Meinshausen, N., Bühlmann, P.: Stability selection. Journal of the Royal Statistical Society: Series B (Statistical Methodology) **72**(4), 417–473 (2010)
10. Guerrero, R., Wolz, R., Rao, A.W., Rueckert, D.: Manifold population modeling as a neuro-imaging biomarker: Application to ADNI and ADNI-GO. NeuroImage **94C**, 275–286 (2014)
11. Ojala, T., Pietikäinen, M., Harwood, D.: A comparative study of texture measures with classification based on featured distributions. Pattern Recognition **29**(1), 51–59 (1996)
12. Rueckert, D., Sonoda, L.I., Hayes, C., Hill, D.L.G., Leach, M.O., Hawkes, D.J.: Nonrigid registration using free-form deformations: Application to breast MR images. IEEE Transactions on Medical Imaging **18**(8), 712–721 (1999)
13. Heckemann, R.A., Ledig, C., Aljabar, P., Gray, K.R., Rueckert, D., Hajnal, J.V., Hammers, A.: Label propagation using group agreement. In: MICCAI 2012 Grand Challenge and Workshop on Multi-Atlas Labeling, pp. 75–78 (2012)

Multi-atlas Context Forests for Knee MR Image Segmentation

Qin Liu[1], Qian Wang[1], Lichi Zhang[1], Yaozong Gao[2,3], and Dinggang Shen[3(✉)]

[1] Med-X Research Institute, School of Biomedical Engineering,
Shanghai Jiao Tong University, Shanghai, China
{liuqin_bme,wang.qian,lichizhang}@sjtu.edu.cn
[2] Department of Computer Science, University of North Carolina at Chapel Hill,
Chapel Hill, USA
yzgao@cs.unc.edu
[3] Department of Radiology and BRIC, University of North Carolina at Chapel Hill,
Chapel Hill, USA
dgshen@med.unc.edu

Abstract. It is important, yet a challenging procedure, to segment bones and cartilages from knee MR images. In this paper, we propose multi-atlas context forests to first segment bones and then segment cartilages. Specifically, for both the bone and cartilage segmentations, we *iteratively* train sets of random forests, based on training atlas images, to classify the individual voxels. The random forests rely on (1) the appearance features directly computed from images and also (2) the context features associated with tentative segmentation results, generated by the previous layer of random forest in the iterative framework. To extract context features, multiple atlases (with expert segmentation) are first registered, with the tentative segmentation result of the subject under consideration. Then, the spatial priors of anatomical labels of registered atlases are computed and used to calculate context features of the subject. Note that these multi-atlas context features will be iteratively refined based on the (updated) tentative segmentation result of the subject. As better segmentation result leads to more accurate registration between multiple atlases and the subject, context features will become increasingly more useful for the training of subsequent random forests in the iterative framework. As validated by experiments on the SKI10 dataset, our proposed method can achieve high segmentation accuracy.

1 Introduction

Osteoarthritis is a very common form of articular disorders among the elderly population. Severe osteoarthritis may cause serious disabilities, which are major social/economic burdens [1]. Knee osteoarthritis is primarily a disease in the knee articular cartilage, which is characterized by cartilage degeneration and morphological changes. Therefore, the quantitative analysis of knee cartilage is vital to study osteoarthritis and also plays an important role in clinical assessment, as well as

© Springer International Publishing Switzerland 2015
L. Zhou et al. (Eds.): MLMI 2015, LNCS 9352, pp. 186–193, 2015.
DOI: 10.1007/978-3-319-24888-2_23

surgical planning of the disease. As magnetic resonance (MR) imaging allows precise visualization of knee joint structures, including cartilage and pathological changes [2], it is increasingly recognized as an optimal modality to evaluate the progression of osteoarthritis. In recent years, there have been many attempts in developing automated methods for knee segmentation [3-8]. As a pioneer work on this problem, Folkesson *et al.* [7] proposed a voxelwise classification approach, in which an approximate nearest-neighbor framework is used for cartilage classification by utilizing derived image features. Koo *et al.* [8] applied support vector machines (SVM) to segment cartilages with multi-contrast MR images. These works assumed that the features of individual voxels were independently and identically distributed. However, this assumption may not be valid, as the anatomical labels of neighboring voxels can be highly correlated. Also, due to (1) low contrasts between cartilage and surrounding tissues (e.g., menisci and muscles) and (2) spatial variation of shapes of cartilages across the subjects, performance of these methods may be limited. Accordingly, Fripp *et al.* [4] developed a hierarchical segmentation scheme, which consisted of three steps, i.e., automatic bone segmentation using a 3D active shape model, bone-cartilage-interface (BCI) extraction, and cartilage segmentation from the BCI using a hybrid deformable model. Although promising results were reported in this work, the search for initial model pose parameters can be very time consuming, even when using a coarse-to-fine searching strategy.

In this paper, we propose a fully automatic learning method for bone and cartilage segmentation. Specifically, we choose random forests to classify individual voxels in each image [9-10]. Furthermore, inspired by auto-context model [11], we cascade a set of iteratively trained random forests to better segment bone and cartilage, using both appearance features and context features. However, in the conventional auto-context model, the tentative segmentation result of the testing subject, in the form of probabilistic classification map, is often directly used to extract context features. This will lead to huge training/testing errors, as the cartilage region is extremely small and difficult to segment. This issue can become even worse for classifiers trained in subsequent iterations from the accumulation of errors.

To alleviate the issue above, we incorporate multiple atlases (with expert segmentation) to extract context features and then derive *multi-atlas context forests* for segmentation. Specifically, multiple atlases are first registered with the subject under consideration according to its tentative segmentation result, which can be obtained with the initially-trained random forest in our iterative framework. Then, the spatial priors of anatomical labels of the registered atlases are computed and used to calculate the context features. In this way, the subsequent random forest can be trained with these context features, as well as with appearance features that are directly extracted from the subject. This will lead to improved segmentation of the subject, which also improves the registration between multiple atlases and the subject as well as the context features that are used for the next random forest. With this iterative training, the segmentation result of the subject can be gradually refined, allowing us to obtain reasonable segmentation result for the subject.

2   Method

In this section, we present our proposed *multi-atlas context forests framework*, by training sets of random forests based on both appearance and context features. In Section 2.1, we elaborate our proposed framework, in which multiple atlases are incorporated to extract context features and derive *context forests*. In Section 2.2, we apply our proposed framework to first segment bones, and then utilize the context information of segmented bones to segment cartilages.

2.1   Multi-atlas Context Forests

The purpose of our *multi-atlas context forests* is to demonstrate that the spatial priors of anatomical labels of the registered atlases can be used to extract context features, when given a tentative segmentation result of the subject. The flowchart of our proposed framework is shown in Fig. 1.

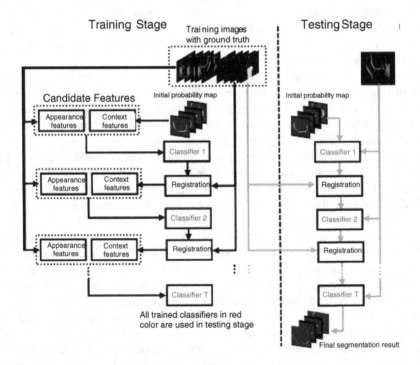

Fig. 1. The flowchart of our *multi-atlas context forests* in both training and testing stages. Data flows are shown by black and green arrows for the two training and testing stages, respectively. *In the training stage*, the classifiers are trained iteratively using both appearance features (from training images) and context features (from the tentative segmentation result of previously trained classifier). *In the testing stage*, the testing subject goes through all iteratively-trained classifiers to obtain the final segmentation result.

In the conventional auto-context method, the context features are often directly extracted from tentative segmentation result (represented with probabilistic classification map) using a set of Haar-like operators. Additional implementation details, regarding feature extraction, are provided in Section 3.1. On the other hand, as cartilage is typically small, its tentative segmentation results are generally too unreliable to provide satisfactory context information. That is, huge training/testing errors may occur and accumulate over sequential classifiers. In this way, the performance of the conventional auto-context method will be often limited for knee (especially cartilage) segmentation.

To overcome these challenges, we propose incorporating multiple atlases and their spatial priors to extract context features. Specifically, we derive subject-specific spatial priors of anatomical labels, based on the tentative segmentation result of the subject under consideration. By introducing multiple atlases to the extraction of context features, our proposed multi-atlas context forests can achieve more accurate segmentations. The details of proposed framework are described below.

- The initial spatial prior of each anatomical label (in the form of probability map for the first iteration) is generated by simply averaging the expert segmentation of all training (atlas) images. Suppose we have N atlases A_i $(i = 1,2,...,N)$ with Boolean segmentation indicators, including S_i^{FB} for femur, S_i^{TB} for tibia, S_i^{FC} for femoral cartilage, and S_i^{TC} for tibial cartilage. For the anatomical label $y \in \{FB, TB, FC, TC\}$, its initial probability map can be denoted as:

$$p_0(y) = \frac{1}{N}\Sigma_i^N S_i^y \tag{1}$$

In the following, we use these generated initial probability maps to extract context features. Along with appearance features, the first random forest can be trained.

- For the j-th iteration, we obtain the tentative segmentation result in the form of probability maps $\{p_j(y)\}$, from the j-th random forest. The conventional auto-context method directly uses $p_j(y)$ to extract context features to train the next classifier. In this work, we register all expert segmentations S_i^y to $\{p_j(y)\}$. Specifically, we convert $\{p_j(y)\}$ into a binary segmentation. Then, the registration is done by diffeomorphic Demons [12]. (Note that the purpose of the registration process is to align the expert segmentation of each atlas with the tentative segmentation result of the subject.) After obtaining the transformations T_i^y via registration, we update $p_j(y)$ as below:

$$p_j(y) \leftarrow \frac{1}{N+1}\left(\Sigma_{i=1}^N (T_i^y \circ S_i^y) + p_j(y)\right) \tag{2}$$

Finally, the new context features can be extracted from updated maps $\{p_j(y)\}$. Then, along with appearance features, we can train the $(j + 1)$-th random forest.

- By repeating the step above, we can train sets of cascaded trained random forests. In the application stage, a testing image can go through all cascaded trained random forests to obtain the final segmentation result.

2.2   Bone and Cartilage Segmentation

In this section, we apply the above *multi-atlas context forests* to segment both bones and cartilages. Although bones and cartilages can be segmented simultaneously using our proposed method, it is more reasonable to first segment bones and then cartilages. The reason is that 1) the size of bone is much larger than that of the cartilage, 2) the cartilage is thin and attached to only a certain area of the bone surface, making it much harder to segment than bone, and 3) the segmentation result of bone provides spatial context information to guide the segmentation of cartilage.

After segmenting the bones of the subject, we register all of the *expert bone segmentation* of each atlas to the bone segmentation result of the subject, as a way of guiding cartilage segmentation via segmented bones. The above-estimated deformable transformations via registration can then be used to warp the *expert cartilage segmentation* of each atlas to the space of the subject. Note that, although the deformable transformations are estimated based on segmented bones, the cartilages of atlases can be warped to align the cartilages of the subject, since all cartilages are thin and closely attached to surfaces of their respective bones. Based on the registered cartilage segmentations of atlases, we can use Eq. 1 to compute the spatial priors of cartilage for the subject. The detailed steps are described below.

- Note that, as mentioned above, each of N atlases, A_i, includes 1) femur segmentation S_i^{FB}, 2) tibia segmentation S_i^{TB}, 3) femoral cartilage segmentation S_i^{FC}, and 4) tibial cartilage segmentation S_i^{TC} ($i = 1, 2, ..., N$). Then, for a test subject I, we can use our proposed method to obtain the segmented bones: S^{FB} and S^{TB}. The, we can register the expert bone segmentation of each atlas, S_i^{FB} and S_i^{TB}, to the segmented bones of subject, S^{FB} and S^{TB}, by following the same registration procedure described in Section 2.1.
- After obtaining the deformable transformation T_i^{Bone} for each atlas, we can warp the expert *cartilage* segmentation of each atlas and then compute the initial spatial priors for the subject as follows:

$$p(y) = \frac{1}{N} \sum_{i=1}^{N} T_i^{Bone} \circ S_i^y, \quad y \in \{FC, TC\}. \tag{3}$$

The spatial priors estimated above can be used to initiate cartilage segmentation of the subject, by using our proposed method in Section 2.1.

3   Experimental Results

The public SKI10 dataset [14] is used to evaluate our proposed method for the segmentation of knee MR images. In particular, we randomly select 30 images for training and 40 for testing. All images were preprocessed by following the strategies in [15], including intensity normalization [7], histogram matching, and affine registration to a common space using FSL toolbox [16]. After each test image is segmented in the common space, the segmentation result is further warped back to its original image space, where the expert segmentation is used as ground truth for quantitative comparison.

For bone segmentation, we compute the *initial* spatial priors of the bones by simply averaging the expert bone segmentations of all atlases. However, for cartilage segmentation, we compute the *initial* spatial priors using Eq. 3, where the segmented bones of the subject are used for aligning the expert cartilage segmentation of each atlas. For comparison purposes, we also defined a downgraded version of our method, which ignores segmented bones in estimating the initial spatial priors of the cartilage in the subject. That is, cartilage of the subject is segmented independently from its segmented bones; in this way, the initial spatial priors of the cartilage are obtained by directly averaging all S_i^y in Eq. 3, without using the estimated deformable transformations.

We use the same settings to iteratively train random forests for bone and cartilage segmentations. In particular, we set the maximum depth of each tree (in the forest) at 32. Each leaf node of the tree has a minimum of 8 samples to avoid over-fitting. Haar-like operators are employed so that they extract both appearance and context features, from 3D patches (with maximum size of 10mm×10mm×10mm) of respective images/maps. Each node can randomly choose features from a Haar-like feature pool, with a total of 3000 features.

3.1   Bone Segmentation

The Dice Similarity Coefficient (DSC) is used to measure the performance of our method, as popularly used for evaluation of segmentation performance. Table 1 shows the segmentation results for bones. Our method is shown to be comparable with state-of-the-art methods in bone segmentation, although datasets and subject numbers are different.

Table 1. Bone segmentation (measured by the mean DSC and the standard deviation) of our method and start-of-the-art methods.

Method	Dataset	Femur DSC	Tibia DSC
Shan et al. [13]	18 SPGR images	97.0%±1.1%	96.7%±1.2%
Wang et al. [5]	OAI (176 images)	94.9%±1.9%	96.0%±2.2%
Fripp et al. [4]	20 FS SPGR images	95.2%±7.2%	95.2%±6.4%
Our method	SKI10 dataset	**97.3%±1.3%**	**97.0%±1.9%**

3.2   Cartilage Segmentation

In Fig. 2, we compare segmentation accuracies of cartilage between our proposed *multi-atlas context forests* (designated by Case 1 in Fig. 2), (1) the conventional auto-context model (Case 2), and (2) the downgraded variant of our method, as described in Section 3.1 (Case 3). Note that, in the first iteration, Case 1 and Case 2 are equivalent with the same experimental results. In general, our method yields the highest segmentation accuracy across all four iterations. Specifically, the improvement of our method (with DSC of 0.811 in the fourth iteration) over Case 2 (0.798) shows that the context features provided by the registered atlases are more effective in improving cartilage segmentation. Meanwhile, the improvement of Case 1 (0.811) over Case 3 (0.801) indicates that the bone segmentation result provides important spatial context guidance for segmentation of cartilage.

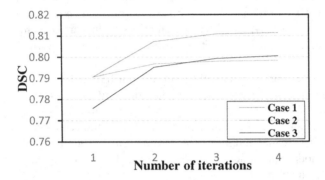

Fig. 2. Comparison on accuracies of cartilage segmentation between our *multi-atlas context forests* (Case 1), the conventional auto-context model (Case 2), and the downgraded variant of our method (Case 3). Here, the mean DSC measures of *femur and tibial cartilages* are reported.

Furthermore, we compare the cartilage segmentation results of our method with the results from state-of-the-art methods in the literature. Table 2 shows the quantitative comparisons. As observed, our method achieves comparable cartilage segmentation accuracy compared to three state-of-the-art methods, although different datasets were used.

Table 2. Cartilage segmentation (measured by the mean DSC and the standard deviation) by our method and start-of-the-art methods.

Method	Dataset	Fem. Cart. DSC	Tib. Cart. DSC
Shan et al. [18]	18 SPGR images	78.2±5.2%	**82.6±3.8%**
Folkesson et al. [7]	139 Esaote C-span images	77.0±8.0%	81.0±6.0%
Lee et al. [17]	SKI10 dataset	**81.8±3.0%**	79.2±4.6%
Proposed method	SKI10 dataset	81.2±3.7%	80.9±3.4%

4   Conclusions

We proposed a novel learning method to segment bone and cartilage in 3D MR images by effectively exploiting the spatial context relation in knee joints. Based on bone segmentation results, we further incorporate the spatial context information of bone to improve the accuracy of cartilage segmentation. Experimental results using the SKI10 dataset demonstrate the effectiveness of our method. Future research will focus on quantitative analysis of articular cartilages.

References

1. Mody, G.M., Brooks, P.M.: Improving Musculoskeletal Health: Global Issues. Best Practice and Research Clinical Rheumatology. **26**, 237–249 (2012)
2. Eckstein, F., Cicuttini, F., Raynauld, J.P., Waterton, J.C., Peterfy, C.: Magnetic Resonance Imaging (MRI) of Articular Cartilage in Knee Osteoarthritis (OA): Morphological Assessment. Osteoarthritis and Cartilage **14**, 46–75 (2006)
3. Heimann, T., Meinzer, H.P.: Statistical Shape Models for 3D Medical Image Segmentation: a Review. Medical Image Analysis **13**, 543–563 (2009)
4. Fripp, J., Crozier, S., Warfield, S.K., Ourselin, S.: Automatic Segmentation and Quantitative Analysis of the Articular Cartilages from Magnetic Resonance Images of the Knee. IEEE Transactions on Medical Imaging **29**, 55–64 (2010)
5. Wang, Q., Wu, D., Lu, L., Liu, M., Boyer, K.L., Zhou, S.K.: Semantic Context Forests for Learning-based Knee Cartilage Segmentation in 3D MR Images. Medical Computer Vision Large Data in Medical Imaging, pp. 105–115 (2014)
6. Vincent, G., Wolstenholme, C., Scott, I., Bowes, M.: Fully Automatic Segmentation of the Knee Joint Using Active Appearance Models. Medical Image Analysis for the Clinic: A Grand Challenge, 224–230 (2010)
7. Folkesson, J., Dam, E.B., Olsen, O.F., Pettersen, P.C., Christiansen, C.: Segmenting Articular Cartilage Automatically Using a Voxel Classification Approach. IEEE Transactions on Medical Imaging, 106–115 (2007)
8. Koo, S., Hargreaves, B., Andriacchi, T., Gold, G.: Automatic segmentation of articular cartilage from MRI: a multi-contrast and multi-dimensional approach. In: Proc. Intl. Soc. Mag. Reson. Med., p. 2546 (2008)
9. Breiman, L.: Random Forests. Springer (2001)
10. Wang, L., Gao, Y., Shi, F., Li, G., Gilmore, J.H., Lin, W., Shen, D.: LINKS: Learning-based Multi-source IntegratioN FrameworK for Segmentation of Infant Brain Images. Neuroimage **108**, 160–172 (2015)
11. Tu, Z., Bai, X.: Auto-context and Its Application to High-level Vision Tasks and 3D Brain Image Segmentation. IEEE Transactions on Pattern Analysis and Machine Intelligence **32**, 1744–1757 (2010)
12. Vercauteren, T., Pennec, X., Perchant, A., Ayache, N.: Diffeomorphic Demons: Efficient Non-parametric Image Registration. NeuroImage **45**, S61–S72 (2009)
13. Shan, L., Zach, C., Charles, C., Niethammer, M.: Automatic Atlas-based Three-label Cartilage Segmentation from MR Images. Medical Image Analysis **18**, 1233–1246 (2014)
14. Heimann, T., Morrison, B.J., Styner, M.A., Niethammer, M., Warfield, S.: Segmentation of knee images: a grand challenge. In: MICCAI Workshop on Medical Image Analysis for the Clinic, pp. 207–214 (2010)
15. Zhang, K., Lu, W., Marziliano, P.: Automatic Knee Cartilage Segmentation from Multi-contrast MR Images Using Support Vector Machine Classification with Spatial Dependencies. Magnetic Resonance Imaging **31**, 1731–1743 (2013)
16. Jenkinson, M., Beckmann, C.F., Behrens, T.E., Woolrich, M.W., Smith, S.M.: FSL. NeuroImage **62**, 782–790 (2012)
17. Lee, S., Shim, H., Park, S.H., Yun, I.D., Lee, S.U.: Learning local shape and appearance for segmentation of knee cartilage in 3D MRI. In: Proceedings of the 4th Medical Image Analysis for the Clinic—A Grand Challenge Workshop (2010)
18. Shan, L., Charles, C., Niethammer, M.: Automatic atlas-based three-label cartilage segmentation from MR Knee Images. In: IEEE Workshop on Mathematical Methods in Biomedical Image Analysis, pp. 241–246 (2010)

Longitudinal Patch-Based Segmentation of Multiple Sclerosis White Matter Lesions

Snehashis Roy[1][(✉)], Aaron Carass[2], Jerry L. Prince[2], and Dzung L. Pham[1]

[1] Center for Neuroscience and Regenerative Medicine,
Henry Jackson Foundation, Bethesda, USA
snehashis.roy@nih.gov
[2] Department of Electrical and Computer Engineering,
The Johns Hopkins University, Baltimore, USA

Abstract. Segmenting T_2-weighted white matter lesions from longitudinal MR images is essential in understanding progression of multiple
sclerosis. Most lesion segmentation techniques find lesions independently
at each time point, even though there are different noise and image contrast variations at each point in the time series. In this paper, we present
a patch based 4D lesion segmentation method that takes advantage of
the temporal component of longitudinal data. For each subject with multiple time-points, 4D patches are constructed from the T_1-w and FLAIR
scans of all time-points. For every 4D patch from a subject, a few relevant
matching 4D patches are found from a reference, such that their convex
combination reconstructs the subject's 4D patch. Then corresponding
manual segmentation patches of the reference are combined in a similar
manner to generate a 4D membership of lesions of the subject patch. We
compare our 4D patch-based segmentation with independent 3D voxel-
based and patch-based lesion segmentation algorithms. Based on ground
truth segmentations from 30 data sets, we show that the mean Dice
coefficients between manual and automated segmentations improve after
using the 4D approach compared to two state-of-the-art 3D segmentation
algorithms.

1 Introduction

Magnetic resonance imaging (MRI) is a widely used noninvasive modality to
image the human brain. Segmentations of T_2-weighted white matter (WM)
lesions from serial MR images provide quantitative information about lesion
evolution, which is associated with the progression and prognosis of MS. Longitudinal information, such as the appearance of new lesions, as well as enlargement
or reduction of lesions over time are routinely used as a clinical measures for
disease progression and response to treatment. Although manual delineations
of lesions are considered as ground truth, they are time consuming, prone to

S. Roy—Support for this work included funding from the Department of Defense
in the Center for Neuroscience and Regenerative Medicine and by the grants
NIH/NINDS R01NS070906.

© Springer International Publishing Switzerland 2015
L. Zhou et al. (Eds.): MLMI 2015, LNCS 9352, pp. 194–202, 2015.
DOI: 10.1007/978-3-319-24888-2_24

extensive inter-rater variability, and impractical for large clinical data sets [1]. Therefore accurate automatic lesion segmentations from longitudinal MR scans are desirable.

There are multiple ways to longitudinally segment lesions from serial MR images. The simplest way is to segment lesions at each time-point independently. Many lesion segmentation techniques are available for segmenting lesions from a single time-point (cf. [2–4]). However, applying 3-D algorithms to 4-D data results in inconsistencies due to differences in noise or intensity variations in lesions between scans. Particularly, in the detection of chronic lesions, it is advantageous to consider multiple time-points to inform the segmentation at a single time-point.

Registration based approaches [5] first register all the time-points to an atlas (or baseline). Once registered, new appearing or shrinking lesions are found by directly comparing voxel-wise intensity changes. Although this is a true "4D" approach, its accuracy depends on that of the registrations, which may not be robust in presence of lesions. Another type of segmentation method relies on intensity models of pairwise subtraction images. Images from two consecutive time-points are first registered. Then a logistic regression model or a statistical threshold is applied on the subtraction image to find significant intensity variations, which leads to incident lesions in the follow-up scan. Several approaches based on time series have also been reported for automatic segmentation of MS lesions. In these methods, temporal derivatives [6] or principal component analysis of the temporal profiles of voxel-wise intensity features are used to characterize the lesion progression in MS. However, they typically need more time-points for stable results, which may not be feasible in a clinical scenario.

In this paper, we propose a supervised 4D method for segmenting MS lesions from serial MR images. We do not employ any pair-wise difference images, but use features from all the time-points simultaneously, thereby producing a longitudinally consistent complete lesion map at every time-point. Instead of using voxel-wise features, we use patch based features, which have been shown to be preferable in many image processing tasks [7–9].

2   Materials and Method

2.1   Dataset

The dataset contains ten subjects, each with three time-points. Each time-point contains a T_1-w MPRAGE and a FLAIR image, scanned at $0.83 \times 0.83 \times 1.1$ mm^3 and $0.83 \times 0.83 \times 2.2$ mm^3 resolution, respectively. Two consecutive scans are separated by approximately one year for all the subjects. Among the 10 subjects, 8 of them were diagnosed with relapsing-remitting MS (RRMS), one with secondary-progressive MS (SPMS), and one with primary-progressive MS (PPMS). Lesions were manually delineated on the 30 time-points to generate binary reference segmentations.

2.2   Method

The algorithm requires at least one subject to be withheld as the training data, called a reference, defined as a $(m + 1)$-tuple of T images, $\{a_1^{(1)}, \ldots, a_1^{(T)}\}, \ldots, \{a_{m+1}^{(1)}, \ldots, a_{m+1}^{(T)}\}$, where $a_1^{(t)}$ to $a_m^{(t)}$ denotes m-channel input MR images, such as T_1-w, T_2-w, PD-w, or FLAIR, for the tth time-point, $t = 1, \ldots, T$. $a_{m+1}^{(t)}$ denotes the manual binary segmentations of lesions. T denotes the total number of time-points. Although we use only MPRAGE and FLAIR sequences in all our experiments (i.e., $m = 2$), any number of sequences can be accommodated in the methodology. Similarly, any number of reference images can be used, as shown in Sec. 3.1. However, we define the notation with just one reference for clarity.

The subject is denoted as an m-tuple of T images, $\{s_1^{(1)}, \ldots, s_1^{(T)}\}, \ldots, \{s_m^{(1)}, \ldots, s_m^{(T)}\}$. Note that the subject and reference need not be registered. MR images $a_k^{(t)}$ and $s_k^{(t)}$, $k = 1, \ldots, m$, are intensity normalized so that the modes of their WM intensities are unity. The WM intensity modes were found automatically based on a smooth kernel density estimator of the histograms.

For every reference MR image, 3D patches are extracted around every voxel, and are transformed into 1D vectors of dimension d. For example, for $3 \times 3 \times 3$ patches, $d = 27$. Patches from multiple time-points are concatenated to form a subject feature vector. Subject features are denoted by $\mathbf{b}(j) \in \mathbb{R}^{mTd \times 1}$, where $d \times 1$ patches from m sequences and T time-points are concatenated. Similarly, a reference MR feature $\mathbf{a}_{\text{MR}}(i) \in \mathbb{R}^{mTd \times 1}$ is the concatenation of patches from m MR images of T time-points $a_1^{(t)}, \ldots, a_m^{(t)}, t = 1, \ldots, T$. Corresponding manually segmented patches are concatenated to form segmentation features $\mathbf{a}_S(i) \in \mathbb{R}^{Td \times 1}$. The elements of $\mathbf{a}_S(i)$ are $\in \{0, 1\}$. i and j denote the voxels in the reference and subject space, $i = 1, \ldots, M, j = 1, \ldots, N$, where M and N are the number of non-zero voxels in the reference and subject, respectively. From now on, we also refer to the MR $(mTd \times 1)$ or segmentation $(Td \times 1)$ feature vectors as a "patch". All MR features are normalized so that their ℓ_2 norms are unity [7]. A reference MR dictionary of patches is defined as $A_{\text{MR}} \in \mathbb{R}^{mTd \times M}$, whose columns are the MR patches $\mathbf{a}_{\text{MR}}(i)$. Similarly a reference segmentation dictionary is defined as $A_S \in \mathbb{R}^{Td \times M}$, whose columns are the segmentation patches $\mathbf{a}_S(i)$. In Sec. 3.1, we will explain a strategy to modify the dictionaries A_{MR} and A_S in order to improve the accuracy and speed of the algorithm.

Since the subject MR contrasts $s_1^{(t)}, \ldots, s_m^{(t)}$ are co-registered, a subject patch $\mathbf{b}(j)$ contains information about temporal trajectories of the lesion evolution around the center voxel j. Given a rich dictionary of patches A_{MR}, we assume that it contains similar looking examples like $\mathbf{b}(j)$. Therefore it is likely that for a given $\mathbf{b}(j)$, a few patches from A_{MR} can be found whose convex combination is $\mathbf{b}(j)$. More specifically,

$$\mathbf{b}(j) \approx A_{\text{MR}}\mathbf{x}(j), \quad \text{for some } \mathbf{x}(j) \in \mathbb{R}^M, ||\mathbf{x}(j)||_0 \ll M \; \forall j, \; \mathbf{x}(j) \geq \mathbf{0}, \quad (1)$$

where $\mathbf{x}(j)$ contains sparse weights for each of the M reference patches in the dictionary A_{MR}. Minimizing the ℓ_0 norm of $\mathbf{x}(j)$ enforces sparsity, which results in only a few patches in A_{MR} contributing to $\mathbf{b}(j)$. The non-negativity constraints in $\mathbf{x}(j)$ enforces similarity in the texture between the subject patch and the contributing reference patches.

Eqn. 1 can be efficiently solved by minimizing the ℓ_1 norm of $\mathbf{x}(j)$. We use an elastic net regularization, which generates $\mathbf{x}(j)$ by minimizing the following objective function,

$$\widehat{\mathbf{x}}(j) = \arg\min_{\mathbf{x}} ||\mathbf{b}(j) - A_{\mathrm{MR}}\mathbf{x}||_2^2 + \lambda_1||\mathbf{x}||_1 + \lambda_2||\mathbf{x}||_2^2, \ \mathbf{x} \geq \mathbf{0}. \qquad (2)$$

The first term is a least squares fitting term enforcing the similarity between the subject patch $\mathbf{b}(j)$ and its reconstruction using the dictionary A_{MR}. The second term is an ℓ_1 regularization enforcing sparsity in $\mathbf{x}$. The third term is a ℓ_2 ridge regularization. Combination of the ℓ_1 and ℓ_2 penalties together enforces a grouping effect, where similar looking patches in the dictionary are chosen while keeping a certain level of sparsity in $\widehat{\mathbf{x}}(j)$. λ_1 and λ_2 are two weights balancing the contributions of ℓ_1 and ℓ_2 terms. We empirically chose $\lambda_1 = \lambda_2 = 0.01$. Once $\widehat{\mathbf{x}}(j)$ is estimated for every subject patch, the lesion membership can be obtained at the jth voxel by combining the segmentation patches $\mathbf{a}_S(i)$ using the same weights applied to the segmentation patches, $\boldsymbol{\mu}(j) = A_S\widehat{\mathbf{x}}(j)$, where $\boldsymbol{\mu}(j)$ is a $Td \times 1$ 4D lesion membership at the jth voxel. Since we are only interested in the WM lesions, the false positives due to FLAIR hyperintensities in the gray matter are removed by multiplying the memberships with WM masks obtained from LesionTOADS [3]. The memberships are thresholded at a threshold to generate hard segmentations, empirically determined in Sec. 3.

2.3   Dictionary Modification

The sparse coefficient vector $\widehat{\mathbf{x}}(j)$ is an $M \times 1$ vector, where M is the number of reference voxels, with typically $M \sim 10^7$. It is computationally expensive to solve Eqn. 2 for N subject patches, where $N \sim 10^7$ as well. It is common practice to subsample the dictionary to reduce its size and thereby reduce computational expense. However, in this case, special consideration must be paid to the way the subsampling is performed in order to sufficiently represent the different ways that lesion voxels may evolve. For T timepoints at a single voxel, there are 2^T possible combinations for a lesion mask to evolve. We therefore create 2^T sub-dictionaries to ensure that every possible lesion evolution time series contains a sufficient number of samples. This is performed as follows. For every $Td \times 1$ reference manual segmentation feature vector $\mathbf{a}_S(i)$, T center voxels from the T time-points are considered. We first characterize a reference feature $\mathbf{a}_S(i)$ (and $\mathbf{a}_{\mathrm{MR}}(i)$) according to the labels of those T center voxels of the T reference manual segmentation patches. Since each element in $\mathbf{a}_S(i) \in \{0,1\}$, there are $(2^T - 1)$ combinations for at least one of the T center voxels being a lesion (i.e., label 1), and one where all center voxels are zero, i.e., normal tissue. Therefore, we divide A_{MR} and A_S into 2^T sub-dictionaries $A_{\mathrm{MR}}(k) \in \mathbb{R}^{mTd \times L_k}, A_S(k) \in \mathbb{R}^{Td \times L_k}, k = 1, \ldots, 2^T$, according to the label types of the center voxels of the manual segmentation patches. L_k is the number of patches in each sub-dictionary, and $\sum_{k=1}^{2^T} L_k = M$.

FLAIR   L-TOADS   3D Patch   4D Patch   Manual

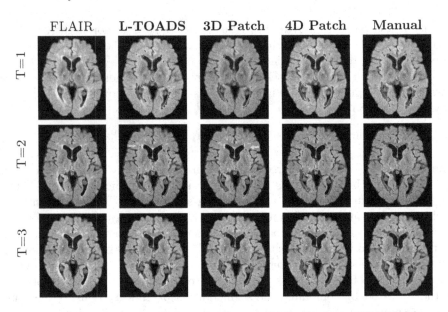

Fig. 1. A comparison of our 4D segmentation method with LesionTOADS [3] and a 3D patch-based method [4] is shown. Individual 3D segmentations sometimes miss or underestimate (yellow arrows) lesions, while our 4D method produces temporally more consistent segmentations.

Instead of using the whole reference dictionary A_{MR} for every subject patch $\mathbf{b}(j)$ in Eqn. 2, we use a kd-tree to find n similar looking MR reference patches from each of the 2^T number of $A_{\mathrm{MR}}(k)$ and combine them in a new subject patch specific dictionary $B_{\mathrm{MR}}(j)$, having $n \times 2^T$ reference patches. Corresponding segmentation patches are combined to form a smaller segmentation dictionary $B_S(j)$ as well. With $T = 3$ in our case, we choose $n = 200$, reducing the number of eligible reference patches from $M \sim 10^7$ to 1600. Eqn. 2 is solved for each subject patch $\mathbf{b}(j)$ using the patch specific dictionary $B_{\mathrm{MR}}(j)$. Then the memberships $\boldsymbol{\mu}(j)$ is obtained with $B_S(j)$. By choosing a small number ($n = 200$) of similar looking patches from each of the sub-dictionaries, the computational burden in Eqn. 2 is reduced by including all possible types of reference lesion patches, therefore keeping the richness of the dictionary.

3   Results

We compare our 4D method with two other methods, a voxel based method LesionTOADS [3] and a 3D patch-based method [4], both of which segment each 3D volume independently of the other longitudinally acquired volumes. Fig. 1 shows segmentations obtained from these three methods. Although the lesion intensity change across time-points are visually imperceptible, both Lesion-TOADS and the 3D patch method sometimes miss or under-estimate (yellow arrows) lesions as shown in Fig. 1. In comparison, our 4D patch method produces a more accurate and temporally consistent segmentation.

Quantitative comparisons between automatic and manual segmentations are carried out using sensitivity, Dice coefficient, lesion true positive rate (LTPR), lesion false positive rate (LFPR), and absolute volume difference (VD), as defined in [2]. Voxel-based overlap measures such as sensitivity and Dice are affected if the lesion volume is small [2], because lesion boundaries are often significantly different between raters. Hence, LTPR and LFPR are lesion count based measures indicating if a lesion is detected in the automated segmentations.

After the membership images ($\boldsymbol{\mu}(j)$ at every voxel) are obtained, they are thresholded to generate a hard segmentation. The optimal threshold is obtained using a cross-validation on two randomly chosen subjects. One of them is treated as test data, and is segmented using the other one as the reference, and vice versa. The maximum average Dice is observed to be 0.734 at a threshold of 0.44. This threshold is used for the remainder of the experiments.

3.1   Number of Reference Images

As mentioned earlier, multiple references can be included in our framework. To include more than one reference image in Eqn. 2, A_{MR} and A_S are populated with patches from all the reference images. Like any supervised method, the performance of our lesion segmentation method depends on the variability of the reference patches such that matching example patches can always be found for any subject patch. Therefore it is expected that the segmentation accuracy will improve by increasing the number of reference images. In this section, we describe an empirical procedure to select the number of reference images. Five subjects are randomly chosen for this experiment. Four subjects are again randomly chosen as potential reference images, and then all five subjects are segmented using one or more of the four references. Then Dice coefficients are averaged over all 15 time-points in each case. Median Dices are 0.468, 0.539, 0.549, and 0.549 for 1–4 references, respectively. Therefore, we used three references to segment all the 10 subjects.

3.2   Quantitative Evaluation

In this section, we compare our 4D method with three references against Lesion-TOADS and a 3D patch-based method on 10 subjects. The 3D patch-based method also uses the same three references. Lesion volumes are often used as clinical measures in MS progression. Hence we have plotted automatically detected lesion volumes (in cc) with respect to the ground truth in Fig. 2(a). Solid blue, magenta, red, and black lines indicate linear fits of LesionTOADS, 3D and 4D patch-based methods, and the unit slope line. The slopes are 0.594, 0.748, and 0.951 for LesionTOADS, 3D and 4D patch-based method, respectively, while the R^2 for the linear fits are 0.488, 0.732, and 0.889, respectively. The intercepts are 6.75, 2.88, and 1.75 cc, respectively. A t-test for the null hypothesis that the intercepts are zero gives p-values 5×10^{-4}, 0.060 and 0.079 for LesionTOADS,

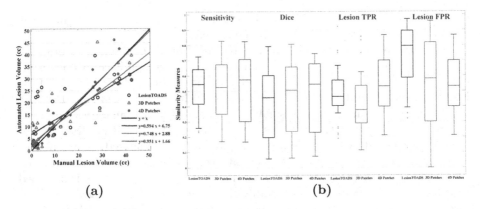

Fig. 2. (a) Scatter plot of manual lesion volumes (in cc) against automated ones are shown for LesionTOADS (blue), 3D patch based (magenta) and 4D patch-based method (red). (b) Boxplots of voxelwise sensitivity, Dice coefficients, lesion true positive rate (LTPR), and lesion false positive rate (LFPR) are shown.

the 3D and the 4D patch-based methods, indicating that LesionTOADS has a significant bias (6.75 cc) in segmentation, while the patch-based methods do not.

Boxplots of sensitivity, Dice coefficients, LTPR, and LFPR, for the 30 time-points, between automatic and manual segmentations are shown in Fig. 2(b). Median sensitivities for LesionTOADS, 3D and 4D patch-based method are 0.546, 0.526, 0.575, respectively, while median Dice coefficients are 0.458, 0.507 and 0.545. Median LTPR are 0.465, 0.379, and 0.532, while median LFPR are 0.795, 0.582, and 0.532, respectively. A Wilcoxon signed-rank test shows significant improvement of the 4D method over LesionTOADS in Dice coefficient and over 3D patch-based method on LTPR ($p < 0.01$). The LFPR for the 4D method is significantly lower than LesionTOADS ($p < 0.01$), but not the 3D patch-based method. The median absolute volume differences are 0.405, 0.539 and 0.284, respectively. Non-parametric testing gives the p-values for VD as 0.03 and 0.07 comparing the 4D method with the LesionTOADS and 3D patch-based method.

4   Discussion

A limitation of the current implementation is that the number of reference time-points must be the same as the number of subject time-points. This may not always be feasible in a clinical setting. If a subject has fewer scans than the reference, then a part of the reference time-points can be used. However, if the subject has more scans than the reference, one possible way is to divide the subject time-points into components having the same number of time-points as the reference. Then each component are segmented separately using the reference, and the corresponding segmentations can be fused.

Like any supervised algorithm, the accuracy of our 4D method depends on the choice of the references. For a subject patch $\mathbf{b}(j)$, a few matching reference patches are extracted from the dictionary A_{MR} in Eqn. 1. We made the underlying assumption that the references are rich enough such that matching patches can always be found. If this assumption is violated, sub-optimal results are obtained. An illustration is shown in Sec. 3.1. Among the randomly chosen four references, one of them had PPMS, while the others had RRMS. Example patches corresponding to relapsing-remitting types of lesions generally observed in RRMS were not abundant in the reference with PPMS. Therefore the Dice coefficient obtained from a single reference (the subject with PPMS) is significantly lower than two references (0.468 vs 0.539, $p = 0.026$), where one of the references was a subject with RRMS. Hence, the references should be chosen carefully so as to include relevant example patches.

Large inter-rater variability are usually observed in MS lesion segmentation [2]. Since lesions are small objects with ambiguous boundaries, overlap measures are generally lower when lesion load is small. We observed a minimum Dice of 0.08 for a subject with very low lesion load. Our Dice and sensitivities are of similar range in magnitude with previously reported 3D lesion segmentation methods [4,10], although the results are not directly comparable because the validations are done on different datasets.

References

1. Garcia-Lorenzo, D., Francis, S., Narayanan, S., Arnold, D.L., Collins, D.L.: Review of automatic segmentation methods of multiple sclerosis white matter lesions on conventional magnetic resonance imaging. Med. Image Anal. **17**(1), 1–18 (2013)
2. Geremia, E., Clatz, O., Menze, B.H., Konukoglu, E., Criminisi, A., Ayache, N.: Spatial decision forests for MS lesion segmentation in multi-channel magnetic resonance images. NeuroImage **57**(2), 378–390 (2011)
3. Shiee, N., Bazin, P.L., Ozturk, A., Reich, D.S., Calabresi, P.A., Pham, D.L.: A Topology-Preserving Approach to the Segmentation of Brain Images with Multiple Sclerosis Lesions. NeuroImage **49**(2), 1524–1535 (2009)
4. Roy, S., He, Q., Carass, A., Jog, A., Cuzzocreo, J.L., Reich, D.S., Prince, J.L., Pham, D.L.: Example based lesion segmentation. In: Proc. of SPIE, vol. 9034, p. 90341Y (2014)
5. Ganiler, O., Oliver, A., Diez, Y., Freixenet, J., Vilanova, J.C., Beltran, B., Ramio-Torrenta, L., Rovira, A., Llado, X.: A subtraction pipeline for automatic detection of new appearing multiple sclerosis lesions in longitudinal studies. Neuroradiology **56**(5), 363–374 (2014)
6. Gerig, G., Welti, D., Guttmann, C.R.G., Colchester, A.C.F., Szekely, G.: Exploring the discrimination power of the time domain for segmentation and characterization of active lesions in serial MR data. Med. Image Anal. **4**(1), 31–42 (2000)
7. Roy, S., Carass, A., Prince, J.L.: Magnetic resonance image example based contrast synthesis. IEEE Trans. Med. Imag. **32**(12), 2348–2363 (2013)
8. Roy, S., Carass, A., Prince, J.L.: Synthesizing MR contrast and resolution through a patch matching technique. In: Proc. of SPIE, vol. 7263, p. 76230j (2010)

9. Wang, L., Shi, F., Gao, Y., Li, G., Gilmore, J.H., Lin, W., Shen, D.: Integration of sparse multi-modality representation and anatomical constraint for isointense infant brain MR image segmentation. NeuroImage **16**(1), 152–164 (2014)
10. Weiss, N., Rueckert, D., Rao, A.: Multiple sclerosis lesion segmentation using dictionary learning and sparse coding. In: Mori, K., Sakuma, I., Sato, Y., Barillot, C., Navab, N. (eds.) MICCAI 2013, Part I. LNCS, vol. 8149, pp. 735–742. Springer, Heidelberg (2013)

Hierarchical Multi-modal Image Registration by Learning Common Feature Representations

Hongkun Ge[1,2], Guorong Wu[1], Li Wang[1], Yaozong Gao[1,2], and Dinggang Shen[1,2(✉)]

[1] Department of Radiology and BRIC,
University of North Carolina at Chapel Hill, Chapel Hill, NC 27599, USA
dinggang_shen@med.unc.edu
[2] Department of Computer Science,
University of North Carolina at Chapel Hill, Chapel Hill, NC 27599, USA

Abstract. Mutual information (MI) has been widely used for registering images with different modalities. Since most inter-modality registration methods simply estimate deformations in a local scale, but optimizing MI from the entire image, the estimated deformations for certain structures could be dominated by the surrounding unrelated structures. Also, since there often exist multiple structures in each image, the intensity correlation between two images could be complex and highly nonlinear, which makes global MI unable to precisely guide local image deformation. To solve these issues, we propose a hierarchical inter-modality registration method by robust feature matching. Specifically, we first select a small set of key points at salient image locations to drive the entire image registration. Since the original image features computed from different modalities are often difficult for direct comparison, we propose to learn their common feature representations by projecting them from their native feature spaces to a common space, where the correlations between corresponding features are maximized. Due to the large heterogeneity between two high-dimension feature distributions, we employ Kernel CCA (Canonical Correlation Analysis) to reveal such non-linear feature mappings. Then, our registration method can take advantage of the learned common features to reliably establish correspondences for key points from different modality images by robust feature matching. As more and more key points take part in the registration, our hierarchical feature-based image registration method can efficiently estimate the deformation pathway between two inter-modality images in a global to local manner. We have applied our proposed registration method to prostate CT and MR images, as well as the infant MR brain images in the first year of life. Experimental results show that our method can achieve more accurate registration results, compared to other state-of-the-art image registration methods.

1   Introduction

Deformable image registration plays a very important role in medical image analysis [1, 2]. According to the number of image modalities used in registration, the deformable registration methods can be categorized into two types: single-modal and multi-modal image registration. For the latter, mutual information (MI) [3] or normalized

© Springer International Publishing Switzerland 2015
L. Zhou et al. (Eds.): MLMI 2015, LNCS 9352, pp. 203–211, 2015.
DOI: 10.1007/978-3-319-24888-2_25

mutual information [4] are widely used, by assuming the existence of statistical relation between intensities of two (multi-modal) images under registration. In the last two decades, MI-based registration methods have achieved many successes in medical imaging area, such as for registration of CT and MR brain images [2].

However, MI-based image registration methods have the following limitations. (1) MI measurement is often estimated from the entire image in order to have sufficient number of intensities to estimate histogram. Since intensity correlation of entire images is often optimized by estimating local deformations point by point, the registration of small structures (e.g., tumor) could be dominated by surrounding large structures, unrelated structures or even background. (2) Since there often exist multiple structures in the images under registration, their intensity correlation could be highly nonlinear and complex, thus making global MI unable to precisely guide local image registration. This can be demonstrated by CT and MR prostate images shown in Fig. 1. Intensities of bladder (blue) and rectum (red) are similar in CT, but different in MR image, in which the intensities of bladder are much brighter than those of rectum. Obviously, it is difficult to find simple intensity correlation to characterize both bladder and rectum.

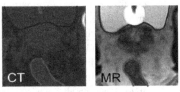

Fig. 1. Example CT and MR prostate images. Red and blue contours are rectum and bladder respectively.

Feature-based image registration is one of possible approaches to overcome the above-mentioned issues in the conventional MI-based registration methods. This registration approach is often driven by the anatomical correspondences hierarchically established between two images, by using image features (e.g., intensities [5]) extracted from a neighborhood of each key point as a morphological signature. However, since image features computed from different modality images are often distributing differently in the feature space, it is difficult to measure feature similarities. As a result, it is not straightforward to apply the feature-based registration framework to multi-modal images by using their native features.

To solve this problem, we propose to learn the common feature representations for two different modality images via Kernel CCA [6]. Specifically, we extract image features from well-registered image pairs at each key point in a multi-resolution manner, for characterizing anatomical structures in different resolutions. For each resolution, we can apply Kernel CCA to find respective nonlinear mappings that maximize the correlation between two different modality features in common space. In this way, the anatomical correspondences between two multi-modal images can be quantitatively measured by feature similarities between the learned common feature representations.

In the application (i.e., image registration) stage, these learned common features can be used for developing a hierarchical feature-based multi-modal image registration method. Specifically, given two new images, we first extract multi-resolution features in their own spaces. Then, we apply Kernel CCA mapping functions in each resolution to transform features into the common space. These common features can be used for correspondence detection. To improve the robustness of correspondence detection and subsequent registration, we initially select only a small number of key points with distinctive features in both images (i.e., salient points at image boundaries and corners), and let them drive correspondence detection by matching the learned common features. After tentatively determining correspondences with these key points, we use thin-plate spline (TPS) to interpolate dense deformation field. To further refine the registration results, we gradually add more and more key points to guide image registration. By using hierarchical strategy, the registration performance can be iteratively improved.

We evaluate the performance of our proposed method for the cases of registering CT and MR prostate images, as well as the first-year infant brain MR images. Compared with several state-of-the-art methods such as MI-based registration method (Elastix [7]) and SyN, our method achieves more accurate registration results, in terms of ROI (Region of Interest) overlap degrees.

2   Method

2.1   Learning Common Feature Representations via Kernel CCA

Suppose we have T pairs of aligned training images, $\{(I_s^{(1)}, I_s^{(2)})|s = 1, ..., T\}$, where we use superscript to denote image modality. At each point v, we consider using intensities of its surrounding image patch as the native image features, i.e., $f_s^{(1)}(v)$ and $f_s^{(2)}(v)$ represent the native features from images $I_s^{(1)}$ and $I_s^{(2)}$, respectively. Patch size is fixed here, but it's straightforward to extend our learning procedure in a multi-resolution manner as we will explain later. We apply a random sampling procedure to obtain M pairs of native features from T pairs of training images. Note that each pair of native image features is extracted at the same anatomical location of two aligned modality images. Furthermore, we reshape native features of each point v into a column vector and thus construct two feature matrices: $X = [x_1, ..., x_i, ..., x_M]^T$ and $Y = [y_1, ..., y_i, ..., y_M]^T$, where the column vectors $x_i = f_s^{(1)}(v)$ and $y_i = f_s^{(2)}(v)$. By assuming L as the total number of image points in each image patch, both X and Y are $M \times L$ matrices. Next step is to learn the common feature representations from X and Y.

Although CCA is widely used to find the linear mapping, we resort to use Kernel CCA since we believe that the relationship between native image features of two modalities is highly nonlinear. Note that Kernel CCA shares the same idea as SVM that maps the data to a high-dimensional space by kernel functions, which is more flexible to deal with complex mapping than linear CCA. Without loss of generality, we use Gaussian kernel ϕ in this paper, where $\phi(a, b) = exp\left(-\|a - b\|^2/2\,\sigma^2\right)$ denotes the Gaussian kernel applied to any two vectors a and b.

First, we compute the kernel matrices for feature matrices X and Y by:

$$K_X = [\phi(x_i, x_j)]_{M \times M}, \ i, j = 1, ..., M \tag{1}$$

$$K_Y = [\phi(y_i, y_j)]_{M \times M}, \ i, j = 1, ..., M \tag{2}$$

Kernel CCA aims to determine the canonical vectors in the mapped feature space, which can be regarded as the basis vectors for projecting the native image features into a common space. The canonical vectors for K_X is defined as $\alpha_{M \times D} = [\alpha_1, ..., \alpha_d, ..., \alpha_D]$, where each α_d is a M-dimensional column vector and D is the minimum rank of matrices K_X and K_Y, i.e., $D = \min(rank(K_X), rank(K_Y))$. Similarly, we define the canonical vectors for K_Y as $\beta_{M \times D} = [\beta_1, ..., \beta_d, ..., \beta_D]$. The optimization function of Kernel CCA is:

$$\text{argmax}_{\alpha_d, \beta_d}(K_X \alpha_d)^T(K_Y \beta_d), \quad d = 1, ..., D$$
$$s.t. \ \alpha_d^T K_X K_X \alpha_d = 1, \ \beta_d^T K_Y K_Y \beta_d = 1. \tag{3}$$

We sequentially solve each pair of α_d and β_d by (1) maximizing the correlation between $K_X \alpha_d$ and $K_Y \beta_d$ across all M training pairs, and (2) requiring α_d to be orthogonal to all previous computed canonical vectors $\alpha_1, ... \alpha_{d-1}$, and also β_d to be orthogonal to all previous computed canonical vectors $\beta_1, ... \beta_{d-1}$. Partial Gram-Schmidt Orthogonalization method can be used here to find the optimal α and β in Eq. 3 [5].

In the testing stage, we first compute the native image features from each testing image. Suppose that we obtain totally N native image features from each of two different modality images under registration. Following the same procedure in the training stage, we stack the native image features into two matrices $P = [p_i]_{N \times L}$ and $Q = [q_i]_{N \times L}$. Then we can get the following kernel matrices:

$$K_{PX} = [\phi(p_i, x_j)]_{N \times M}, \ i = 1, ..., N, \ j = 1, ..., M \tag{4}$$

$$K_{QY} = [\phi(q_i, y_j)]_{N \times M}, \ i = 1, ..., N, \ j = 1, ..., M \tag{5}$$

After that, it is straightforward to transform the native image features P and Q to the common space by using the learned canonical vectors, $\widetilde{P} = K_{PX}\alpha$, $\widetilde{Q} = K_{QY}\beta$, where $\widetilde{P} = [\tilde{p}_i]_{N \times D}$ and $\widetilde{Q} = [\tilde{q}_i]_{N \times D}$ are common feature presentations for two different modality images. Note, if p_i and q_j are located at corresponding structure, $\tilde{p}_i$ and $\tilde{q}_j$ are supposed to be similar after mapping, though p_i and q_j could be very different.

Multi-resolution Implementation. To improve discrimination power of features, we learn the common features in a multi-resolution manner. Specifically, we use different Gaussian kernels to smooth each original image. Thus, although we fix the patch size in extracting native features, we can capture *not only* local *but also* global features. We apply Kernel CCA in each resolution independently to obtain the respective common feature representations.

2.2   Hierarchical Feature-Based Multi-modal Image Registration

Based on the learned common feature representations, we propose a hierarchical feature-based multi-modal image registration method, by iterating the following 3 steps until convergence (or reaching a certain number of iterations).

1) Key Point Selection. We first average and normalize gradient magnitude values over the entire image. These values are roughly considered as the importance of each point in registration. Based on this importance map, a small set of key points with higher importance values can be sampled. It is clear from Fig. 2(a) that the key points are more concentrated at rich-edge areas, where importance values are high. Furthermore, we employ a hierarchical mechanism for selecting key points. Fig. 2(a) shows the selected key points from different stages. Purple points are selected in the initial stages, while red and green voxels are gradually selected and added in the subsequent stages after relaxing the key-point selection criterion.

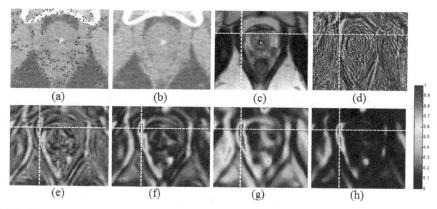

Fig. 2. Illustration of key points selection and feature matching in identifying the correspondence of a CT point in the MR prostate image. The similarity maps using linear CCA feature, high-, middle-, low-, and multi-resolution kernel CCA features are shown in (d)-(h), respectively.

2) Robust Feature Matching. For each key point, we search for its corresponding point in another image by comparing feature similarity. Here, we use the Euclidian distance between common features as the similarity measure. Since we learn the common feature representations in a multi-resolution manner, we can detect correspondences from coarse to fine scales. A typical feature matching result is shown in Fig. 2, where one CT image point (indicated by a red cross in Fig. 2(b)) is compared w.r.t. all points in MR image (Fig. 2(c)). Fig. 2(e)-(g) show the respective similarity maps by using high-, middle-, and low-resolution features, where red and blue denote high and low similarities, respectively. The integrated similarity using multi-resolution features is shown in Fig. 2(h). Fig. 2(d) illustrates the similarity map using the linear CCA features. It is clear that (1) the learned common features by Kernel CCA can accurately guide feature matching for finding the matched anatomical structure while features by linear CCA are not able to do so; and (2) multi-resolution feature representations have more discrimination power than any of single-resolution features and thus can make the image registration more robust to superficial matches.

3) Hierarchical Estimation of Deformation Field. Given the tentatively estimated correspondences on key points, we consider the selected key points as the control points in the entire image domain, and then apply TPS to interpolate the dense deformation field. Thus, all image points can have their deformations immediately. Note that we here allow only the key points steering the entire registration, while other points only following the deformations of nearby key points. Since the key points can establish correspondences more reliably than others, our hierarchical deformation estimation mechanism can make our registration method robust against noise. After two images are approximately registered, we gradually add more and more key points to join the registration by sampling more key points.

3   Experiments

3.1   MR/CT Prostate Image Registration

In this section, we apply our hierarchical multi-modal image registration method for MR and CT prostate images used in radiation therapy. Since MR image has much better contrast in soft tissues, it is relatively easy to manually label the prostate in MR image. Thus, the key step in radiation therapy is to transfer the prostate label from MR image to CT image by MR/CT image registration. We divide the whole dataset to 10 groups and applied 5-fold cross-validation (where, in each fold, 8 groups for training and another 2 groups for testing). Each group contains both CT and MR prostate images from the same patient with size 153×193×50 and resolution 1×1×1mm^3.

In the training stage, we carefully register MR image to CT image with human intervention, for each pair of training images. To obtain middle- and low-resolution images, we apply Gaussian smoothing on the original image with kernel sigma 1.5 and 2.5, respectively. For each training patient, we randomly choose 2,000 image patches with size 7×7×5 for the original, middle- and low-resolution images. Unless otherwise mentioned, the same parameters are used in the following experiments. Here, we compare with the MI-based registration method in Elastix software package.

Typical registration results by MI-based method and our proposed feature-based registration method are shown in Fig. 3. The yellow contours in four images are prostate/rectum boundaries obtained from same CT image as reference. The red contours denote corresponding structures in original MR image before registration (Fig. 3(b)) and two registered MR images by Elastix (Fig. 3(c)) and our method (Fig. 3(d)), respectively. Apparently, contours on the registered MR image by our method (Fig. 3(d)) are much closer to reference contours of CT image than by MI-based method, suggesting more accurate registration by our method. For quantitative evaluation, the mean and variance of prostate DICE ratio of Elastix is 0.8249± 0.0735, while proposed method achieves 0.8718 ± 0.0458, which is almost 5.7% improvement over Elastix.

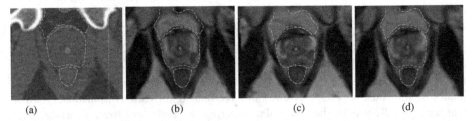

(a)   (b)   (c)   (d)

Fig. 3. Example of CT and MR registration by our method and MI-based method. (a) CT image used as reference; (b) Original MR image; (c) Registered MR image by MI-based method in Elastix; (d) Registered MR image by our method.

3.2   Image Registration for Infant Brain MR Images in the First Year of Life

Accurate registration of infant brain images is very important in many brain development studies [8]. Due to rapid maturation and myelination of brain tissues in the first year of life, the intensity contrast of gray and white matter undergoes dramatic changes. As a result, the conventional image registration methods, even working well for adult brains, have limited performance for infant brain images in the first year of life.

In this section, we demonstrate the registration performance of our proposed method on the most challenging registration task, i.e., registering the 6-month-old infant brain images whose image contrasts between white matter (WM) and gray matter (GM) are the poorest in the first year [9] (Fig. 4(a)). In detail, we implement the registration between 6-month-old and 12-month-old brain images across different subjects, in which 6-month-old images are used as reference space. The dataset includes 11 subjects and each subject contains both 6-month-old and 12-month-old MR T1 images with size 256×256×198 and resolution 1×1×1mm^3. Specifically, the first step is to learn common feature representations between 6-month-old and 12-month-old images. In each cross validation, 9 subjects are chosen as training images, in which 6-month-old and 12-month-old images of the same subjects are carefully registered via their segmented images, while other remaining two subjects serve as the testing subjects. Specifically, the 6-month-old image from one testing subject acts as the target image, while the 12-month-old image from another testing subject acts as the moving image. The whole process above (of our cross validation) is repeated 10 times for evaluation.

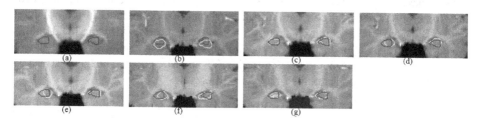

Fig. 4. Typical registration results by 5 different methods. (a) A 6-month-old image. (b) A 12-month-old image. (c-g) Five registration results of warping 12-month-old image to 6-month-old image by our proposed method with/without Kernel CCA (c-d), SyN (e), Demons (f), and Elastix (g), respectively. Yellow contours in (b-g) denote the hippocampal boundaries of 12-month-old image in the original (b) and warped (c-g) spaces, while red contours in all images indicate the *same* hippocampal boundaries of 6-month-old image in different spaces.

Since we have the manual tissue segmentations (WM, GM, and CSF (Cerebral-Spinal Fluid)) and also manual segmentation of hippocampus, we can quantitatively evaluate the registration performance based on both tissue and ROI overlap ratios. Table 1 presents the statistics of tissue DICE and ROI overlap ratio, compared with state-of-the-art Elastix (MI-based), diffeomorphic Demons, and SyN. As we can see, our proposed method achieves the best results over other counterpart registration methods. It is worth noting that our method improves DICE ratio by 2.56% over the second best method, which is also statistically significant under paired t-test (p<0.05). To further evaluate the performance of feature representations learned by Kernel CCA, we directly use native features, i.e., image intensities, instead of Kernel CCA features in our proposed method for comparison. As we can see, our proposed method with Kernel CCA achieves higher DICE ratio than that without Kernel CCA, which demonstrates the capability of using Kernel CCA features for guiding registration. Fig. 4 shows typical registration results by 5 different methods. Again, it is apparent that our proposed method with Kernel CCA (Fig. 4(c)) produces the most accurate results.

Table 1. Comparison of tissue DICE and hippocampus overlap ratio by 5 different methods.

Method	WM	GM	CSF	Hippocampus
Elastix (MI-based)	63.24 ± 2.34	72.34 ± 1.24	41.98 ± 5.82	47.03±6.38
Demons	63.08 ± 2.65	70.96 ± 1.70	46.47 ± 4.42	58.33 ±7.65
SyN	65.03 ± 2.61	73.79 ± 1.53	49.17 ± 4.20	59.65 ±7.49
Proposed without KCCA	65.37 ± 1.96	72.15 ± 1.41	42.96 ± 2.22	55.27 ± 7.93
Proposed with KCCA	**67.59**± 2.54	**75.07**± 1.67	**50.02**± 6.10	**61.30** ±5.88

4   Conclusion

We have presented a novel hierarchical feature-based multi-modal image registration method. To address the significant difference between native image features of multi-modal images, we employ Kernel CCA to learn common feature representations for maximizing the statistical correlation of transformed native features in the common space. By using these common features, we further develop a hierarchical multi-modal image registration procedure through robust feature matching. We have shown promising results of our method in registering CT and MR prostate images, as well as the infant MR brain images in the first year of life.

References

1. Maintz, J., Viergever, M.: A survey of medical image registration. Medical Image Analysis **2**, 1–36 (1998)
2. Pluim, J.P.W., Maintz, J.B.A., Viergever, M.A.: Mutual-information-based registration of medical images: a survey. IEEE Transactions on Medical Imaging **22**, 986–1004 (2003)
3. Wells, I., William, M., Viola, P., Atsumi, H., Nakajima, S., Kikinis, R.: Multi-modal volume registration by maximization of mutual information. Medical Image Analysis **1**, 35–51 (1996)
4. Knops, Z.F., Maintz, J.B.A., Viergever, M.A., Pluim, J.P.W.: Normalized mutual information based registration using k-means clustering and shading correction. Medical Image Analysis **10**, 432–439 (2006)
5. Wu, G., Kim, M., Wang, Q., Shen, D.: S-HAMMER: Hierarchical Attribute-Guided, Symmetric Diffeomorphic Registration for MR Brain Images. Human Brain Mapping **35** (2014)

6. Hardoon, D.R., Szedmak, S., Shawe-Taylor, J.: Canonical Correlation Analysis: An Overview with Application to Learning Methods. Neural Computation **16**, 2639–2664 (2004)

7. Klein, S., Staring, M., Murphy, K., Viergever, M.A., Pluim, J.P.W.: elastix: a toolbox for intensity based medical image registration. IEEE Transaction on Medical Imaging **29**, 196–205 (2010)

8. Li, G., Wang, L., Shi, F., Lyall, A.E., Lin, W., Gilmore, J.H., Shen, D.: Mapping longitudinal development of local cortical gyrification in infants from birth to 2 years of age. The Journal of Neuroscience **34**, 4228–4238 (2014)

9. Wang, L., Shi, F., Gao, Y., Li, G., Gilmore, J.H., Lin, W., Shen, D.: Integration of sparse multi-modality representation and anatomical constraint for isointense infant brain MR image segmentation. NeuroImage **89**, 152–164 (2014)

Semi-automatic Liver Tumor Segmentation in Dynamic Contrast-Enhanced CT Scans Using Random Forests and Supervoxels

Pierre-Henri Conze[1]([✉]), François Rousseau[2], Vincent Noblet[1], Fabrice Heitz[1], Riccardo Memeo[3], and Patrick Pessaux[3]

[1] ICube, Université de Strasbourg, CNRS, Fédération de Médecine Translationnelle de Strasbourg (FMTS), Strasbourg, France
conze@unistra.fr
[2] Institut Mines-Télécom, Télécom Bretagne, INSERM, LATIM, Brest, France
[3] Department of Hepato-Biliary and Pancreatic Surgery, Nouvel Hôpital Civil, Institut Hospitalo-Universitaire de Strasbourg, Strasbourg, France

Abstract. Pre-operative locoregional treatments (PLT) delay the tumor progression by necrosis for patients with hepato-cellular carcinoma (HCC). Toward an efficient evaluation of PLT response, we address the estimation of liver tumor necrosis (TN) from CT scans. The TN rate could shortly supplant standard criteria (RECIST, mRECIST, EASL or WHO) since it has recently shown higher correlation to survival rates. To overcome the inter-expert variability induced by visual qualitative assessment, we propose a semi-automatic method that requires weak interaction efforts to segment parenchyma, tumoral active and necrotic tissues. By combining SLIC supervoxels and random decision forest, it involves discriminative multi-phase cluster-wise features extracted from registered dynamic contrast-enhanced CT scans. Quantitative assessment on expert groundtruth annotations confirms the benefits of exploiting multi-phase information from semantic regions to accurately segment HCC liver tumors.

1 Introduction

Hepato-cellular carcinoma (HCC) is the most common type of liver cancer and the third most frequent cause of cancer-related death. Pre-operative locoregional treatments (PLT) tend to downstage HCC tumors by necrosis. Standard evaluation scores (RECIST, mRECIST, EASL or WHO) used to predict the response to PLT do not provide fully satisfactory results [1]. A more efficient HCC patient follow-up is reached through tumor necrosis (TN) rate which provides more significant correlation with survival rates.

To overcome inter-expert variability induced by visual qualitative assessment, we present a computed-aided diagnosis method for TN rate computation. Assessing TN remains an open issue due to a wide variability of shape, size, location, contour aspect and intensity of HCC tumors. It requires the segmentation of healthy liver parenchyma as well as tumoral active and necrotic areas (Fig. 4).

© Springer International Publishing Switzerland 2015
L. Zhou et al. (Eds.): MLMI 2015, LNCS 9352, pp. 212–219, 2015.
DOI: 10.1007/978-3-319-24888-2_26

For this task, dynamic contrast-enhanced images provide discriminative information since HCC is characterized by arterial enhancement followed by venous washout in response to contrast agent injection [2].

Dynamic contrast-enhanced images have been recently exploited for HCC liver tumor segmentation via extraction of *multi-phase voxel-wise* features used in level sets [3], k-means [4] or graph cuts [5]. These multi-phase features capture the dynamic in response to agent injection and tend to build a full perfusion model from low temporal resolution data (Fig. 3*b*). However, to reach a better accuracy, user interaction appears necessary since arterial enhancement and venous washout depend on contrast agent kinetic and injection protocol [2]. In this direction, tumor extraction has been covered in an interactive perspective for single-phase images [6,7] by relying on supervised ensemble learning with *single-phase voxel-wise* features including spatial characteristics. Although more appropriate, such strategy is voxel-wise as in [3–5] and therefore requires a significant amount of interaction while relying on a limited spatial context

In this work, we propose to exploit robust *multi-phase cluster-wise* features extracted from registered multi-phase contrast-enhanced CT scans by combining clustering and supervised ensemble learning. Performing interactive learning and prediction on semantic regions allow tumor segmentation to take advantage of discriminative dynamic information at an extended spatial extent. Moreover, it ensures weak interactions efforts for practitioners. This method applied to TN rate estimation is a key step toward accurate PLT response assessment.

2   Methodology

2.1   Traditional Approach: *Single-Phase Voxel-Wise* Random Forest

In an interactive setting for image segmentation, the user usually defines manually a set of K labeled voxels $\boldsymbol{S} = \{\boldsymbol{v}_k, c(\boldsymbol{v}_k)\}_{k \in \{1,...,K\}}$ where $c(\boldsymbol{v}_k) \in \{c_1, ..., c_N\}$ is the label at voxel $\boldsymbol{v}_k$ with N the total class number. The set $\boldsymbol{S}$, referred as *training data*, is used to build a voxel/label mapping model whose aim is to predict the label $c(\boldsymbol{v})$ of each test voxel $\boldsymbol{v}$. In the context of ensemble learning methods, random decision forests [8] have grown in popularity due to their ability to offer a unified framework for many machine learning tasks [9].

A random decision forest consists of T independent trees made of both *internal nodes* which split input data according to binary tests and *terminal nodes* which reach all together a final data partition. At each internal node, the split sends voxels to left and right children nodes. For this task, the associated binary test focuses on a randomly subset $\hat{\theta}(\boldsymbol{v})$ of the visual features $\theta(\boldsymbol{v})$ extracted for input voxels $\boldsymbol{v}$ and halve the input dataset according to:

$$h(\boldsymbol{v}, \theta) = \begin{cases} \text{true, if } \tau_{low} < \hat{\theta}(\boldsymbol{v}) < \tau_{up} \\ \text{false, otherwise} \end{cases} \tag{1}$$

where $\hat{\theta}(\boldsymbol{v})$ is compared to thresholds τ_{low} and τ_{up}. In the context of tumor segmentation, methods relying on random decision forest such as [7,10] usually focus on one single image and therefore involve *single-phase* visual features $\theta(\boldsymbol{v})$.

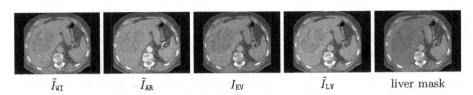

$$\tilde{I}_{\text{WI}} \qquad \tilde{I}_{\text{AR}} \qquad I_{\text{EV}} \qquad \tilde{I}_{\text{LV}} \qquad \text{liver mask}$$

Fig. 1. Registered multi-phase input data ($\tilde{I}_{\text{WI}}$, $\tilde{I}_{\text{AR}}$, I_{EV} and $\tilde{I}_{\text{LV}}$) obtained from dynamic contrast-enhanced CT scans with associated liver segmentation mask.

During training, each tree takes the *training voxel* set S as input and optimizes its own internal nodes ($\{\tau_{low}, \tau_{up}, \hat{\theta}(v)\}$) via information gain maximization [9] to obtain the most discriminative binary tests with respect to S. After this optimization, each leaf node l_t of the tth tree receives a partition S_{l_t} of the training data S and produces an entire class probability distribution: $\text{p}_{l_t}(c_i|S)$ $\forall i \in \{1, ..., N\}$. To predict the label $c(v)$ of a given *test voxel* v with associated single-phase features $\theta(v)$, v is injected into each optimized tree which makes it reaches a leaf node l_t per tree following split rules. For each label c_i, we get:

$$\text{p}(c(v) = c_i) = \frac{1}{T}\sum_{t=1}^{T}\text{p}_{l_t}(c(v) = c_i|S) = \frac{1}{T}\sum_{t=1}^{T}\frac{|\{v_k, c(v_k)\} \in S_{l_t} \mid c(v_k) = c_i|}{|S_{l_t}|}$$

(2)

The final prediction of $c(v)$ corresponds to the label c_i maximizing $\text{p}(c(v) = c_i)$:

$$c(v) = \arg\max_{c_i} \text{p}(c(v) = c_i) \tag{3}$$

2.2   Proposed Methodology: *Multi-phase Cluster-Wise Random Forest*

From Voxels to Semantic Regions. In the traditional approach (Sec. 2.1), voxels are acting without inter-dependencies which may result in a lack of spatial consistency regarding classification results. Features are sometimes explicitly related to spatial context [7,10] but spatial extent remains limited. *A-posteriori* regularization techniques such as conditional random field (CRF) [11] would more accurately introduce spatial constraints but it strongly increases computational complexity. Moreover, such voxel-wise learning-based approaches require a significant amount of interaction for the end-user to get a large enough training set. To reduce interaction efforts and intrinsically introduce spatial consistency, we perform random forest on training and test *semantic regions* instead of voxels.

Exploiting Multi-phase Input Data. Since practitioners focus HCC diagnosis on the association of both arterial hypervascularity and venous washout [2], we propose to take full advantage of *multi-phase* contrast-enhanced CT scans. In practice, for a given examination, a contrast agent is injected to the patient and CT scans are acquired at different phases : before injection (WI) but also after at

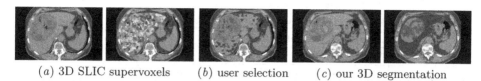

(a) 3D SLIC supervoxels   (b) user selection   (c) our 3D segmentation

Fig. 2. Semi-automatic tumor segmentation with *multi-phase cluster-wise* random forest: by performing user interaction (b) and learning on 3D supervoxels (a), it segments parenchyma (*blue*), active (*red*) and necrotic (*green*) areas of the 3D liver volume (c).

arterial (AR), early venous (EV) and late venous (LV) phases. Each examination consists in a set of images $S_I = \{I_{\text{WI}}, I_{\text{AR}}, I_{\text{EV}}, I_{\text{LV}}\}$ which are warped with respect to I_{EV} since I_{EV} exhibits greater inter-class contrasts than other acquisitions. The set of registered multi-phase images (Fig. 1) is $S_{\tilde{I}} = \{\tilde{I}_{\text{WI}}, \tilde{I}_{\text{AR}}, I_{\text{EV}}, \tilde{I}_{\text{LV}}\}$ where $\tilde{\ }$ denotes warped scans. To obtain $S_{\tilde{I}}$ from S_I, we apply a symmetric diffeomorphic non-rigid registration based on the variational formulation of [12]. A liver segmentation mask (Fig. 1) is assumed to be available at EV phase.

Proposed Protocol. Our interactive tumor segmentation method translates in *multi-phase cluster-wise* random forest classification for TN rate estimation. $N = 3$ classes are considered: parenchyma, active and necrotic areas.

First, the liver volume is over-segmented using a 3D extension of the simple linear iterative clustering (SLIC) superpixel algorithm [13]. Starting from all the voxels belonging to the liver mask in I_{EV}, SLIC provides a set of K_R 3D compact clusters $R = \{r_i\}_{i \in \{1,\ldots,K_R\}}$ (Fig. 2a). Then, the interactive training cluster selection occurs. Instead of brushing strokes on many voxels, the practitioner has only to select and label a subset of R (Fig. 2b). We claim that such interaction is more suitable for clinical practice due to its simplicity and its possible integration in multi-examination training. It results in a *training* cluster set $S = \{r_j, c(r_j)\}_{j \subset \{1,\ldots,K_R\}}$ combining cluster r_j with groundtruth labels $c(r_j) \in \{c_1, c_2, \ldots, c_N\}$. A random forest is then built based on the training set S via a training procedure for which internal nodes are optimized with respect to *multi-phase cluster-wise* visual features $\theta(r_j)$ assigned to each cluster r_j.

Test clusters r ($r \in R \backslash S$) are then propagated into the forest to get a label prediction $c(r)$ (Fig. 2c) based on their own *multi-phase cluster-wise* features. Finally, the TN rate τ is computed as follows: $\tau = \frac{\sum_r |r| . \mathbf{1}_{c(r)=c_1}}{\sum_r |r| . [\mathbf{1}_{c(v)=c_0} + \mathbf{1}_{c(v)=c_1}]}$ where $|r|$ is the number of voxels in cluster r, c_0 and c_1 active and necrosis labels.

Multi-phase Cluster-Wise Features. The accuracy of our method is related to the ability of the features to discriminate the different tissues. We assign to each semantic region, r, 20 *multi-phase cluster-wise* visual features divided into 3 groups (Fig. 3a). The two first groups introduce spatial characteristics in terms of intensity and gradient magnitude at the cluster spatial extent. In both cases and for each phase, mean and standard deviation values are computed among all voxels of r. Thus, we quantify intrinsic intensity, visual homogeneity, textural

Related to	*Multi-phase cluster-wise* features	Nb
Spatial intensity	mean intensity including BL	4
	standard deviation	4
Spatial gradient	mean gradient magnitude	4
	standard deviation	4
Multi-phase	peak enhancement (PE)	1
	area under enhancement curve (AUC)	1
	inter-phase diff. $\Delta_{EV/AR}$, $\Delta_{LV/EV}$	2

(a)

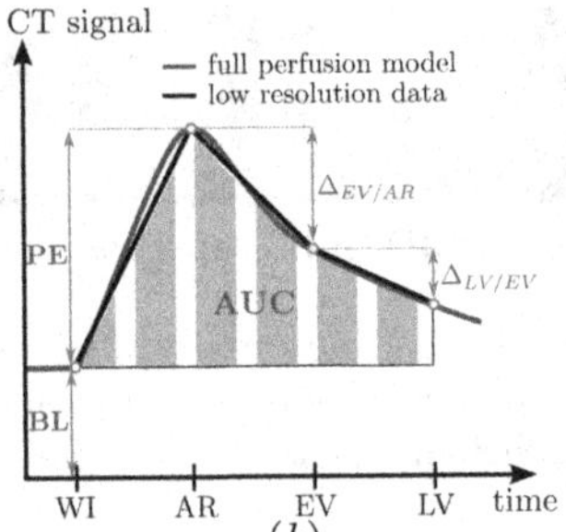

CT signal — full perfusion model — low resolution data — $\Delta_{EV/AR}$ — $\Delta_{LV/EV}$ — PE — AUC — BL — WI   AR   EV   LV   time

(b)

Fig. 3. *Multi-phase cluster-wise* features involved into random forest (*a*) to discriminate the different tissues and illustration of dynamic features (*b*).

information and texture-scale repartition. The third group fully exploits dynamic contrast-enhanced data by combining several multi-phase intensity information averaged among the voxels of r: dynamic features used in [3–5] including peak enhancement (PE) and area under curve (AUC) (Fig. 3*b*) to which is added inter-phase intensity differences $\Delta_{EV/AR}$ and $\Delta_{LV/EV}$ since PE only compares WI and AR. The baseline pre-contrast (BL) (Fig. 3*b*) is taken into account with intensity features. These dynamic features discriminate clusters based on their own dynamic characterized by arterial enhancement and venous washout.

3   Results

Evaluation on Clinical Data. The protocol has been tested on data collected from 7 examinations $\{e_1, e_2, \ldots, e_7\}$ performed on patients with HCC. Each examination results in a set of dynamic contrast-enhanced CT scans including I_{WI}, I_{AR} and I_{EV} with additional I_{LV} for e_1 and e_2. For each e_i, 6 equally reparted 2D axial slices have been selected in I_{EV} to cover the tumor spatial extent and labeled by 4 experts in hepato-digestive surgery to reach groundtruth (GT) segmentation masks delimitating parenchyma, active and necrotic tissues. Manual segmentation is performed on temporally averaged images over all phases. It results in a database of 42 slices with associated fused GT masks obtained by fusing all the expert annotations with STAPLE [14]. This database has been created since, to our knowledge, no such data is freely available.

Each examination e_i is processed independently. For each one, we extract among all the 3D SLIC clusters those overlapping the annotated 2D axial slices. Among these clusters, we identify those whose intersection with annotated slices has a predominant GT label (consensus over at least 95% of voxels). This predominant label is assigned to the 3D cluster as its own GT label. Finally, 1/3 of these labeled 3D SLIC clusters are randomly selected (to simulate user interaction) and used to train our *multi-phase cluster-wise* random forest (*MpCl*-RF). Once trained, the forest is employed to classify all the remaining 3D SLIC clusters. We provide comparisons with *single-phase voxel-wise* (*SpVx*), *single-phase cluster-wise* (*SpCl*) and *multi-phase voxel-wise* (*MpVx*) random forest (RF). To make comparisons possible, training for *Sp/MpVx* focus on voxels belonging to clusters selected for training in *Sp/MpCl*. Each forest contains $T = 100$ trees.

Features differ for each method. Cluster-wise strategies assign to clusters the features of Fig. 3 for *MpCl* and a modified set for *SpCl* since multi-phase features are ousted and spatial intensity and gradient ones only focus on I_{EV}. In voxel-wise, *MpVx* assigns to voxels intrisic and spatially averaged (3^3 windows) intensity and gradient at each phase as well as PE, AUC, $\Delta_{EV/AR}$ and $\Delta_{LV/EV}$ whereas *SpVx* only involves intrisic and averaged intensity and gradient in I_{EV}.

SpVx, SpCl, MpVx and *MpCl* are quantitatively assessed via TN rate error $\Delta\tau = |\tau - \tau_{GT}|$ comparing estimated and GT TN rates and *DICE* coefficients between obtained and fused GT masks for parenchyma, active and necrotic tissues: $DICE_{prcm}$, $DICE_{activ}$ and $DICE_{necro}$. To be less sensitive to the variability due to RF random aspects, results for each e_i are averaged over 10 realizations.

Discussion. We present in Tab. 1 a comparative assessment of the 4 methods through $\Delta\tau$ and *DICE* coefficients averaged over the whole database. Segmentation results are displayed on Fig. 4 with corresponding fused GT mask (one slice per examination). The comparative study reveals better results using *MpCl*-RF. It obtains the smallest $\Delta\tau$ with 5.26 and the highest *DICE* for parenchyma, active and necrotic areas with 74.4, 71.9 and 93.3. In comparison, *MpVx*-RF reaches equivalent $DICE_{necro}$ but less accurate $\Delta\tau$, $DICE_{activ}$ and $DICE_{prcm}$. According to visual results (Fig. 4), *MpVx*-RF allows an obvious worst spatial consistency while requiring more interaction efforts compared to *MpCl*-RF.

The comparison between single and multi-phase approaches confirms that exploiting multi-phase CT images instead of one single scan significantly improves the results with gains of *DICE* around 8.6 (11.2), 8.1 (6.8) and 3.6 (6.9) resp. for cluster and voxel-based strategies. The significant differences between *Sp/MpCl*-RF tend to justify the use of robust multi-phase features when making RF working on clusters since a classification error on one single cluster can have a strong impact on the accuracy. In addition, the averaged maximum inter-expert variability computed over the GT masks provided by the 4 experts is 21.2 ± 15.2

Table 1. Quantitative comparisons of *single-phase voxel-wise* (*SpVx*), *single-phase cluster-wise* (*SpCl*), *multi-phase voxel-wise* (*MpVx*) and the proposed *multi-phase cluster-wise* (*MpCl*) random forest (RF) through TN rate error and *DICE* coefficients averaged over the whole database. Best results are emphasized in bold.

methods	*SpVx*-RF	*SpCl*-RF	*MpVx*-RF	***MpCl*-RF**
$\Delta\tau$	6.40 ± 2.85	9.13 ± 4.78	6.60 ± 3.32	$\mathbf{5.26 \pm 3.90}$
$DICE_{activ}$	54.3 ± 17.2	65.8 ± 15.3	65.5 ± 12.4	$\mathbf{74.4 \pm 12.6}$
$DICE_{necro}$	65.0 ± 21.6	63.8 ± 25.8	71.8 ± 17.6	$\mathbf{71.9 \pm 19.5}$
$DICE_{prcm}$	80.5 ± 13.1	89.7 ± 4.90	87.4 ± 9.00	$\mathbf{93.3 \pm 3.08}$

test slice $Sp\,Vx$-RF $SpCl$-RF $Mp\,Vx$-RF   **$MpCl$-RF**   fused GT

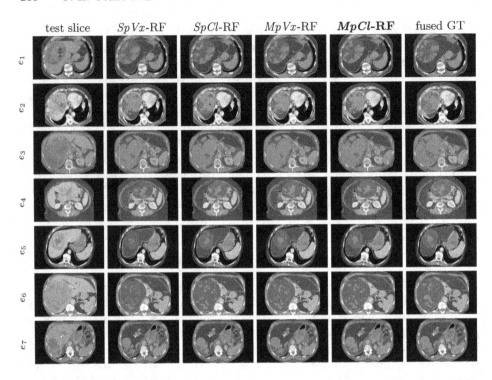

Fig. 4. HCC liver tumor segmentation results via *single-phase voxel-wise* ($Sp\,Vx$), *single-phase cluster-wise* ($SpCl$), *multi-phase voxel-wise* ($Mp\,Vx$) and the proposed *multi-phase cluster-wise* ($MpCl$) random forest (RF) with groundtruth (GT) masks. Parenchyma, active and necrotic areas are respectively in blue, red and green.

in TN rate. This significant variability reinforces the necessity to work toward an efficient computed-aided diagnosis method dedicated to TN rate estimation in order to overcome the bias induced by visual qualitative assessment.

4   Conclusion

In this work, we addressed the semi-automatic evaluation of pre-operative locoregional treatments (PLT) response for hepato-cellular carcinoma (HCC). Toward this goal, we proposed a method that estimates the tumor necrosis (TN) rate from dynamic contrast-enhanced CT scans. While ensuring weak interaction efforts for practitioners, it accurately segments parenchyma, active and necrotic tissues. Our approach applies random forest on supervoxels and involves robust multi-phase cluster-wise features. Quantitative assessment on clinical data confirms the benefits of exploiting dynamic information extracted from multi-phase images at a cluster spatial extent. Multi-examination learning would deserve further investigation to make the proposed strategy becoming fully automatic. More generally, it could be easily applied to other tumor types, organs and modalities.

Acknowledgments. This work received the financial support from Fondation Arc, www.fondation-arc.org.

References

1. Ronot, M., Bouattour, M., Wassermann, J., Bruno, O., Dreyer, C., Larroque, B., Castera, L., Vilgrain, V., Belghiti, J., Raymond, E., et al.: Alternative response criteria (Choi, EASL and mRECIST) versus RECIST 1.1 in patients with advanced hepatocellular carcinoma treated with Sorafenib. The Oncologist (2014)
2. Ronot, M., Vilgrain, V.: Hepatocellular carcinoma: Diagnostic criteria by imaging techniques. Best Practice & Research Clinical Gastro-enterology 28(5) (2014)
3. Lee, J., Cai, W., Singh, A., Yoshida, H.: Estimation of necrosis volumes in focal liver lesions based on multi-phase hepatic CT images. In: Virtual Colonoscopy & Abdominal Imaging. Computational Challenges & Clinical Opportunities (2011)
4. Raj, A., Juluru, K.: Visualization and segmentation of liver tumors using dynamic contrast MRI. In: Conference of Engineering in Medicine and Biology (2009)
5. Fang, R., Zabih, R., Raj, A., Chen, T.: Segmentation of liver tumor using efficient global optimal tree metrics graph cuts. In: Yoshida, H., Sakas, G., Linguraru, M.G. (eds.) Abdominal Imaging. Computational and Clinical Applications. LNCS, vol. 7029, pp. 51–59. Springer, Heidelberg (2012)
6. Shimizu, A., Narihira, T., Furukawa, D., Kobatake, H., Nawano, S., Shinozaki, K.: Ensemble segmentation using Adaboost with application to liver lesion extraction from a CT volume. In: Workshop on 3D Segmentation in the Clinic (2008)
7. Geremia, E., Menze, B.H., Clatz, O., Konukoglu, E., Criminisi, A., Ayache, N.: Spatial decision forests for ms lesion segmentation in multi-channel mr images. In: Medical Image Computing and Computer-Assisted Intervention (2010)
8. Breiman, L.: Random Forests. Machine learning 45(1), 5–32 (2001)
9. Criminisi, A., Shotton, J., Konukoglu, E.: Decision forests: A unified framework for classification, regression, density estimation, manifold learning and semi-supervised learning. Foundations and Trends in Computer Graphics and Vision 7(2–3) (2012)
10. Cuingnet, R., Prevost, R., Lesage, D., Cohen, L.D., Mory, B., Ardon, R.: Automatic detection and segmentation of kidneys in 3D CT Images using random forests. In: Ayache, N., Delingette, H., Golland, P., Mori, K. (eds.) MICCAI 2012. LNCS, vol. 7512, pp. 66–74. Springer, Heidelberg (2012)
11. Bauer, S., Nolte, L.-P., Reyes, M.: Fully automatic segmentation of brain tumor images using support vector machine classification in combination with hierarchical conditional random field regularization. In: Fichtinger, G., Martel, A., Peters, T. (eds.) MICCAI 2011. LNCS, vol. 6893, pp. 354–361. Springer, Heidelberg (2011)
12. Beg, M., Miller, M., Trouvé, A., Younes, L.: Computing large deformation metric mappings via geodesic flows of diffeomorphisms. International Journal of Computer Vision (2005)
13. Achanta, R., Shaji, A., Smith, K., Lucchi, A., Fua, P., Susstrunk, S.: Slic superpixels compared to state-of-the-art superpixel methods. IEEE Transactions on Pattern Analysis and Machine Intelligence 34(11), 2274–2282 (2012)
14. Warfield, S.K., Zou, K.H., Wells, W.M.: Simultaneous truth and performance level estimation (STAPLE): an algorithm for the validation of image segmentation. IEEE Transactions on Medical Imaging 23(7), 903–921 (2004)

Flexible and Latent Structured Output Learning
Application to Histology

Gustavo Carneiro[1]([⊠]), Tingying Peng[2], Christine Bayer[3], and Nassir Navab[2]

[1] ACVT, University of Adelaide, Adelaide, Australia
Gustavo.Carneiro@adelaide.edu.au
[2] CAMP, Technical University of Munich, Munich, Germany
[3] Department of Radiation Oncology, Technical University of Munich,
Munich, Germany

Abstract. Malignant tumors that contain a high proportion of regions deprived of adequate oxygen supply (hypoxia) in areas supplied by a microvessel (i.e., a microcirculatory supply unit - MCSU) have been shown to present resistance to common cancer treatments. Given the importance of the estimation of this proportion for improving the clinical prognosis of such treatments, a manual annotation has been proposed, which uses two image modalities of the same histological specimen and produces the number and proportion of MCSUs classified as normoxia (normal oxygenation level), chronic hypoxia (limited diffusion), and acute hypoxia (transient disruptions in perfusion), but this manual annotation requires an expertise that is generally not available in clinical settings. Therefore, in this paper, we propose a new methodology that automates this annotation. The major challenge is that the training set comprises weakly labeled samples that only contains the number of MCSU types per sample, which means that we do not have the underlying structure of MCSU locations and classifications. Hence, we formulate this problem as a latent structured output learning that minimizes a high order loss function based on the number of MCSU types, where the underlying MCSU structure is flexible in terms of number of nodes and connections. Using a database of 89 pairs of weakly annotated images (from eight tumors), we show that our methodology produces highly correlated number and proportion of MCSU types compared to the manual annotations.

Keywords: Weakly supervised training · Latent structured output learning · High order loss function

1 Introduction

The majority of human tumours contain chronic (limitations in oxygen diffusion) and acute (local disturbances in perfusion) hypoxic regions, which lead to poor

Gustavo Carneiro thanks the Alexander von Humboldt Foundation (Fellowship for Experienced Researchers). This work was partially supported by the Australian Research Council Projects funding scheme (project DP140102794).

© Springer International Publishing Switzerland 2015
L. Zhou et al. (Eds.): MLMI 2015, LNCS 9352, pp. 220–228, 2015.
DOI: 10.1007/978-3-319-24888-2_27

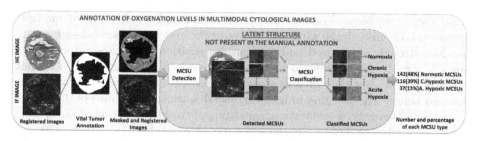

Fig. 1. Manual annotation using the HE and IF images as inputs and producing a count and proportion of the MCSU types present in the histological specimen.

clinical prognosis in treatments based on radiotherapy and chemotherapy [1]. While chronic hypoxia (CH) promotes the death of normal and tumor cells [2], acute hypoxia (AH) leads to tumor aggressiveness, so it is important to estimate the number and proportion of hypoxic regions in tumors to improve the clinical prognosis of such treatments [1]. Matei et al. [2] proposed a manual annotation of the number and proportion of hypoxic regions using (immuno-)fluorescence (IF) and hematoxylin and eosin (HE) stained images of a histological specimen, involving the following steps (Fig. 1): 1) registration of the IF and HE images; 2) delineation of the vital tumor region; 3) detection of microcirculatory supply units (MCSU), which are areas supplied by microvessels; 4) classification of MCSUs into normoxia (N - normal oxygenation supply), CH or AH; and 5) computation of the number and proportion of MCSU types. This annotation requires expertise that is generally not available in clinical settings, which makes it a good candidate for automation. A major hurdle is that this annotation [2] contains only the final number and proportion of MCSU types, without indication of MCSU locations, sizes and labels (an MCSU has size of around $200\mu m$ and class appearance as defined in Fig. 2). Therefore, this is a weakly supervised and multi-class structured learning problem that is formulated in this paper as a latent structured output problem [3] that minimizes a high order loss function [6] based on the mismatch between the manual and automated estimation of the number of MCSU types, where this latent structure is flexible in terms of the connections and number of MCSUs.

Literature Review: Although new, our problem is similar the segmentation of brain structures [7–9], involving a detection of sparse structures and multi-class classification. However, different from our problem, the segmentation of brain structures is formulated as a strongly supervised problem, where it is possible to use the position and shape priors. The detection of lymph nodes [10] also deals with the identification of sparse structures without priors. In contrast to our problem, lymph node detection is strongly supervised and concerns a binary

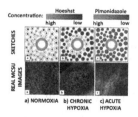

Fig. 2. MCSU classes appearance [2].

classification problem. The automated detection and localization of multiple organs [11,12] also deals with sparse detection and multi-class classification, but it is strongly supervised and one can use position and shape priors. There are a few problems formulated as weakly supervised latent structured output learning [13–15], but they present some differences compared to our problem, as detailed below. The tracking of indistinguishable translucent objects [13] uses a stronger and lower level annotation, consisting of the identification of the objects before and after occlusion. In the semantic segmentation [14,15], images are annotated with a set of classes, where the pixel-level annotation is not available, but these methodologies use lower level loss functions and deal with non-sparse segmentation problems.

Contributions: Our contribution is a new weakly supervised latent structured output learning methodology for the detection and multi-class classification of sparse structures in multimodal cytological images that is trained with the minimization of a high order loss function, where the main novelty is the flexible structure of the latent MCSU structure in terms of number of nodes and connections. In addition, this is the first methodology for the automated classification of oxygenation levels in multimodal cytological images. We analised a database of 89 pairs of IF and HE images (from eight tumors), where 16 pairs of images from two tumors were for training local MCSU multi-class classifiers, and 73 pairs of images from six tumors were for training and testing the latent structured output learning methodology. Using a leave-one-tumor-out cross validation experiment, we obtain a high correlation between the manual and automated annotations in terms of the number and proportion of MCSU types.

2 Methodology

Our methodology depends on a dataset $\mathcal{D} = \{(\mathbf{x}_n, \mathbf{v}_n, \mathbf{y}_n)\}_{n=1}^{N}$, where $\mathbf{x} = \{\mathbf{x}^{(\mathrm{IF})}, \mathbf{x}^{(\mathrm{HE})}\}$ is the input IF and HE images, with $\mathbf{x}^{(\mathrm{IF})}, \mathbf{x}^{(\mathrm{HE})} : \Omega \to \mathbb{R}$ ($\Omega \in \mathbb{R}^2$ denotes the image lattice), $\mathbf{v} : \Omega \to \{0,1\}$ is the vital tumor mask (Fig. 1), and $\mathbf{y} \in \mathcal{Y} \subseteq \mathbb{N}^3$ denotes the annotation of the number of normotic (N), chronic hypoxic (CH) and acute hypoxic (AH) MCSUs. The hidden structure is represented by the graph $\mathcal{G}(\mathcal{V}, \mathcal{E})$, where the nodes in $\mathcal{V}$ denote the MCSUs and edges in $\mathcal{E}$ represent their connections, and each node is associated with a label $c \in \{1,2,3,4\}$ (1 stands for N, 2 for CH, 3 for AH and 4 for Necrosis). We include the class Necrosis (Ne) because the vital tumor mask $\mathbf{v}$ often includes necrotic regions that must be processed during learning and inference. The structure and labeling of this graph are formed by an algorithm parametrized by the latent variable $h \in \mathcal{H}$ and the output variable $\mathbf{y}$, as described below (see Fig. 3).

2.1 Inference and Learning

We formulate our problem as a latent structured support vector machine parameterized by $\mathbf{w}$, where the inference optimizes the following objective function:

$$(\mathbf{y}^*, h^*) = \arg \max_{\mathbf{y} \in \mathcal{Y}, h \in \mathcal{H}} \mathbf{w}^\top \Psi(\mathbf{x}, \mathbf{y}, h). \qquad (1)$$

In (1), we have $\Psi(\mathbf{x}, \mathbf{y}, h) = [f_1^{(1,1)}, ..., f_4^{(1,1)}, ..., f_1^{(1,K)}, ..., f_4^{(1,K)}, f^{(2,1)}, ..., f^{(2,L)}]$, where $f_c^{(1,k)} = \sum_{v \in \mathcal{V}} \delta(m_v(\mathbf{y}) - c) \phi^{(1,k)}(c, \mathbf{x}; \theta^{(1,k)})$ with $m_v(\mathbf{y}) \in \{1, 2, 3, 4\}$ denoting the label of node $v \in \mathcal{V}$ estimated with $\mathbf{y}$ as described below in (3), $\delta(.)$ is the Dirac delta function and $k \in \{1, ..., K\}$ with $\phi^{(1,k)}(c, \mathbf{x}; \theta^{(1,k)}) = -\log P^{(k)}(c|\mathbf{x}_v, \theta^{(1,k)})$ representing the kth unary potential function defined below in (3) and representing the negative log probability of assigning class c to node v, and $f^{(2,l)} = \sum_{(v,t) \in \mathcal{E}} \phi^{(2,l)}(c_v, c_t, \mathbf{x}; \theta^{(2,l)})$ for $l \in \{1, ..., L\}$ with $\phi^{(2,1)}(c_v, c_t, \mathbf{x}; \theta^{(2,l)}) = (1 - \delta(c_v - c_t)) g(c_v, c_t, \mathbf{x}; \theta^{(2,l)})$ representing the binary potential function that measures the compatibility (indicated by $g(.)$) between nodes v and t when their labels are different (indicated by the Dirac $\delta(.)$). We consider the following binary potentials: 1) $g(c_v, c_t, \mathbf{x}; \theta^{(2,1)}) = 1/\|\mathbf{p}_v - \mathbf{p}_t\|$ (where $\mathbf{p}_v \in \Omega$ denotes the position of node v in the image), 2) $g(c_v, c_t, \mathbf{x}; \theta^{(2,2)}) = 1/\|\mathbf{r}_v - \mathbf{r}_t\|$ (where $\mathbf{r}_v = [P^{(k)}(c_v|\mathbf{x}, \theta^{(1,k)})]_{c_v \in \{1, ..., 4\}, k \in \{1, ..., K\}} \in \mathbb{R}^{4 \times K}$ is a vector of the classifier responses for each class in node v); and 3) $g(c_v, c_t, \mathbf{x}; \theta^{(2,3)}) = 1/(\|\mathbf{p}_v - \mathbf{p}_t\| \times \|\mathbf{r}_v - \mathbf{r}_t\|)$.

The learning procedure is formulated as [4]:

$$\begin{aligned} \underset{\mathbf{w}, \{\xi_n\}_{n=1}^N}{\text{minimize}} \quad & \frac{1}{2}\|\mathbf{w}\|^2 + \frac{C}{N} \sum_{n=1}^N \xi_n \\ \text{subject to} \quad & \max_{h_n \in \mathcal{H}} \mathbf{w}^\top \Psi(\mathbf{x}_n, \mathbf{y}_n, h_n) - \mathbf{w}^\top \Psi(\mathbf{x}_n, \widehat{\mathbf{y}}_n, \widehat{h}_n) \geq \Delta(\mathbf{y}_n, \widehat{\mathbf{y}}_n) - \xi_n \\ & \xi_n \geq 0, \forall \widehat{\mathbf{y}}_n \in \mathcal{Y}, \forall \widehat{h}_n \in \mathcal{H}, n = 1, ..., N, \end{aligned} \quad (2)$$

where ξ_n are the slack variables and $\Delta(\mathbf{y}_n, \widehat{\mathbf{y}}_n) = \sum_{c=1}^3 |\mathbf{y}_n(c) - \widehat{\mathbf{y}}_n(c)|$ measures the loss between annotations $\mathbf{y}_n$ and $\widehat{\mathbf{y}}_n$. The problem in (2) is solved by the following concave-convex procedure [16]: 1) estimation of the latent variable value consistent with annotations and current estimate for $\mathbf{w}$, as in $\max_{h_n \in \mathcal{H}} \mathbf{w}^\top \Psi(\mathbf{x}_n, \mathbf{y}_n, h_n)$; and 2) new estimation of $\mathbf{w}$ using (2) given $\{h_n\}_{n=1}^N$ from step 1. Note that the estimation of $\mathbf{w}$ is based on the cutting plane algorithm [17] that iteratively solves a loss augmented inference problem that inserts a new constraint in the set of most violated constraints with $(\widehat{\mathbf{y}}_n, \widehat{h}_n) = \arg\max_{\mathbf{y} \in \mathcal{Y}, h \in \mathcal{H}} \Delta(\mathbf{y}_n, \mathbf{y}) + \mathbf{w}^\top \Psi(\mathbf{x}, \mathbf{y}, h)$. The inference used for this loss augmented problem and (1) is based on graph cuts (GC) [18], where the high order loss function $\Delta(\mathbf{y}_n, \widehat{\mathbf{y}}_n)$ is integrated into GC based on the decomposition of [6].

2.2 The Flexible and Latent Structure $\mathcal{G} = (\mathcal{V}, \mathcal{E})$

The flexible and latent structure represented by the graph $\mathcal{G} = (\mathcal{V}, \mathcal{E})$ is needed to built $\Psi(.)$ in (1) and (2). The estimation of $\mathcal{G}$ starts with the detection and classification of microvessel pixels (leftmost image in Fig. 3-(b)) using the IF and HE images (Fig. 3-(a)). We define a variable $\mathbf{t} : \Omega \to \{0, 1\}$, where $\mathbf{t}_i = 1$ if the red channel of the IF image at $i \in \Omega$ is larger than $\tau = 0.1$ (from the range $[0, 1]$), otherwise $\mathbf{t}_i = 0$ (see yellow dots in the first image of Fig. 3-(b)). Using the sketches in Fig. 2, we annotate image samples for training the following multiclass classifiers: 1) Adaboost [19], 2) linear SVM [20], 3) random forest [21], and 4) deep convolutional neural networks [22]. The features used by these classifiers

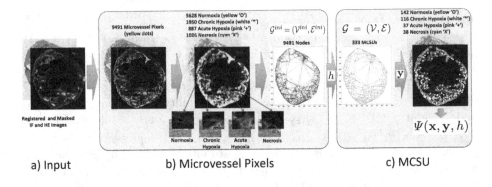

Fig. 3. Building and labeling $\mathcal{G}$. From the IF/HE images (a), microvessel pixels are detected, classified and structured in an initial graph (b), which is modified to represent the MCSU structure (c) that are then used to form $\Psi(.)$ for (1) and (2).

are composed of the pixel values extracted from a patch $\mathbf{x}_i$ of size $200\mu m$, where $\mathbf{t}_i = 1$. Note that, as explained above, the class Ne must be added, where in general, a necrotic patch comprises a red center with black pixels around it in the IF image and a dark purple color in the HE image. This process results in four classifiers: $\{P^{(k)}(c|\mathbf{x}_i, \theta^{(1,k)})\}_{k=1}^{K}$ (with $K = 4$). We show the results from a majority voting process of the four classifiers in the middle image of Fig. 3-(b). We can then form an initial graph using the microvessel pixels, with $\mathcal{G}^{ini} = (\mathcal{V}^{ini}, \mathcal{E}^{ini})$, with $\mathcal{V}^{ini} = \{i|\mathbf{t}_i = 1\}$, and the edges $\mathcal{E}^{ini}$ defined by Delaunay triangulation (rightmost image in Fig. 3-(b)).

The graph $\mathcal{G} = (\mathcal{V}, \mathcal{E})$ is built and labeled using h and $\mathbf{y}$, as follows: 1) estimate the graph structure by running a minimum spanning tree clustering algorithm [23] over the graph $\mathcal{G}^{ini}$, where the edge weight between nodes i and j is defined as $\|\mathbf{p}_i - \mathbf{p}_j\| \times \|\mathbf{r}_i - \mathbf{r}_j\|$ ($\mathbf{p}_i$ is the 2-D position of i and $\mathbf{r}_i$ is the response from the classifiers - this emphasizes that nearby microvessel pixels that have similar classifier responses must be in the same MCSU), and each cluster $\mathcal{C}$ must have a diameter smaller than $h \times 200\mu m$, with $h \in [0.5, 2]$ (this diameter is measured by $\max_{i,j \in \mathcal{C}} \|\mathbf{p}_i - \mathbf{p}_j\|$ with $\mathcal{C} = \{i|i \in \mathcal{V}^{ini}\}$ denoting the set of $\mathcal{G}^{ini}$ nodes belonging to the same cluster); and 2) assuming $\{\mathcal{C}_v\}_{v=1}^{|\mathcal{V}|}$ are the clusters for the nodes $v \in \mathcal{V}$ from step (1), the graph labeling (to be used by $\Psi(.)$ in (1) and (2)) uses the annotation $\mathbf{y}$ as follows:

$$\underset{\mathbf{M}}{\text{minimize}} \quad -\|\mathbf{M} \odot \mathbf{P}\|_F^2 + \sum_{c=1}^{3} \left(\mathbf{y}(c) - \|\mathbf{M} \odot \mathbf{E}_c\|_F^2\right)^2 \tag{3}$$

$$\text{subject to} \quad \mathbf{1}_4^\top \mathbf{M} = \mathbf{1}_{|\mathcal{V}|}^\top, \ \mathbf{M} \in \{0,1\}^{4 \times |\mathcal{V}|},$$

where $\mathbf{P} \in \mathbb{R}^{4 \times |\mathcal{V}|}$, with $\mathbf{P}(c, v) = \prod_{k=1}^{K} P^{(k)}(c|\mathbf{x}_v, \theta^{(1,k)})$ for $c \in \{1, 2, 3, 4\}$ and $v \in \mathcal{V}$ (note that $P^{(k)}(c|\mathbf{x}_v, \theta^{(1,k)}) = \prod_{i \in \mathcal{C}_v} P^{(k)}(c|\mathbf{x}_i, \theta^{(1,k)})$ in (1)), $\mathbf{E}_1 = [\mathbf{1}_{|\mathcal{V}|}, \mathbf{0}_{|\mathcal{V}|}, \mathbf{0}_{|\mathcal{V}|}, \mathbf{0}_{|\mathcal{V}|}]^\top \in \{0,1\}^{4 \times |\mathcal{V}|}$ denotes a matrix with ones in first row and zeros elsewhere (similarly for $c = 2, 3$ with ones in rows 2 and 3), $\mathbf{1}_N$ and $\mathbf{0}_N$ represent a size N column vector of ones or zeros, $\|.\|_F$ denotes the Frobenius norm, $\odot$ represents the Hadamard product, and the summation varies from 1 to 3 because $\mathbf{y}$ has the annotation for three classes only. The optimization in (3) minimizes the objective function by maximizing the label assignment probability and minimizing the difference between the number of MCSU classes in $\mathbf{M}$ and in the variable $\mathbf{y}$. We relax the second constraint to $\mathbf{M} \in [0, 1]$ to make the original integer programming problem feasible. The edge set $\mathcal{E}$ is obtained with Delaunay triangulation (left in Fig. 3-(c)). Note that $\mathbf{M}$ in (3) contains the label of each node $v \in \mathcal{V}$ needed in (1), with $m_v(\mathbf{y}) = \arg\max_{c \in \{1,\ldots,4\}} \mathbf{M}(c, v)$ (right in Fig. 3-(c)). The discrepancy in the number of microvessel pixels and MCSUs shown in Fig. 3(b)-(c) is due to the fact that MCSUs are formed by a set of microvessel pixels, where MCSUs could have been cut in different directions (parallel, oblique, or transversal) during material preparation, and also because MCSUs can vary in size.

3 Materials and Methods

We use the material from [2], consisting of five xenografted human squamous cell carcinoma lines of the head and neck (FaDu), which were transplanted subcutaneously into the right hind leg of nude mice. Each whole tumor cryosection was scanned and photographed using AxioVision 4.7 and the multidimensional and mosaix modules. The IF images of tumor cryosections were prepared with three separate stainings: Pimonidazole was used for visualizing hypoxia (green regions), CD31 for microvessels (red regions), and Hoechst 33342 for perfusion stain (blue). Next, the cover slip was removed to stain the same slice with HE. In total, there are 89 pairs of IF and HE images from eight tumors, where 16 pairs from two tumors are used for training the classifiers $\{P^{(k)}(c|\mathbf{x}_i, \theta^{(1,k)})\}_{k=1}^4$, and the remaining 73 pairs from six tumors for training and testing our proposed weakly supervised latent structured output learning methodology. We run a six-fold cross validation experiment, leaving one tumor out in each run. These pairs of IF and HE images are registered [24] and downsampled such that the resolution is approximately $10\mu m$ per pixel, and a manually delineated mask is used to mark the vital tumor tissue (Fig. 1).

The estimation of $\mathbf{y}^*$ and h^* in (1) and the loss augmented inference in (2) to estimate $\widehat{\mathbf{y}}_n$ and $\widehat{h}_n$ are based on graph cut (alpha-expansion) [18] with $\mathcal{H} = \{0.5, 1, 1.5, 2\}$. We compare our results with an ideal method based on an observed structured SVM, where h is set with a value that best approximates the manually annotated number of MCSUs (that is, h is treated as observed in this ideal method), as in $h^* = \arg\min_h \|\mathbf{1}^\top \mathbf{y} - |\mathcal{V}|\|$, where $|\mathcal{V}|$ is the number of MCSUs in $\mathcal{G}$ (Sec. 2.2). This result produced by this ideal method can be seen as the best case scenario for our latent structured output learning problem. Finally, the quantitative experiment measures the correlation of the percentage and counting of MCSU types between manual and automated annotations in the test sets, using Bland Altman plots [25], which shows the number of samples, sum of squared error (SSE), Pearson r-value squared, linear regression, and p-value.

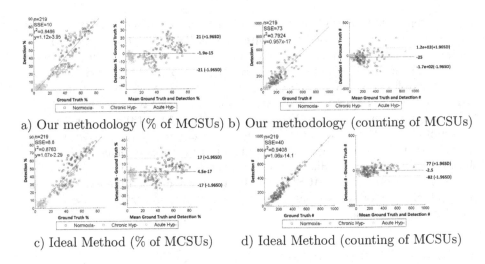

a) Our methodology (% of MCSUs)   b) Our methodology (counting of MCSUs)

c) Ideal Method (% of MCSUs)   d) Ideal Method (counting of MCSUs)

Fig. 4. Bland Altman graphs of the percentage (left) and counting (right) results for the proposed methodology (top) and the ideal method with observed h (bottom).

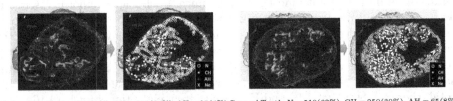

Ground Truth: N = 473(72%), CH = 158(24%), AH = 25(4%) Ground Truth: N = 510(62%), CH = 250(30%), AH = 65(8%)

Detection: N = 423(75%), CH = 111(20%), AH = 29(5%)   Detection: N = 484(67%), CH = 196(27%), AH = 47(6%)

Fig. 5. Automated annotations produced by the proposed methodology. Please see additional results on the supplementary material.

4   Results

Figure 4 (a-b) shows the Bland Altman plots for the proposed methodology for the percentage and counting of MCSU classes, which can be compared to the ideal method in Fig. 4(c-d). In all cases in Fig. 4, the correlation coefficient (r^2) is around 0.8 and above with p-values significantly smaller than 0.01, showing strong correlation results. Finally, Fig. 5 shows examples (using different tumors from the test set) of the annotations produced by our proposed methodology.

5   Discussion and Conclusion

Fig. 4 shows that the proposed methodology produces a result that is comparable to the ideal method (with a "known" h) in the case of percentage of MCSU classes. In the case of counting the MCSU types, our methodology presents a larger variance, but a similar bias. Nevertheless, the correlation coefficient obtained for both cases (MCSU percentage and counting) is large, with values around 0.8 and above and p-values $<< 0.01$, indicating strong correlation results. The qualitative results in Fig. 5 show that our final classification results are similar to the ground truth annotation. These results provide evidence that our approach is potentially useful in a clinical setting for the automated annotation of oxygenation levels in multimodal cytological images.

References

1. Bayer, C., Vaupel, P.: Acute versus chronic hypoxia in tumors. Strahlentherapie und Onkologie **188**(7), 616–627 (2012)
2. Maftei, C.A., et al.: Changes in the fraction of total hypoxia and hypoxia subtypes in human squamous cell carcinomas upon fractionated irradiation: evaluation using pattern recognition in microcirculatory supply units. Radiotherapy and Oncology **101**(1), 209–216 (2011)
3. Yu, C.N.J., Joachims, T.: Learning structural svms with latent variables. In: ICML, pp. 1169–1176 (2009)
4. Kumar, M.P.: Weakly Supervised Learning for Structured Output Prediction. PhD thesis, Ecole Normale Supérieure de Cachan (2014)
5. Lou, X., Hamprecht, F.: Structured learning from partial annotations (2012). arXiv preprint arXiv:1206.6421
6. Pletscher, P., Kohli, P.: Learning low-order models for enforcing high-order statistics. In: AISTATS, pp. 886–894 (2012)
7. Carneiro, G., et al.: Semantic-based indexing of fetal anatomies from 3-d ultrasound data using global/semi-local context and sequential sampling. In: CVPR (2008)
8. Patenaude, B., et al.: A bayesian model of shape and appearance for subcortical brain segmentation. Neuroimage **56**(3), 907–922 (2011)
9. Tu, Z., et al.: Brain anatomical structure segmentation by hybrid discriminative/generative models. TMI **27**(4), 495–508 (2008)
10. Barbu, A., et al.: Automatic detection and segmentation of lymph nodes from ct data. TMI **31**(2), 240–250 (2012)
11. Pauly, O., Glocker, B., Criminisi, A., Mateus, D., Möller, A.M., Nekolla, S., Navab, N.: Fast multiple organ detection and localization in whole-body MR dixon sequences. In: Fichtinger, G., Martel, A., Peters, T. (eds.) MICCAI 2011, Part III. LNCS, vol. 6893, pp. 239–247. Springer, Heidelberg (2011)
12. Zhou, S.K.: Discriminative anatomy detection: Classification vs regression. Pattern Recognition Letters **43**, 25–38 (2014)
13. Fiaschi, L., et al.: Tracking indistinguishable translucent objects over time using weakly supervised structured learning. In: CVPR (2014)
14. Mahapatra, D., et al.: Weakly supervised semantic segmentation of crohn's disease tissues from abdominal mri. In: ISBI (2013)
15. Quellec, G., et al.: Weakly supervised classification of medical images. In: ISBI (2012)
16. Yuille, A.L., Rangarajan, A.: The concave-convex procedure. Neural Computation **15**(4), 915–936 (2003)
17. Joachims, T., et al.: Cutting-plane training of structural svms. Machine Learning **77**(1), 27–59 (2009)

18. Boykov, Y., Veksler, O., Zabih, R.: Fast approximate energy minimization via graph cuts. TPAMI **23**(11), 1222–1239 (2001)
19. Zhu, J., et al.: Multi-class adaboost. Statistics and Its (2009)
20. Tsochantaridis, I., et al.: Support vector machine learning for interdependent and structured output spaces. In: ICML (2004)
21. Breiman, L.: Random forests. Machine Learning **45**(1), 5–32 (2001)
22. Krizhevsky, A., Sutskever, I., Hinton, G.E.: Imagenet classification with deep convolutional neural networks. In: NIPS (2012)
23. Grygorash, O., Zhou, Y., Jorgensen, Z.: Minimum spanning tree based clustering algorithms. In: ICTAI (2006)
24. Peng, T., Yigitsoy, M., Eslami, A., Bayer, C., Navab, N.: Deformable registration of multi-modal microscopic images using a pyramidal interactive registration-learning methodology. In: Ourselin, S., Modat, M. (eds.) WBIR 2014. LNCS, vol. 8545, pp. 144–153. Springer, Heidelberg (2014)
25. Altman, D.G., Bland, J.M.: Measurement in medicine: the analysis of method comparison studies. The statistician, 307–317 (1983)

Identifying Abnormal Network Alterations Common to Traumatic Brain Injury and Alzheimer's Disease Patients Using Functional Connectome Data

Davy Vanderweyen[2], Brent C. Munsell[1(✉)], Jacobo E. Mintzer[4], Olga Mintzer[5], Andy Gajadhar[1], Xun Zhu[2], Guorong Wu[3], Jane Joseph[2], and Alzheimers Disease Neuroimaging Initiative

[1] Department of Computer Science, College of Charleston, Charleston, SC, USA
munsellb@cofc.edu
[2] Department of Neurosciences, Medical University of South Carolina, Charleston, SC, USA
[3] Department of Radiology and BRIC, University of North Carolina at Chapel Hill, Chapel Hill, NC, USA
[4] Clinical Biotechnology Research Institute, Roper St. Francis Hospital, Charleston, SC, USA
[5] Ralph H. Johnson VA Medical Center, Charleston, SC, USA

Abstract. The objective of this study is to determine if patients with traumatic brain injury (TBI) have similar pathological changes in brain network organization as patients with Alzheimer's disease (AD) using functional connectome data reconstructed from resting-state fMRI (rsfMRI). To achieve our objective a novel machine learning technique is proposed that uses a top-down reverse engineering approach to identify abnormal network alterations in functional connectome data that are common to patients with AD and TBI. In general, if the proposed machine learning approach classifies a TBI connectome as AD, then this suggests a common network pathology exists in the connectomes of AD and TBI. The advantage of proposed machine learning technique is twofold: 1) existing longitudinal TBI imaging data is not required, and 2) the potential risk of a TBI patient converting to AD later in life does not require a lengthy and potentially expensive longitudinal imaging study. Experiments are provided that show the AD pathology learned by our connectome-based machine learning technique is able to correctly identify TBI patients with 80% accuracy. In summary, this research may lead to early interventions that can dramatically increase the quality of life for TBI patients who may convert to AD.

1 Introduction

Recent epidemiological studies [6,14] have shown that traumatic brain injury (TBI) is a risk factor for the development of Alzheimer's disease (AD) later in life. Furthermore, the long-term accumulation of both amyloid beta peptide

© Springer International Publishing Switzerland 2015
L. Zhou et al. (Eds.): MLMI 2015, LNCS 9352, pp. 229–237, 2015.
DOI: 10.1007/978-3-319-24888-2_28

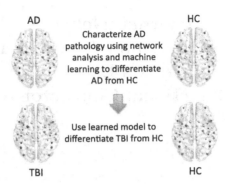

Fig. 1. Basic concept of proposed study. A top-down reverse engineering approach is used to uncover similar pathological changes expressed in the functional connectome of patients with AD and TBI. If the learned classification model identifies a TBI connectome as AD, then this suggests a common network pathology exists in the connectomes of patients with AD and TBI.

deposition and tau pathology, both widely accepted markers of AD pathology, may alter the functional network organization of the brain [3]. Improvements in computational analyses of neuroimaging data now permit the assessment of whole brain maps of functional connectivity, commonly referred to as the *brain connectome* [9]. In particular, resting-state function magnetic resonance imaging (rsfMRI) is a popular paradigm to image the brains intrinsic functional organization while an individual is alert and awake but not engaged in any particular cognitive task. Over the last several years machine learning techniques have been applied on the brain connectome reconstructed from fMRI data to better understand the pathology of patients that suffer from AD [11,12,15] and/or TBI [1,2]. However, little to no research has been performed that evaluates if TBI patients have similar abnormal network alterations, or *pathological changes*, in brain network organization as patients with AD based only functional connectome data, i.e. no EEG, demographic, or biospecimen is included. This research is vitally important for patients suffering from TBI that may have served in the military, or played in a contact sport (such as American football or soccer) where concussions are common, in that, understanding how the pathology expressed in the connectomes of patients with AD is similar to the pathology expressed in the connectomes of patients with TBI may provide crucial information about the risk of converting to AD later in life.

Unfortunately, identifying the level of risk of young Veterans with TBI who may convert to AD is very difficult problem because: 1) existing longitudinal TBI brain imaging data is generally not available, and 2) conducting a longitudinal study that collects and analyzes rsfMRI imaging data over 20 year (or more) period to better understand pathological changes in brain network organization is an expensive and laborious undertaking. To overcome these limitations, a novel machine learning technique is proposed that uses a top-down reverse engineering approach to a discover if a common network pathology exists in the function connectomes of patients with AD and TBI. As illustrated in Fig. 1, in the proposed approach a AD connectome-based classification pipeline is first constructed that uses graph theory based connectivity analysis [7] to identify pathological changes in brain regions capable of differentiating patients with AD from healthy controls (HC). Next, the trained AD classification pipeline is then used to classify patients with TBI. In general, if the classification pipeline recognizes TBI connectomes as AD, then this suggests a common network pathology exists in the connectomes of patients with AD and TBI.

2   Materials and Methods

2.1   Participants

Alzheimer's and healthy control rsfMRI data were obtained from the Alzheimers Disease Neuroimaging Initiative (ADNI) imaging database[1], and TBI rsfMRI data were obtained from the Department of Defense (DoD) ADNI imaging database[2]. In the AD group we studied 15 patients who were diagnosed with AD, in the TBI group we studied 14 patients who were diagnosed with TBI, and the HC group included 40 subjects. The average age (in years) of the AD group is 72, TBI group is 69, and HC group is 71.

2.2   rsfMRI Data Acquisition

All rsfMRI brain scans were gathered by three GE MRI models (Signa HDxt, Discovery MR750, and Discovery MR750w), and a Siemens TrioTim scanner. All GE scanners used an EP/GR pulse sequence with parameters TE=30 ms, flip angle=90°, number of slices=48, slice thickness= 3.3 mm, spatial resolution=$3.28 \times 3.28 \times 3.3$ mm^3, 160 volumes, and matrix=64×64. They only differed in the TR (Discovery MR750=2900 ms; Discovery MR750w=3520 ms; Signa HDxt=2925 ms). The Siemens scanner used an EP pulse sequence with parameters TE=30 ms, TR=3000 ms, flip angle=80°, number of slices=48, slice thickness=3.3 mm, spatial resolution=$3.31 \times 3.31 \times 3.3$ mm^3, 140 volumes, and matrix=64×57.

2.3   rsfMRI Data Preprocessing

The preprocessing steps recommended by [5] for graph theory based connectivity analysis using FSL^3 were followed. Preprocessing steps include slice timing correction, motion correction (MCFLIRT) with rigid-body alignment, geometric distortion correction (FUGUE), and grand mean intensity scaling normalization. Preprocessed images are resampled to 3 mm^3 isotropic voxels and registered to

---

[1] adni.loni.usc.edu

[2] http://www.adni-info.org/DOD.aspx

[3] http://www.fmrib.ox.ac.uk/fsl

MNI space and then parcellated using a 264 region atlas [4]. Regression using FSL is applied to remove effects of global signal and head motion. Regressors include global signal (using a whole-brain mask), and head motion [5]. The residual image from this regression step is then band-pass filtered (.009 to .08 Hz) and spatially smoothed (FWHM=6 mm). After preprocessing, rsfMRI signal is extracted in each of the 264 regions-of-interest (ROIs) defined in the Power atlas using FSLs "Featquery" function. Each ROI is represented by a 10 mm diameter sphere.

2.4   Functional Connectome Reconstruction

Using the atlas ROIs, a $m \times m$ functional connectivity matrix C is reconstructed for each subject where $m = 264$. *In general graph terms, the functional connectivity matrix is a weighted adjacency matrix that represents a fully connected undirected graph.* More specifically, each matrix element reflects the functional connection between two nodes (ROIs), and is found by computing the correlation between two discrete time-series rsfMRI signals. Correlations between two discrete time-series rsfMRI signals is calculated using the partial correlation measure that includes a shrinkage operation [8].

2.5   Node-Based Connectome Feature Vector

The next step is to convert the correlation values defined in C to a m dimension node-based connectome feature vector $\mathbf{a}_i^v = (a_{i1}^v, \ldots, a_{im}^v)$ using one of the two graph-theoretic measures (denoted by v) outlined below.

Betweenness Centrality: Is a global measure that represents the fraction of shortest paths that go through a particular node (or brain region) defined in the connectome. The betweenness centrality measure for node i is $a_i = \frac{1}{(N-1)(N-2)} \sum_{h,j \in N} \frac{\rho_{hj}^i}{\rho_{hj}}$, where $h \neq j$, $h \neq i$, $j \neq i$, The number of shortest path between node h and j is represented by ρ_{hj}, the number of these shortest paths going through node i is represented by ρ_{hj}^i, and N is the total number of the nodes in the network. This measure normalized to a value in $[0\ 1]$, where $(N-1)(N-2)$ is the highest score attainable in the network.

Clustering Coefficient: Is a measure of local influence or connectivity that determines which nodes (or brain regions) are most central to a local neighborhood of nodes. The clustering coefficient for node i is $a_i = \frac{2t_i}{k_i(k_i-1)}$, where k_i is the number of nodes adjacent to node i, and t_i is the number of 3-clique subgraphs adjacent to node i.

2.6   Alzheimer's Disease Classification Pipeline

The trained classification pipeline defines two sequential components: 1) *Node feature selection* and 2) *SVM classifier*. The specifics of each trained pipeline component, and how pipeline classification performance is assessed are provided below.

Node-Base Connectome Feature Selection: Given a $n \times m$ training data matrix $A^v = [\mathbf{a}_1^v, \mathbf{a}_2^v, \ldots, \mathbf{a}_n^v]$ of n subjects (combination of AD and HC), where row vector is a node-base connectome feature vector for subject i derived using graph measure v (see Section 2.5), and $\mathbf{y} = (y_1, y_2, \ldots, y_n)$ is a n dimension vector that defines the binary group label for each subject in the training data set (i.e. the paired diagnosis information for row vector $\mathbf{a}_i^v$ is y_i). A least squares linear regression algorithm with a ℓ_1 regularization term, i.e. LASSO [10], is used to find a sparse m dimension weight vector $\mathbf{x}$ that minimizes

$$\min_x \frac{1}{2} \|A^v \mathbf{x} - \mathbf{y}\|_2^2 + \lambda \|\mathbf{x}\|_1 ,$$

where $\lambda \|\mathbf{x}\|_1$ is the ℓ_1 regularization (sparsity) term. The above equation is optimized using the LeastR function in the Sparse Learning with Efficient Projections software package[4]. After optimization, $\mathbf{x}$ has weight values in [0 1] where > 0 indicate network nodes that contribute to the clinical outcome. In general, $\mathbf{x}$ is referred to as the sparse representation of training data set. In our approach weight values greater than zero are set to one, therefore the resulting sparse representation becomes a binary mask. That is, a network node is turned on (value of 1) or turned off (value of 0). A new $n \times m$ sparse training matrix $\tilde{A}^v = [\tilde{\mathbf{a}}_1^v, \ldots, \tilde{\mathbf{a}}_n^v]$ is created, where row vector $\tilde{\mathbf{a}}_i^v = (a_{i1}^v x_1, a_{i2}^v x_2, \ldots, a_{im}^v x_m)$. For the results reported in Section 3.1, the value of λ was set to 0.1.

AD Classifier: $\tilde{A}^v$ and $\mathbf{y}$ are used to train a linear two-class SVM classifier based on the LIBSVM library[5]. Once the SVM classifier is trained, the outcome functional connectome not included in the training data set can be predicted as follows: 1) Compute $\mathbf{a}^v$ the node-based connectome feature vector using graph measure v. 2) Create sparse feature vector $\tilde{\mathbf{a}}_i^v$ by applying learned binary weights. 3) Calculate the predicted class label $y = \sum_{i=1}^{m} \alpha_i k(\phi_i, \tilde{\mathbf{a}}^v) + b$, where $k(\cdot)$ is the inner product of two vectors, and α_i is the weight, ϕ_i is the support vector, and b is the bias that defines the linear hyper-plane (decision boundary) learned by the SVM classifier. The sign of the calculated prediction value (i.e., $y \geq 0$ or $y < 0$) determines the class label (i.e. group) the test subject belongs to.

Performance Assessment: Classification performance of the proposed pipeline is assessed using a leave-on-out cross-validation (LOOCV) strategy that iteratively removes one subject from the population as the test subject, and the remaining subjects are used for training. Using the combined 2-by-2 confusion matrix results of each test subject, classification performance is reported using the specificity=TP/(TP+FN), sensitivity=TN/(FP+TN), positive predictive value (PPV)=TP/(TP+FP), negative predictive value (NPV)=TN/(TN+FN),

---

[4] http://www.public.asu.edu/~jye02/Software/SLEP
[5] http://www.csie.ntu.edu.tw/~cjlin/libsvm

and accuracy=(TP+TN)/(TP+FN+FP+TN) measures, where TP = true positive, TN = true negative, FP = false positive, FN = false negative.

2.7 TBI Connectome Classification Using AD Pipeline

If a population of n subjects is used to assess AD classification performance, then a set of n trained AD pipelines $\{P_i^v\}_{i=1}^n$ are created by the LOOCV strategy described in Section 2.6, where $P_i^v = \{\mathbf{x}, \alpha_i, \phi_i, b_i\}$ is the trained AD pipeline at iteration i, v is the graph measure, vector $\mathbf{x}_i$ is the learned sparse representation at iteration i, and the learned SVM classifier parameters at iteration i are scalar b_i and vectors α_i and ϕ_i. Given the AD trained pipelines, and a set of k node-based connectome feature vectors $\{\mathbf{t}_j^v\}_{j=1}^k$ that represent subjects diagnosed with TBI, **Algorithm 1** is used to assess TBI classification performance. In particular, the *classify* function on *line-4* returns a 0 value if TBI subject j is classified as HC using AD pipeline i, and returns a value of 1 if classified as AD.

Algorithm 1. TBI connectomes classified as AD

1: $p \leftarrow$ zeros $(1, n)$ ▷ create an array of n elements initialized to zero.
2: **for** $i \leftarrow 1$ **to** n **do**
3:      **for** $j \leftarrow 1$ **to** k **do**
4:          $p(i) \leftarrow p(i) + $ *classify* $(\mathbf{t}_j^v, P_i^v)$ ▷ $\mathbf{t}_j^v = (t_{j1}^v, \ldots, t_{jm}^v)$ is a m dimension node-based connectome feature vector.
5:      **end for**
6:      $p(i) \leftarrow p(i)/k$
7: **end for**
8: *statistics*(p) ▷ compute the mean, stdev, and variance.

On *line-6* the total number of TBI subjects classified as AD is then normalized by the number total number of TBI subject in the population, where 0 indicates all TBI subjects are classified as HC, and 1 indicates all TBI subjects are classified as AD. When the outer for-loop completes the mean, standard deviation, and variance is computed by the *statistics* function using the values in array p.

3 Results

3.1 AD Classification Results

In this experiment, the total number of subjects in the connectome data set is 55, including 15 AD patients and 40 HCs. The binary class labels used to train the classification pipeline are 1=AD and 0=HC. Table 1 shows the LOOCV results for each graph measure. The best performance PPV=86% and ACC=82% is achieved by a classification pipeline trained using node-based features derived from the clustering coefficient algorithm.

Table 1. AD vs. HC classification results for two different graph measures. The highest performance measures are shown in bold font.

Graph measure	SEN	SPE	PPV	NPV	ACC
Betweenness	**86%**	57%	43%	**92%**	65%
Clustering coefficient	40%	**98%**	**86%**	81%	**82%**

The total number of non-zero network nodes (i.e. brain regions) $|\mathbf{x}_t|$ selected by the LASSO algorithm that can differentiate AD from HC patients is 44. Specifically, $\mathbf{x}_t = \bigcup_{f=1}^{55} \mathbf{x}_f$ is the union of each learned sparse representation for each LOOCV fold. Using a two-sample t-test with $\alpha = 0.05$, a paired[6] p-value is calculated for each non-zero network node in $\mathbf{x}_t$ and then sorted in ascending order, where the null hypothesis represents data that are independent random samples from normal distributions with equal means and equal but unknown variances. The top 10 non-zero nodes with the smallest p-values, i.e., those with the greatest difference between the two groups, are listed and visualized in Fig. 2 using the Brainnet viewer [13] software package.

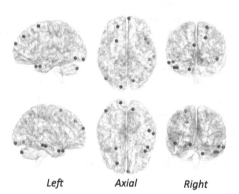

Region	Description
106	R Dorsomedial prefrontal
82	R Temporal pole
178	L Superior frontal gyrus
9	R Medial temporal gyrus
104	L Dorsolateral prefrontal
154	L Lateral secondary visual cortex
128	R Anterior medial temporal
11	R Inferior temporal gyrus
142	L Primary visual cortex
184	R Superior semilunar lobule of cerebellum

Left   Axial   Right

Fig. 2. The top 10 nodes (or brain regions) with the smallest p-value (i.e., nodes with the greatest difference between AD and HC patients). The p-values are calculated using a two-sample t-test. Note: the brain regions are defined using the Power atlas, and are represented by the red nodes.

3.2   TBI Connectome Classification Resutls Using AD Pipeline

In this experiment, the total number of TBI subjects in the connectome data set is 14. Table-2 shows the results for each graph measure using the assessment strategy outlined in Algorithm 1 in Section 2.7. The best TBI classification performance is achieved by a AD pipeline trained using node-based features derived from the clustering coefficient algorithm.

---

[6] Corresponded nodes between the AD and HC groups.

Table 2. TBI classification results using trained AD pipeline for two different node-based graph measures. The highest performance measures are shown in bold font.

Graph measure	mean	stdev	variance
Betweenness	63%	14%	1.9%
Clustering coefficient	**80%**	13%	1.8%

4   Discussion

In this paper a novel machine learning approach is presented that uses a pipeline trained with AD connectome data to classify connectomes of patients with TBI. Specifically, using graph theory network based network analysis a classification pipeline capable of recognizing abnormal network alterations, or pathological changes, found in functional connectomes of patients with AD reconstructed from rsfMRI is trained, then the trained pipeline is used to classify connectomes of patients with TBI also reconstructed from rsfMRI. Our general hypothesis is, a common network pathology exists in the connectomes of patients with AD and TBI. Based on TBI classification results in Table-2, this supports our hypothesis. Even though the number of subjects (AD and HC) used to train the AD classification pipeline are small, we feel our findings are clinically important, and when larger rsfMRI data sets become available the proposed approach may significantly advance AD outcome forcasting in the context of patients that convert from TBI to AD later in life. Lastly, a common problem encountered during the training procedure is to over fit the constructed model to connectome data acquired from the same MRI scanner at the same site. As a result, when given unseen connectome data derived from subjects scanned using a different scanner or a different site, the over fit model could be too specific and may adversely affect TBI classification performance. The results in Table-2 suggest the trained AD classification pipeline appears to robust to site and/or scanner differences.

References

1. Han, K., Mac Donald, C.L., Johnson, A.M., Barnes, Y., Wierzechowski, L., Zonies, D., Oh, J., Flaherty, S., Fang, R., Raichle, M.E., et al.: Disrupted modular organization of resting-state cortical functional connectivity in us military personnel following concussive mildblast-related traumatic brain injury. Neuroimage **84**, 76–96 (2014)
2. Messé, A., Caplain, S., Pélégrini-Issac, M., Blancho, S., Lévy, R., Aghakhani, N., Montreuil, M., Benali, H., Lehéricy, S.: Specific and evolving resting-state network alterations in post-concussion syndrome following mild traumatic brain injury. PloS one **8**(6), e65470 (2013)
3. Mormino, E.C., Smiljic, A., Hayenga, A.O., H. Onami, S., Greicius, M.D., Rabinovici, G.D., Janabi, M., Baker, S.L., Yen, I.V., Madison, C.M., Miller, B.L., Jagust, W.J.: Relationships between beta-amyloid and functional connectivity in different components of the default mode network in aging. Cerebral Cortex (2011)
4. Power, J.D., Barnes, K.A., Snyder, A.Z., Schlaggar, B.L., Petersen, S.E.: Spurious but systematic correlations in functional connectivity MRI networks arise from subject motion. Neuroimage **59**(3), 2142–2154 (2012)

5. Power, J.D., Mitra, A., Laumann, T.O., Snyder, A.Z., Schlaggar, B.L., Petersen, S.E.: Methods to detect, characterize, and remove motion artifact in resting state fMRI. Neuroimage **84**, 320–341 (2014)
6. Qureshi, S.U., Kimbrell, T., Pyne, J.M., Magruder, K.M., Hudson, T.J., Petersen, N.J., Yu, H.J., Schulz, P.E., Kunik, M.E.: Greater prevalence and incidence of dementia in older veterans with posttraumatic stress disorder. J. Am. Geriatr. Soc. **58**(9), 1627–1633 (2010)
7. Rubinov, M., Sporns, O.: Weight-conserving characterization of complex functional brain networks. Neuroimage **56**(4), 2068–2079 (2011)
8. Schäfer, J., Strimmer, K.: A shrinkage approach to large-scale covariance matrix estimation and implications for functional genomics. Statistical applications in genetics and molecular biology **4**(1) (2005)
9. Sporns, O.: The human connectome: origins and challenges. Neuroimage **80**, 53–61 (2013)
10. Tibshirani, R.: Regression shrinkage and selection via the lasso. Journal of the Royal Statistical Society, Series B **58**, 267–288 (1994)
11. Wang, J., Zuo, X., Dai, Z., Xia, M., Zhao, Z., Zhao, X., Jia, J., Han, Y., He, Y.: Disrupted functional brain connectome in individuals at risk for alzheimer's disease. Biological Psychiatry **73**(5), 472–481 (2013)
12. Wee, C.Y., Yap, P.T., Zhang, D., Denny, K., Browndyke, J.N., Potter, G.G., Welsh-Bohmer, K.A., Wang, L., Shen, D.: Identification of MCI individuals using structural and functional connectivity networks. NeuroImage **59**(3), 2045–2056 (2012)
13. Xia, M., Wang, J., He, Y.: BrainNet Viewer: a network visualization tool for human brain connectomics. PLoS ONE **8**(7), e68910 (2013)
14. Yaffe, K., Vittinghoff, E., Lindquist, K., Barnes, D., Covinsky, K.E., Neylan, T., Kluse, M., Marmar, C.: Posttraumatic stress disorder and risk of dementia among US veterans. Arch. Gen. Psychiatry **67**(6), 608–613 (2010)
15. Zhao, X., Liu, Y., Wang, X., Liu, B., Xi, Q., Guo, Q., Jiang, H., Jiang, T., Wang, P.: Disrupted small-world brain networks in moderate alzheimer's disease: a resting-state fmri study. PloS one **7**(3), e33540 (2012)

Multimodal Multi-label Transfer Learning for Early Diagnosis of Alzheimer's Disease

Bo Cheng, Mingxia Liu, and Daoqiang Zhang[✉]

Department of Computer Science and Engineering,
Nanjing University of Aeronautics and Astronautics, Nanjing 210016, China
dqzhang@nuaa.edu.cn

Abstract. Recent machine learning based studies for early Alzheimer's disease (AD) diagnosis focus on the joint learning of both regression and classification tasks. However, most of existing methods only use data from a single domain, and thus cannot utilize the intrinsic useful correlation information among data from correlated domains. Accordingly, in this paper, we consider the joint learning of multi-domain regression and classification tasks with multimodal features for AD diagnosis. Specifically, we propose a novel multimodal multi-label transfer learning framework, which consists of two key components: 1) a multi-domain multi-label feature selection (MDML) model that selects the most informative feature subset from multi-domain data, and 2) multimodal regression and classification methods that can predict clinical scores and identify the conversion of mild cognitive impairment (MCI) to AD patients, respectively. Experimental results on the Alzheimer's Disease Neuroimaging Initiative (ADNI) database show that the proposed method help improve the performances of both clinical score prediction and disease status identification, compared with the state-of-the-art methods.

1 Introduction

Alzheimer's disease (AD) is characterized by the progressive impairment of neurons and their connections, which leads to the loss of cognitive function and the ultimate death. It is reported that an estimated 700,000 older Americans will die with AD, and many of them will die from complications caused by AD in 2014 [1]. Thus, for timely therapy that might be effective to slow the disease progression, it is important for early diagnosis of AD and its early stage, i.e., mild cognitive impairment (MCI). Recently, many machine learning methods based on multimodal biomarkers have been used for early diagnosis of AD [2-5]. These multimodal data include the structural brain atrophy measurements from magnetic resonance imaging (MRI) scans, brain of functional changes by using the fluorodeoxyglucose positron emission tomography (FDG-PET), and pathological amyloid depositions measured through cerebrospinal fluid (CSF). Existing studies have shown that fusing multimodal biomarkers can provide complementary information for learning models, which helps improve the performances compared to methods using single-modality biomarkers [2-5].

In the literature, rather than only identifying disease status in classification problems, several studies begin to predict continuous clinical scores from brain images

© Springer International Publishing Switzerland 2015
L. Zhou et al. (Eds.): MLMI 2015, LNCS 9352, pp. 238–245, 2015.
DOI: 10.1007/978-3-319-24888-2_29

[3,6,13], such as Alzheimer's Disease Assessment Scale-Cognitive subscale (ADAS-Cog) and Mini-Mental State Examination (MMSE). It is worth nothing that, predicting clinical scores helps evaluate the stage of AD pathology and predict future progression [3,13]. On the other hand, some recent studies have indicated that the tasks of identifying disease status and predicting clinical scores are highly correlated, and the joint learning of regression and classification tasks can help alleviate the small-sample-size problem [3,7,8]. In these methods, the tasks of identifying disease status and predicting clinical scores are considered as different learning tasks, and multi-task learning methods are used to combine those different learning tasks.

However, most of existing studies on the joint learning of regression and classification only focus on using data from a single learning domain, and thus cannot utilize the intrinsic useful correlation information among data from different learning domains. In machine learning community, transfer learning provides an effective solution to deal with the problem involving multiple learning domains of data, and it assumes that the different learning domains have a certain correlation [15]. More recently, several studies have developed transfer learning-based methods for MCI converters (MCI-C) prediction, by treating AD/NC as auxiliary domain to help the learning problem in target domain of MCI-C/MCI non-converters (MCI-NC) [4,9,10]. Although these methods demonstrate that transfer learning methods yield better performance than conventional single-domain based methods, the underlying correlation among different domains is seldom considered in their learning models.

Inspired by the above problems, in this paper, we propose a novel multimodal multi-label transfer learning framework to jointly learn multi-domain regression and classification tasks by using multimodal data. Specifically, we first propose a Multi-Domain Multi-Label feature selection (MDML) method based on transfer learning and multi-label learning, which is used to select the most informative feature-subset from multi-domain data. Then, we employ the multi-kernel support vector machine (M-SVM) for classification and the multi-kernel relevance vector regression machine (M-RVR) for regression, which are used to identify MCI-C patients and to predict clinical scores, respectively. We validate the efficacy of our proposed method on both single-modality and multimodal data (including MRI, FDG-PET and CSF) from the ADNI database.

2 Method

In this section, we introduce our proposed multimodal multi-label transfer learning framework. Specifically, in Section 2.1, we first develop a multi-domain multi-label (MDML) feature selection method for selecting the most discriminative features. Then, in Section 2.2, we employ the multimodal regression and classification methods to predict clinical scores and identify the conversion of MCI to AD patients, respectively.

2.1 Multi-domain Multi-label Feature Selection

In the early AD diagnosis, it is very important to find discriminative brain regions from brain images (e.g., MRI and PET images). In the literature, Lasso-based sparse learning methods are widely used for feature selection to identify the most informative multimodal biomarkers [11], and have been shown effective in improving the classification performance. On the other hand, some studies suggest that the tasks of identifying disease status and predicting clinical scores are highly correlated. However, traditional Lasso-based methods cannot capture the intrinsic useful correlation information among different label groups (e.g., class labels and clinical score labels). For addressing that problem, we propose a sparse multi-label group Lasso model, by incorporating the underlying correlation information into the learning process.

Assume we have a training set $\mathbf{X} = \{\mathbf{x}_n\}_{n=1}^N \in \mathbb{R}^{N \times F}$ with N samples, where $\mathbf{x}_n \in \mathbb{R}^F$ is a sample with F features. Denote the label matrix for the training data as $\mathbf{Y} = [\mathbf{y}^1, ..., \mathbf{y}^l, ..., \mathbf{y}^L] \in \mathbb{R}^{N \times L}$, where $\mathbf{y}^l = \{y_n^l\}_{n=1}^N \in \mathbb{R}^N$ is the l-th type of labels and L is the number of label groups. In this study, there are three different label groups ($L = 3$), including 1) class labels $\mathbf{y}^1$, 2) MMSE score labels $\mathbf{y}^2$, and 3) ADAS-Cog score labels $\mathbf{y}^3$. Let $\mathbf{W} \in \mathbb{R}^{F \times L}$ represent the weight matrix, with the row vector $\mathbf{w}_f$ denoting the coefficient vector associated with f-th feature across different label groups. Then, our proposed sparse multi-label group Lasso model is formulated as follows:

$$\min_{\mathbf{W}} \frac{1}{2} \|\mathbf{Y} - \mathbf{XW}\|_F^2 + \lambda_1 \|\mathbf{W}\|_{1,1} + \lambda_2 \|\mathbf{W}\|_{2,1} \tag{1}$$

where the second term $\|\mathbf{W}\|_{1,1} = \sum_{f=1}^F \sum_{l=1}^L |w_{f,l}|$ can select a discriminative subset of samples relevant self-label group, and the last term $\|\mathbf{W}\|_{2,1} = \sum_{f=1}^F \|\mathbf{w}_f\|_2$ is a 'group sparsity' regularizer that is used to simultaneously select a common feature subset relevant to all label groups. In addition, λ_1 and λ_2 are two regularization parameters that control the relative contributions of those three terms in Eq. (1). Here, the term $\|\cdot\|_F$ is the Frobenius norm of a matrix. By using a specific optimization algorithm [12,14] for solving the optimization problem of Eq. (1), we can get the sparse weight matrix $\mathbf{W}$, where features corresponding to those non-zero coefficients in $\mathbf{W}$ will be selected. In this way, we can find a common feature subset corresponding to all label groups.

Although the sparse multi-label group Lasso model can extract useful correlation information among different label groups, it only addresses the issue of single-domain learning. In the single-domain learning, we separately adopt the sparse multi-label group Lasso model to handle the multiple related domain data and get the multiple weight matrices $\{\mathbf{W}^1, ..., \mathbf{W}^d, ..., \mathbf{W}^D\}$, where D is the number of related learning domains with an index $d \in \{1, \cdots, D\}$, thus it cannot utilize the intrinsic useful correlation information among multiple related learning domains. To join the multiple related learning domain data, we extend the sparse multi-label group Lasso model to a multi-domain multi-label learning (MDML) model, which is formulated as follows:

$$\min_{\mathbf{W}} \frac{1}{2} \sum_{d=1}^D \|\mathbf{Y}^d - \mathbf{X}^d \mathbf{W}^d\|_F^2 + \lambda_1 \sum_{d=1}^D \|\mathbf{W}^d\|_{1,1} + \lambda_2 \sum_{d=1}^D \|\mathbf{W}^d\|_{2,1} + \\ \lambda_3 \sum_{l=1}^L \sum_{d=1}^{D-1} \|\mathbf{w}^{l,d} - \mathbf{w}^{l,d+1}\|_F^2 \tag{2}$$

where $\lambda_1, \lambda_2, \lambda_3 > 0$ are the regularization parameters that control the relative contributions of the four terms, and the last term $\|\mathbf{w}^{l,d} - \mathbf{w}^{l,d+1}\|_F^2$ is adopted to keep the temporal smoothness of multi-weight vector $\mathbf{w}^{l,d}$ among multiple related learning domains [6]. We propose to solve the optimization problem of Eq. (2) by the accelerated gradient method (AGM) [12]. In this study, there are two learning domains (i.e., $D = 2$, AD/NC subjects as the related learning domain, and MCI-C/MCI-NC subjects as the target domain).

2.2   Multimodal Regression and Classification

After MDML feature selection on the multi-domain training data, we will employ the multimodal regression and classification methods for combining with multimodal features in the target domain. Similar to the works in [2,3], in our multimodal multi-label transfer learning framework, we use the multi-kernel learning method to combine multimodal features. Specifically, we adopt the multi-kernel support vector machine (M-SVM) [3] to identify the MCI-C patients and employ the multi-kernel relevance vector machine regression (M-RVR) [2] method to predict the clinical scores.

Given M sets of data extracted from different modalities, we first compute the multimodal kernel matrixes $\{\mathbf{K}^{(1)}, \ldots, \mathbf{K}^{(m)}, \ldots, \mathbf{K}^{(M)}\}$. Then, we use the multi-kernel learning method to define a new integrated kernel function for two subjects in the m-th modality (i.e., $\mathbf{x}_a^{(m)}$ and $\mathbf{x}_b^{(m)}$) as follows:

$$k(\mathbf{x}_a, \mathbf{x}_b) = \sum_{m=1}^{M} c_m k^{(m)}(\mathbf{x}_a^{(m)}, \mathbf{x}_b^{(m)}) \qquad (3)$$

where $k^{(m)}$ denotes the kernel function for the m-th modality, and c_m denotes the weight for the m-th modality. From Eq. (3), we can achieve the integrated target domain kernel matrix $\mathbf{K} = \sum_{m=1}^{M} c_m \mathbf{K}^{(m)}$. To find the optimal values for weights c_m, we constrain them so that $\sum_m c_m = 1, 0 \leq c_m \leq 1$ and then adopt a *coarse-grid search* through cross-validation on the training data, which has been shown effective in extensive studies [2,3].

3   Experiments

In this section, we evaluate the effectiveness of our proposed multimodal multi-label transfer learning framework on multimodal data (including MRI, PET and CSF) from the Alzheimer's Disease Neuroimaging Initiative (ADNI) database. In the following, we first introduce the experimental settings, and then show the experimental results and discussion.

3.1   Experimental Settings

In our experiments, the baseline ADNI subjects with all corresponding MRI, PET, CSF, MMSE, and ADAS-Cog data are included, which leads to a total of 202 subjects (including 51 AD subjects, 99 MCI subjects, and 52 normal controls (NCs)). For the 99 MCI subjects, it includes 43 MCI converters and 56 MCI non-converters. We use 51 AD and 52 NC subjects as related learning domain, and 99 MCI subjects as target domain. Similar to [3], we adopt an image pre-processing procedure for all MRI and PET images to extract ROI-based features. In addition, three CSF biomarkers are also used in this study, namely CSF $A\beta_{42}$, CSF t-tau, and CSF p-tau. As a result, for each subject, we have 93 features derived from MRI images, 93 features generated from PET images, and 3 features obtained from CSF biomarkers.

To evaluate the performance of different learning methods, we use a 10-fold cross-validation strategy and repeat this process 10 times to compute the average classification accuracy, sensitivity, specificity, and AUC (Area Under the ROC Curve) value. We also adopt the popular root-mean-square error (RMSE) and the correlation coefficient (CORR) as regression performance measures. In particular, for classifying MCI-C and MCI-NC, we use the 10-fold cross-validation on 99 MCI subjects, and we use the 10-fold cross-validation on all 202 subjects for regression. The SVM classifier is implemented using the LIBSVM toolbox (http://www.csie.ntu.edu.tw/~cjlin/libsvm/), with a linear kernel and a default value for the parameter C ($C = 1$). The regularization parameters (i.e., λ_1, λ_2 and λ_3) can be chosen from the range of Ω^1 by an inner 10-fold cross-validation on the training data. The RVM regression is implemented using Sparse Bayesian toolbox (http://www.miketipping.com/), with the Gaussian kernel with the width parameter selected from range $\{2^1, 2^2, 2^3, 2^4, 2^5, 2^6, 2^7, 2^8\}$ that can be determined by an inner 10-fold cross-validation on the training data. In particular, the multi-kernel combination weights are determined via a grid search with range from 0 to 1 and step size 0.1 on the training data. In addition, we also perform the same feature normalization scheme as in [3] in our experiments.

3.2 Results

In the experiments of MCI-C vs. MCI-NC classification, we compare our proposed method with SVM/M-SVM, Lasso, ML-gLasso and Multi-task feature selection (MTFS) [3] methods by using both single-modality data and multimodal data, with results shown in Table 1. It is worth noting that, SVM and M-SVM denote methods using SVM for single-modality and M-SVM for multimodal data without feature selection, respectively. At the same time, Lasso, ML-gLasso, MTFS and MDML denote methods using corresponding feature selection (i.e., Lasso, ML-gLasso, MTFS and MDML) algorithms and adopting SVM/M-SVM methods for classification. In Fig. 1, we also present the ROC curves achieved by different methods for multimodal case. As we can see from Table 1 and Fig. 1, our proposed MDML method consistently achieves better results than SVM/M-SVM, Lasso, MTFS and ML-gLasso methods in terms of all performance measures, which validates the efficacy of our MDML method on using AD and NC subjects as related learning domain. Specifically, in multimodal case, our proposed MDML method can achieve a classification accuracy of 0.787, which is significantly better than M-SVM, Lasso, MTFS and ML-gLasso methods which achieve only 0.638, 0.673, 0.717 and 0.716, respectively.   In addition, our proposed ML-gLasso method also achieves better results than SVM/M-SVM, and Lasso methods. It implies that multi-label learning can effectively utilize the intrinsic useful correlation information from multi-label groups.

---

^{1} $\Omega \in \{0.00001, 0.0001, 0.0005, 0.001, 0.004, 0.007, 0.01, 0.02, 0.03, 0.05, 0.06, 0.08, 0.1, 0.2, 0.4, 0.6, 0.8\}$

Table 1. Comparison of performance of four methods for MCI-C vs. MCI-NC classification using different modalities. (ACC=Accuracy, SEN=Sensitivity, SPE = Specificity, ML-gLasso= Multi-Label group Lasso).

Modality	Method	ACC	SEN	SPE	AUC
MRI+PET+CSF	M-SVM	0.638	0.588	0.677	0.683
	Lasso	0.673	0.739	0.588	0.728
	ML-gLasso	0.716	0.763	0.654	0.761
	MTFS	0.717	0.768	0.649	0.766
	MDML	**0.787**	**0.822**	**0.738**	**0.843**
MRI	SVM	0.539	0.476	0.577	0.554
	Lasso	0.636	0.675	0.583	0.696
	ML-gLasso	0.688	0.722	0.643	0.715
	MTFS	0.667	0.703	0.619	0.718
	MDML	**0.732**	**0.761**	**0.694**	**0.774**
PET	SVM	0.580	0.521	0.625	0.612
	Lasso	0.609	0.651	0.554	0.662
	ML-gLasso	0.642	0.680	0.593	0.635
	MTFS	0.629	0.668	0.578	0.624
	MDML	**0.700**	**0.732**	**0.659**	**0.749**

Table 2. Comparison of performance of four methods for prediction of MMSE/ ADAS-Cog scores using different modalities, respectively.

Modality	Method	MMSE		ADAS-Cog	
		RMSE	CORR	RMSE	CORR
MRI+PET+CSF	M-RVR	2.171	0.526	4.753	0.623
	Lasso	2.039	0.622	4.550	0.686
	mLasso	2.003	0.647	4.415	0.714
	MTFS	1.975	0.655	4.346	0.708
	MDML	**1.963**	**0.663**	**4.258**	**0.725**
MRI	RVR	2.312	0.449	5.422	0.474
	Lasso	2.179	0.514	5.239	0.509
	mLasso	2.128	0.541	5.071	0.552
	MTFS	2.104	0.557	5.004	0.570
	MDML	**2.085**	**0.565**	**4.928**	**0.588**
PET	RVR	2.327	0.387	4.946	0.583
	Lasso	2.215	0.488	4.651	0.646
	mLasso	2.131	0.538	4.494	0.676
	MTFS	2.115	0.551	4.414	0.690
	MDML	**2.094**	**0.561**	**4.314**	**0.704**

On the other hand, our proposed method can be used to predict the clinical scores. Accordingly, in the second group of experiments, we compare our MDML method with RVR/M-RVR, Lasso, mLasso and MTFS [3] methods for both single-modality and multimodal cases. It is worth noting that, for MDML method, without related learning domain can be used for the prediction of clinical scores. In addition, the mLasso feature selection is a variant of ML-gLasso, which has no $L_{1,1}$-norm regularization term and only selects a common feature subset relevant to all label types. Table 2 shows their prediction performance for MMSE/ADAS-Cog scores using different modalities. Similar to the classification experiments, we first use Lasso, mLasso, MTFS and MDML methods to perform feature selection, and then adopt RVR for single-modality and M-RVR for multimodal for regression, respectively. Note that RVR/M-RVR methods denote using RVR or M-RVR method without feature selection for MMSE/ADAS-Cog scores prediction. From Table 2, one can observe that our proposed MDML method consistently achieves better results than RVR/M-RVR, Lasso, mLasso and MTFS methods, which further validates the efficacy of our MDML method.

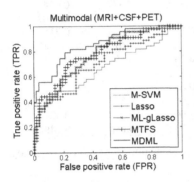

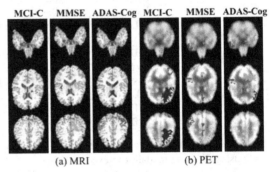

Fig. 1. ROC curves achieved by different methods using multimodal data.

Fig. 2. Stable brain regions identified by MDML method on (a) MRI and (b) PET images. Here, 'MCI-C' is MCI-C vs. MCI-NC classification, and 'MMSE'/'ADAS-Cog' are MMSE/ADAS-Cog scores prediction, respectively.

Finally, in Fig. 2, we visually show the brain regions selected by our MDML method with the highest frequency of occurrence by MDML on MRI and PET images, respectively. Here, to get these features (i.e., brain regions), we count the frequency of each feature and selected across all folds and all runs (i.e., a total of 100 times), and then regard those features as stable features. As can be seen from Fig. 2, our proposed MDML method successfully finds out the most discriminative brain regions (e.g., hippocampal, amygdala, temporal lobe, precuneus, and insula) [3, 11].

4   Conclusion

This paper addresses the problem of jointly exploiting the use of related learning domain data and multi-label group information for early diagnosis of AD. By integrating multi-label learning and transfer learning, we develop a multi-domain multi-label feature selection (MDML) for acquiring the useful correlation information among different learning domains and multi-label groups, and then employ multi-kernel support vector machine for classification and multi-kernel relevance vector machine for regression, respectively. Experimental results on the ADNI database validate the efficacy of our proposed method.

Acknowledgements. This paper is supported by National Natural Science Foundation of China under grant numbers 61422204 and 61473149, by the Jiangsu Natural Science Foundation for Distinguished Young Scholar under grant number BK20130034, by the NUAA Fundamental Research Funds under grant number NE2013105, and by the Scientific and Technological Research Program of Chongqing Municipal Education Commission under Grant KJ1501014.

References

1. Alzheimer's Association: 2014 Alzheimer's disease facts and figures. Alzheimer's & Dement **10**(47), 92 (2014)
2. Cheng, B., Zhang, D., Chen, S., Kaufer, D.I., Shen, D.: Semi-supervised multimodal relevance vector regression improves cognitive performance estimation from imaging and biological biomarkers. Neuroinformatics **11**, 339–353 (2013)
3. Zhang, D., Shen, D.: Multi-modal multi-task learning for joint prediction of multiple regression and classification variables in Alzheimer's disease. NeuroImage **59**, 895–907 (2012)
4. Young, J., Modat, M., Cardoso, M.J., Mendelson, A., Cash, D., Ourselin, S.: Accurate multimodal probabilistic prediction of conversion to Alzheimer's disease in patients with mild cognitive impairment. NeuroImage: Clinical **2**, 735–745 (2013)
5. Westman, E., Muehlboeck, J.S., Simmons, A.: Combining MRI and CSF measures for classification of Alzheimer's disease and prediction of mild cognitive impairment conversion. NeuroImage **62**, 229–238 (2012)
6. Zhou, J., Liu, J., Narayan, V.A., Ye, J.: Modeling disease progression via multi-task learning. NeuroImage **78**, 233–248 (2013)
7. Zhu, X., Suk, H., Shen, D.: A novel matrix-similarity based loss function for joint regression and classification in AD diagnosis. NeuroImage **100**, 91–105 (2014)
8. Wang, H., Nie, F., Huang, H., Risacher, S., Saykin, A.J., Shen, L.: Identifying AD-sensitive and cognition-relevant imaging biomarkers via joint classification and regression. In: Fichtinger, G., Martel, A., Peters, T. (eds.) MICCAI 2011, Part III. LNCS, vol. 6893, pp. 115–123. Springer, Heidelberg (2011)
9. Filipovych, R., Davatzikos, C.: Semi-supervised pattern classification of medical images: application to mild cognitive impairment (MCI). NeuroImage **55**, 1109–1119 (2011)
10. Cheng, B., Zhang, D., Shen, D.: Domain transfer learning for MCI conversion prediction. In: Ayache, N., Delingette, H., Golland, P., Mori, K. (eds.) MICCAI 2012, Part I. LNCS, vol. 7510, pp. 82–90. Springer, Heidelberg (2012)
11. Ye, J., Farnum, M., Yang, E., Verbeeck, R., Lobanov, V., Raghavan, N., Novak, G., DiBernardo, A., Narayan, V.A.: Sparse learning and stability selection for predicting MCI to AD conversion using baseline ADNI data. BMC Neurology **12**, 1471-2377-1412-1446 (2012)
12. Nemirovski, A.: Efficient Method s in Convex Programming (2005)
13. Wang, Y., Fan, Y., Bhatt, P., Davatzikos, C.: High-dimensional pattern regression using machine learning: from medical images to continuous clinical variables. NeuroImage **50**, 1519–1535 (2010)
14. Liu, J., Ji, S., Ye, J.: SLEP: sparse learning with efficient projections. Arizona State University (2009). http://www.public.asu.edu/~jye02/Software/SLEP
15. Pan, S.J., Yang, Q.: A survey on transfer learning. IEEE Transactions on Knowledge and Data Engineering **22**, 1345–1359 (2010)

Soft-Split Sparse Regression Based Random Forest for Predicting Future Clinical Scores of Alzheimer's Disease

Lei Huang[(✉)], Yaozong Gao, Yan Jin[(✉)], Kim-Han Thung, and Dinggang Shen

Department of Radiology and BRIC, School of Medicine,
University of North Carolina at Chapel Hill, Chapel Hill, NC 27599, USA
{leihuang,yzgao}@cs.unc.edu,
{yjinz,khthung,dinggang_shen}@med.unc.edu

Abstract. In this study, we propose a novel sparse regression based random forest (RF) to predict future clinical scores of Alzheimer's disease (AD) with the baseline scores and the MRI features. To avoid the stair-like decision boundary caused by axis-aligned split function in the conventional RF, we present a supervised method to construct the oblique split function by using sparse regression to select the informative features and transform the original features into the target-like features that are more discriminative. Then, we construct the oblique splitting function by applying the principal component analysis (PCA) on the transformed target-like features. Furthermore, to reduce the negative impact of potential mis-split induced by the conventional "hard-split", we further introduce the "soft-split" technique, in which both left and right nodes are visited with certain weights given a test sample. The experiment results show that sparse regression based RF alone can improve the prediction performance of the conventional RF. And further improvement can be achieved when both of the techniques are combined.

1 Introduction

Alzheimer's disease (AD) is known as the most common types of dementia and also a slow progressive neurodegenerative disorder. Many studies have used a variety of imaging features to identify AD patients [1-4]. However, to make a conclusive diagnosis of AD, invasive biopsy confirmation is required that is often inconvenient and expensive. Thus, different clinical scores, such as Mini-Mental State Exam (MMSE), Clinical Dementia Rating (CDR), and Alzheimer's Disease Assessment Scale (ADAS), have been designed to measure the cognitive status of patients. Many studies have shown the correlations between these clinical scores with AD progression [5]. Usually, the neurodegeneration caused by AD begins several years before the onset of the disease and therefore medical intervention is more effective if it starts at an earlier stage. Consequently, a variety of studies have been done to predict the AD

This work was supported by the National Institute of Health grants EB006733, EB008374, EB009634, AG041721, MH100217, and AG042599.

L. Zhou et al. (Eds.): MLMI 2015, LNCS 9352, pp. 246–254, 2015.
DOI: 10.1007/978-3-319-24888-2_30

progression measured by clinical scores based on some predictive biomarkers and risk factors obtained from magnetic resonance imaging (MRI), cerebrospinal fluid (CSF) and baseline clinical scores [6-7].

In this study, we formulate the prediction of AD progression as a regression task, where the MRI and the baseline clinical scores are used as input features, and the future AD clinical scores are used as output targets. Due to the outstanding performance of random forest (RF) [8] in high-dimensional tasks, we utilize RF as our base regression model. RF is an ensemble learning model that consists of multiple decision or regression trees. In RF, each regression tree is generated by recursively creating tree nodes. In each node, training samples are split into two sub-training datasets by a split function, which can be an axis-aligned split function or oblique split function.

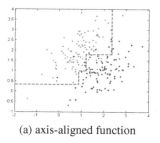

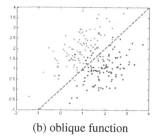

(a) axis-aligned function   (b) oblique function

Fig. 1. A decision boundary generated by (a) an axis-aligned and (b) an oblique split function.

As the name suggests, the axis-aligned split function uses only one feature at a time to separate the feature space of training samples by a hyper-plane that is aligned to the feature axes (Fig. 1(a)). Although it is efficient to compute in the training stage, it generates unsmooth blocky decision boundary in the feature space. That boundary is usually different from the real situation and tends to result in poor generalization performance. In contrast, the oblique split function uses multiple features and a hyper-plane oblique to the axis is learned (Fig. 1(b)), thus improves the former by generating smoother and more complex boundary for better generalization. However, it has much more parameters than the axis-aligned function, especially when dealing with high-dimensional features. Therefore, it becomes impractical to find the optimal splitting boundary merely by exhaustive search, which is commonly used in RF.

In order to overcome the aforementioned problems, we propose a novel sparse regression based RF by utilizing the LASSO (Least Absolute Shrinkage and Selection Operator) regression that plays a supervised role to select the informative features instead of exhaustive search when learning the oblique split function. In the meanwhile, LASSO regression also maps the original features into the target-like features, which are expected to be more discriminative, thus being better suited for splitting the samples. Afterwards, an oblique hyper-plane can be easily found by principal component analysis (PCA) in the mapped feature space.

Furthermore, we introduce a new technique "soft-split". Note that the conventional RF makes "hard-split" (i.e., going either left or right) at each split node and thus assigns each test sample with only one path from the root to a leaf. This splitting strategy works well when there is a clear separation, but it may result in a mis-split if the test sample is located close to the splitting boundary. Instead, soft-split takes the ambiguity of those hard-to-split samples into consideration. At each split, we allow the sample to go to both left and right child nodes with an assigned weight, which depends on the distance of this sample to the learned splitting decision boundary. Finally, we predict each sample as the weighted average of the statistics in all leaf nodes it visits.

We then apply our method to jointly predicting multiple AD-related clinical scores of the subjects from our dataset at multiple future time points from the baseline scores and the MRI derived features. The performance of our method will be compared with other state-of-art regression methods in the field.

2   Method

2.1   Random Forest

The training stage of RF is to generate multiple diverse decision trees, e.g., T trees. For the ith tree, a subset of training data $D_i \subset D$ is randomly sampled with replacement from the entire data set D. Then, starting from the root node, each node in the tree is trained recursively. Taking the jth node as an example, a split function is generated to split the training samples in the jth node of the ith tree, $D_{i,j}$, into the left and right child nodes with samples $D_{i,j}^L$ and $D_{i,j}^R$. To learn the split function, given a feature set Γ, random-sampling is applied to selecting a subset of features $\Gamma_{i,j} \subset \Gamma$. For the axis-aligned function, only one feature and the corresponding threshold are learned as the splitting parameters for each split function:

$$f(x|w,t) = H(w^T x - t), \quad s.t. \ x \in D_{i,j}, \|w\|_0 = 1 \tag{1}$$

where $x \in \mathbb{R}^{|\Gamma_{i,j}| \times 1}$ is a feature vector, $w \in \mathbb{R}^{|\Gamma_{i,j}| \times 1}$, $\|w\|_0 = \sum_{i=0}^{|\Gamma_{i,j}|} 1_{w_i \neq 0} = 1$ indicates that only one feature is selected, and $H(\cdot)$ is a Heaviside function. $H(a) = 1$, when $a > 0$ and 0, otherwise. t is the threshold or the intercept of the hyperplane.

Therefore, $D_{i,j}^L = \{x \in D_{i,j} | f(x|w,t) = 0\}$, $D_{i,j}^R = \{x \in D_{i,j} | f(x|w,t) = 1\}$.

Similarly, the oblique split function is formulated without the $\|w\|_0 = 1$ constraint.

$$f(x|w,t) = H(w^T x - t), \quad s.t. \ x \in D_{i,j} \tag{2}$$

To find the optimal candidates of the feature and the threshold, the purity of the sample set after the split is often used as a criterion. For regression, the increase of purity is usually measured by the reduction of variance:

$$I_{w,t} = V(D) - \sum_{k \in \{L,R\}} \frac{|D^k|}{|D|} V(D^k) \tag{3}$$

$$V(D) = \frac{1}{|D|} \sum_{(x,y) \in D} \left\| y - \frac{1}{|D|} \sum_{(x,y) \in D} y \right\|_2^2 \tag{4}$$

where $V(D)$ is the total target variance in dataset D and (x, y) means a pair of feature and target vectors for a sample. Finally, the training process of each split function can be described as: $f(x|w, t) = \arg\max_{w,t} I_{w,t}$.

In this way, each node will continue to split until it reaches a predefined stop criterion, and then the statistics (e.g., mean) of the target vectors in the inseparable subset will be stored in the leaf nodes for prediction at the testing stage.

The testing process of RF is similar to the training process. By recursively passing a test sample to the left or the right child node, the test sample will finally reach a leaf node, where the saved statistics of the training samples (the mean in our case) can be retrieved as the prediction result of this tree for the test sample. In the end, the prediction result of RF is obtained by averaging the predictions of all decision trees in the forest.

2.2 Sparse Regression in Random Forest

The conventional RF uses exhaustive search to find the optimal splitting parameters w and t. However, the magnitude of the search space grows exponentially along the dimension of w, resulting in the optimization of the oblique split function computationally demanding in practice. Therefore, even though a few studies reported that the oblique function outperformed the axis-aligned function [9], it is still not preferred in real applications.

To learn the oblique split function in a feasible way, we propose to utilize the LASSO regression and PCA to learn w under the supervised setting. During the training stage, we first map the original feature space into the target space with the LASSO regression, thus producing the target-like features. Since the target-like features are more correlated with the regression target, they tend to be more discriminative to separate the sample set than the original features. Specifically, at each node, we first randomly resample a feature subset $\Gamma' \subset \Gamma$ from all of the feature variables. Then the new feature vectors $\{x | x \in \mathbb{R}^{|\Gamma'| \times 1}\}$ and the d-dimensional target vectors $\{y | y \in \mathbb{R}^{d \times 1}\}$ are used as the inputs for the LASSO regression:

$$B^{\text{opt}} = \arg\min_B \sum_{(x,y) \in D} \|y - B^T x\|_2^2 + \lambda \|B\|_1 \tag{5}$$

where $B \in \mathbb{R}^{|\Gamma'| \times d}$ is the sparse coefficient matrix and λ is the regularization parameter that controls the sparsity of B. $\|B\|_1$ is the L_1 norm of B. Once we obtain the sparse coefficient matrix B for the node, we can generate the mapped target-like feature $\widetilde{y} = B^T x$, where $\widetilde{y} \in \mathbb{R}^{d \times 1}$.

To maximize the variance reduction for the optimal split function $f(x|w, t)$, we use PCA to calculate the maximum variance direction of the mapped target-like features $\widetilde{y}$'s and estimate the first principal component $p \in \mathbb{R}^{d \times 1}$. The best splitting hyper-plane is the one orthogonal to the maximum variance direction. Thus, now our split function can be formulated as:

$$f(x|w, t) = H(p^T \widetilde{y} - t) = H(p^T B^T x - t) \tag{6}$$

By comparing Eq. (2) with Eq. (6), we can readily see that:

$$w = (p^T B^T)^T = Bp \qquad (7)$$

From Eq. (7), w can be solved analytically. Now the only unknown parameter is the intercept t of the hyper-plane, which is a scalar and can be feasibly determined by exhaustive search. That is, we randomly sample a set of hyper-planes orthogonal to the maximum variance direction p, and pick the one that leads to the maximum variation reduction as defined in Eq. (2).

2.3   Soft Split in Random Forest

At the testing stage, the traditional hard-split (either going to the left or the right child node) works well when the samples can be well separated by the split function. However, in practice the regression targets of the training samples may highly overlap. Possibly, many "hard-to-split" samples lie very close to the splitting hyper-plane. It is very likely that even though they are located on one side of the hyper-plane, they may belong to the other side due to the fluctuation of noise. The conventional hard-split tends to overlook this fact, resulting in the misclassification of the test sample to a wrong side and leading to inaccurate prediction.

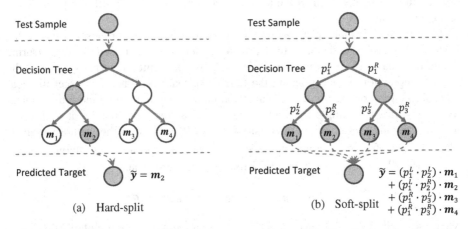

Fig. 2. A testing procedure of (a) the hard-split and (b) the soft-split decision tree. The paths connecting those blue nodes are the paths that the test sample goes through during each procedure. p_i^L and p_i^R denote the splitting weights at the ith node, respectively, and m_k is the statistics of the training samples in the kth leaf node.

To solve this problem, here we introduce the concept of "soft-split". When a test sample reaches a split node, instead of passing it to only one child node, it will be passed to both children with certain weights. Consequently, unlike the conventional RF where each test sample is predicted with the information from one leaf node, the soft-split technique predicts the test sample by linearly fusing the information from multiple leaf nodes it visits with non-zero weights. Mathematically, at each split node, the weights of a test sample that passes into the left and right child nodes are determined by a function of its distance to the learned splitting hyper-plane:

$$p^L = \text{sigmoid}(r) = \frac{1}{1+e^{-sr}}, \ p^R = 1 - p^L \tag{8}$$

where p^L and p^R are the weights of this test sample (represented by its feature subset x) being assigned to the left and right nodes, respectively, r is the signed distance of this sample to the splitting hyper-plane (represented by w and t), and s is a parameter that controls the slope of the sigmoid function. We can see from Eq. (8) that the larger the distance r to the splitting hyper-plane, the more extreme the weights are, i.e., toward 0 or 1. For those hard-to-split samples that are often located closely to the splitting hyper-plane, the left and the right nodes tend to be assigned the similar weights. By combining Eq. (2), Eq. (6), and Eq. (8), the soft-split sparse regression based oblique split function can be formulated as follows:

$$f(x|w,t) = \text{sigmoid}(w^T x - t) = \text{sigmoid}(p^T B^T x - t) \tag{9}$$

Now, $D_{i,j}^L = \left\{ x \in D_{i,j} \middle| f(x|w,t) > c \right\}$ and $D_{i,j}^R = \left\{ x \in D_{i,j} \middle| 1 - f(x|w,t) > c \right\}$, where c denotes the pruning threshold. Soft-split will be replaced by hard-split if either p^L or p^R is smaller than c so that computing efficiency can be improved.

With soft-split, a test sample will go through both the left and right child nodes with certain weights until it reaches the bottom of the tree. Then the weight of each leaf node is calculated as the multiplication of all weights along the path from the root node to itself. The prediction value of the test sample by this tree is the weighted average of the statistics of all leaf nodes with non-zero weights. The comparison between the traditional hard-split and the proposed soft-split is illustrated in Fig. 2.

3   Experiment Results

The dataset we used was downloaded from the Alzheimer's Disease Neuroimaging Initiative (ADNI) database (http://adni.loni.usc.edu/). At the baseline, 805 individuals participated in the study, including 226 normal control subjects (NC), 393 mild cognitive impairment subjects (MCI), and 186 AD subjects. Longitudinal clinical data such as MRI scans and clinical scores were obtained at the baseline and every 12 months after the baseline. Due to the dropouts, the sample size decreased as the study continued. In our experiments, we jointly predict the four clinical scores (MMSE, CDR-SOB, CDR-Global, and ADAS) at the 12th (201 NC, 351 MCI, 149 AD), 24th (192 NC, 289 MCI, 122 AD), 36th (172 NC, 221 MCI, 9 AD) and 48th (51 NC, 50 MCI, 2 AD) month after the baseline by using the MRI features and the baseline scores. The MRI features were the average gray matter volumes from 90 ROIs transferred from the AAL atlas [10].

Here, we compared our proposed methods, i.e., sparse oblique RF (oRF-L1) and sparse oblique RF with soft-split (oRF-L1-soft), with other RF models (the traditional axis-aligned RF, oblique RF with ridge regularization (oRF-L2) [6], and oRF-L2 with soft-split (oRF-L2-soft)) for their performance of future clinical scores prediction.

The prediction performance was measured by the 10-fold cross validation. The RF parameters were selected as follows: the number of trees = 10, the number of candidate for the search of the optimal hyper-plane intercept t = 10, the number of randomly sampled feature variables at each node = 60, the lower bound of sample size in each node = 3, the number of randomly drawn samples in each tree = 720, and the upper bound of tree depth = 20. The weight λ for sparse regression (Eq. 5) and the slope s of the sigmoid function in soft-split (Eq. 8) were automatically determined by two-fold cross validation on the training set. The experiment results are listed in Table 1.

Table 1. The performance comparison between the proposed methods (oRF-L1 and oRF-L1-soft) and other RF models (RF, oRF-L2, and oRF-L2-soft).The best results are shown in bold.

Month	Score / Method	Average Absolute Error				Pearson's Correlation Coefficient			
		MMSE	CDR-SOB	CDR-G	ADAS	MMSE	CDR-SOB	CDR-G	ADAS
12	RF	1.778	0.724	0.142	3.426	0.807	0.840	0.813	0.840
	oRF-L2	1.764	0.743	0.154	3.440	0.800	0.829	0.798	0.828
	oRF-L2-soft	1.722	0.737	0.158	3.444	0.816	0.836	0.805	0.833
	oRF-L1	1.744	0.692	**0.137**	3.422	0.813	0.849	0.823	0.842
	oRF-L1-soft	**1.674**	**0.685**	0.146	**3.275**	**0.826**	**0.855**	**0.830**	**0.852**
24	RF	2.118	0.998	**0.222**	4.298	0.809	0.835	0.804	0.828
	oRF-L2	2.117	1.030	0.229	4.194	0.810	0.833	0.802	0.827
	oRF-L2-soft	2.093	1.020	0.236	4.098	0.820	0.845	0.812	0.839
	oRF-L1	2.101	1.014	0.226	4.227	0.809	0.841	0.804	0.828
	oRF-L1-soft	**2.043**	**0.979**	0.229	**4.070**	**0.822**	**0.852**	**0.816**	**0.841**
36	RF	2.028	0.975	0.223	3.964	0.765	0.785	0.778	0.789
	oRF-L2	2.009	0.912	0.223	3.887	0.775	0.825	0.788	0.800
	oRF-L2-soft	1.950	0.894	0.224	3.753	0.792	0.842	0.806	0.819
	oRF-L1	1.838	0.893	**0.215**	3.770	0.821	0.831	0.802	0.824
	oRF-L1-soft	**1.808**	**0.883**	0.220	**3.653**	**0.832**	**0.843**	**0.813**	**0.836**
48	RF	1.939	1.160	0.250	3.653	0.742	0.653	0.679	0.731
	oRF-L2	1.871	0.998	0.243	3.785	0.731	0.717	0.689	0.697
	oRF-L2-soft	1.830	1.006	0.244	3.729	0.747	0.722	0.693	0.708
	oRF-L1	1.693	**0.977**	**0.236**	3.635	0.800	0.738	0.718	0.745
	oRF-L1-soft	**1.656**	0.978	0.240	**3.564**	**0.804**	**0.746**	**0.725**	**0.752**

To compare the performances of our methods with other regression models, we also conducted the same experiments with support vector machine (SVM,) LASSO regression and ridge regression. The experiment results are listed in Table 2. In previous studies, Duchesne et al. [11] used baseline MRI, age, gender and years of education as features to predict the MMSE scores at the 12th month (75 NC, 49 MCI, 75 AD) and only achieved the correlation of 0.31. Stonnington et al. [12] used only MRI and CSF as features to predict the baseline clinical scores (122 NC, 351 MCI, 113 AD) and achieved the correlation of 0.48 for MMSE, and 0.57 for ADAS.

From the results above, oRF-L1 outperformed RF and oRF-L2, based on both average absolute error and Pearson's correlation coefficient. The performance of oRF-L1-soft was further improved. Our methods also outperformed the results from SVM, LASSO and ridge regression and the previous studies in terms of Pearson's correlation coefficient.

Table 2. The comparison between the proposed methods with SVM, LASSO regression and ridge regression in terms of average Pearson's correlation coefficients across all 4 future time points. The best results are shown in bold.

	MMSE	CDR-SOB	CDR-G	ADAS
LASSO	0.775	0.793	0.777	0.802
Ridge	0.789	0.799	0.781	0.809
SVM	0.786	0.788	0.775	0.793
oRF-L1	0.811	0.815	0.787	0.810
oRF-L1-soft	**0.821**	**0.824**	**0.796**	**0.820**

4 Conclusion

We proposed a novel sparse regression based RF with soft-split to predict the clinical scores in AD at future time points with the baseline scores and the MRI features. Sparse regression with PCA provided an efficient way to locate the oblique split function in RF. The soft-split technique assigned the weights to both child nodes to handle the hard-to-split samples. The combination of both strategies outperformed other state-of-art regression methods. More importantly, the proposed framework can be extended to a general regression tool to predict other regression tasks, not only limited to the AD clinical score prediction.

References

1. Li, J., Jin, Y., Shi, Y., Dinov, I.D., Wang, D.J., Toga, A.W., Thompson, P.M.: Voxelwise spectral diffusional connectivity and its applications to alzheimer's disease and intelligence Prediction. In: Mori, K., Sakuma, I., Sato, Y., Barillot, C., Navab, N. (eds.) MICCAI 2013, Part I. LNCS, vol. 8149, pp. 655–662. Springer, Heidelberg (2013)
2. Zhan, L., et al.: Comparison of nine tractography algorithms for detecting abnormal structural brain networks in Alzheimer's disease. Front. Aging Neurosci. **7**, 48 (2015)
3. Zhan L., et al.: Multiple stages classification of alzheimer's disease based on structural brain networks using generalized low rank approximations (GLRAM). In: MICCAI Computation Diffusion MRI, Mathematics and Visualization, pp. 35–44 (2014)
4. Jin Y., et al.: Automated multi-atlas labeling of the fornix and its integrity in Alzheimer's disease. In: Proc IEEE Int Symp Biomed Imaging, pp. 140–143 (2015)
5. Petrella, J.R., et al.: Neuroimaging and early diagnosis of Alzheimer disease: a look to the future. Radiology **226**(2), 315–336 (2003)
6. Zhu, X., et al.: Matrix-similarity based loss function and feature selection for Alzheimer's disease diagnosis. In: IEEE Conf on CVPR, pp. 3089–3096 (2014)
7. Zhu, X., Suk, H.-I., Shen, D.: A novel multi-relation regularization method for regression and classification in AD diagnosis. In: Golland, P., Hata, N., Barillot, C., Hornegger, J., Howe, R. (eds.) MICCAI 2014, Part III. LNCS, vol. 8675, pp. 401–408. Springer, Heidelberg (2014)

8. Breiman, L.: Random forests. Machine learning **45**(1), 5–32 (2001)
9. Menze, B.H., Kelm, B., Splitthoff, D.N., Koethe, U., Hamprecht, F.A.: On oblique random forests. In: Gunopulos, D., Hofmann, T., Malerba, D., Vazirgiannis, M. (eds.) ECML PKDD 2011, Part II. LNCS, vol. 6912, pp. 453–469. Springer, Heidelberg (2011)
10. Tzourio-Mazoyer, N., et al.: Automated anatomical labeling of activations in SPM using a macroscopic anatomical parcellation of the MNI MRI single-subject brain. Neuroimage **15**(1), 273–289 (2002)
11. Duchesne, S., et al.: Relating one-year cognitive change in mild cognitive impairment to baseline MRI features. Neuroimage **47**(4), 1363–1370 (2009)
12. Stonnington, C.M., et al.: Predicting clinical scores from magnetic resonance scans in Alzheimer's disease. Neuroimage **51**(4), 1405–1413 (2010)

Multi-view Classification for Identification of Alzheimer's Disease

Xiaofeng Zhu[1], Heung-Il Suk[2], Yonghua Zhu[3], Kim-Han Thung[1],
Guorong Wu[1], and Dinggang Shen[1(✉)]

[1] Department of Radiology and BRIC,
University of North Carolina, Chapel Hill, USA
dgshen@med.unc.edu
[2] Department of Brain and Cognitive Engineering,
Korea University, Seoul, Republic of Korea
[3] School of Computer, Electronics and Information,
Guangxi University, Nanning, China

Abstract. In this paper, we propose a multi-view learning method using Magnetic Resonance Imaging (MRI) data for Alzheimer's Disease (AD) diagnosis. Specifically, we extract both Region-Of-Interest (ROI) features and Histograms of Oriented Gradient (HOG) features from each MRI image, and then propose mapping HOG features onto the space of ROI features to make them comparable and to impose high intra-class similarity with low inter-class similarity. Finally, both mapped HOG features and original ROI features are input to the support vector machine for AD diagnosis. The purpose of mapping HOG features onto the space of ROI features is to provide complementary information so that features from different views can *not only* be comparable (*i.e.,* homogeneous) *but also* be interpretable. For example, ROI features are robust to noise, but lack of reflecting small or subtle changes, while HOG features are diverse but less robust to noise. The proposed multi-view learning method is designed to learn the transformation between two spaces and to separate the classes under the supervision of class labels. The experimental results on the MRI images from the Alzheimer's Disease Neuroimaging Initiative (ADNI) dataset show that the proposed multi-view method helps enhance disease status identification performance, outperforming both baseline methods and state-of-the-art methods.

1 Introduction

Alzheimer's Disease (AD) is the most popular form of dementia among the elderly population. It is estimated that there are around 90 million AD patients in the world, with the number of AD patients expected to reach 300 million by 2050 [8,12]. In this regard, it is very interesting and important to find an accurate biomarker for the diagnosis of AD and its prodromal stage, *i.e.,* Mild Cognitive Impairment (MCI). For the past few decades, neuroimaging has been widely used to investigate AD-related pathologies in the spectrum between cognitive normal and AD [7,17], where various machine learning techniques have been designed

© Springer International Publishing Switzerland 2015
L. Zhou et al. (Eds.): MLMI 2015, LNCS 9352, pp. 255–262, 2015.
DOI: 10.1007/978-3-319-24888-2_31

for the analysis of complex patterns in neuroimaging data, as well as identification of a subject's clinical status. For example, Cuingnet *et al.* embedded a graph-based regularization operator into Support Vector Machine (SVM) for the identification of AD [2], while Wang *et al.* designed a sparse Bayesian multi-task learning model to adaptively investigate the dependence of AD subjects, for improving the AD diagnosis performance [10].

Since multi-modality data (including Magnetic Resonance Imaging (MRI), Positron Emission Tomography (PET), and CerebroSpinal Fluid (CSF) biomarkers) are often acquired in applications and have been shown to provide complementary information for AD diagnosis [4,5,11,13,16], a great number of research use multi-modality data for AD diagnosis and obtain significant performance improvements, compared to the methods that use a single modality data [9,15,19]. For example, Zhang *et al.* designed an approach that conducts AD diagnosis by directly concatenating features of multiple modalities of data including MRI data, PET data, and CSF data, as their method outperformed other methods with individual modality data, such as MRI data or PET data [13,18]. However, to the best of our knowledge, very few previous works have focused on the identification of AD with multi-view or visual features of neuroimaging data.

In this paper, we propose a new multi-view learning method using multiple representations of MRI images for AD diagnosis, via the following three stages: 1) *Image processing.* We extract both Region-Of-Interest (ROI) features and 3-dimensional Histograms of Oriented Gradient (HOG) [6] features from given MRI images. 2) *Multi-view learning.* A new multi-view learning method is designed to map HOG features onto the space of ROI features, by ensuring high similarity for samples with the same label, while low similarity for samples with different labels. This makes classes well separated. 3) *AD classification.* Both the mapped HOG features and the original ROI features are fed into a SVM classifier to identify AD.

Compared to conventional methods (*e.g.*, the multi-modality method [13] and the single-view method [9]) for AD diagnosis, this work has the following contributions.

- We extract both HOG features and ROI features from only MRI images to form multi-view features, rather than conventional multi-modality methods using both MRI images and PET images [13]. That is, multi-modality methods need to pay additional for PET images, whereas no additional payments are required for our method. In practice, the ANDI dataset provides more MRI images (*e.g.*, more than 800) than PET images (*e.g.*, only about 400), and has been indicated that less training data can easily result in underfitting [9].
- Few studies focus on AD diagnosis via visual features, such as HOG, even though HOG features and ROI features can provide complementary information. It has been shown that ROI features, *e.g.*, the average of gray matter volume within a brain region, are robust to the noise but are less diverse for AD diagnosis [13]. In contrast, HOG features can output multiple bi-dimensional histograms for a brain region to reflect the change of blocks

within a brain region, so HOG features are good at reflecting small or subtle changes within brain, though vulnerable to noises [6].

– Compared to learning common space among different views like Canonical Correlation Analysis (CCA) [14], the proposed method learns the mappings from the HOG feature space to the ROI feature space, with the guidance of learning high intra-class similarity and low inter-class similarity.

2   Approach

2.1   Notations

We denote matrices as boldface uppercase letters, vectors as boldface lower-case letters, and scalars as normal italic letters, respectively. For a matrix $\mathbf{X} = [x_{ij}]$, its i-th row and j-th column are denoted as $\mathbf{x}^i$ and $\mathbf{x}_j$, respectively. The Frobenius norm and the transpose operator of a matrix $\mathbf{X}$ are denoted as $\|\mathbf{X}\|_F = \sqrt{\sum_i \|\mathbf{x}^i\|_2^2} = \sqrt{\sum_j \|\mathbf{x}_j\|_2^2} = \sqrt{\sum_{i,j} x_{ij}^2}$ and $\mathbf{X}^T$, respectively.

2.2   Image Processing

The ROI feature can be regarded as the global feature, as it is obtained by averaging gray matter tissue volume within a brain region. The ROI feature has been indicated to be robust to noise but very coarse in sense, such as the lack of reflecting small or subtle changes involved in brain diseases [9]. However, disease-related structural/functional changes may occur in multiple brain regions [13]. Therefore, the simple ROI representation may not effectively capture diseased-related pathologies. In contrast, the HOG feature decomposes a 3D image into a grid of small squared 3D cells, where a bi-dimensional histogram of gradient along spatial and orientation bins is computed and then returns a descriptor for each cell [6]. The HOG feature considers the diversity of each cell and can be regarded as the local feature. In this work, we simultaneously extract ROI features (*i.e.*, global features) and HOG features (*i.e.*, local features) from an MRI image to form a multi-view representation for AD diagnosis. To do this, we use 830 MRI images (including 198 ADs, 403 MCIs and 229 Normal Controls (NC)) from ADNI database[1]. Additionally, we select 124 progress MCIs (pMCI) and 118 stable MCIs (sMCI) from 403 MCIs to conduct the binary classification pMCI vs. sMCI[2].

More specifically, we first preprocessed the MRI images by performing spatial distortion, skull-stripping, and cerebellum removal, sequentially, and then segmented the MRI images into gray matter, white matter, and cerebrospinal fluid. Furthermore, the MRI images were parcellated into 93 ROIs based on a Jacob template, by non-rigid brain registration. We finally computed the gray matter tissue volumes of the ROIs as the ROI features.

---

[1] Please refer to 'http://adni.loni.usc.edu/' for up-to-date information.

[2] In ADNI, these numbers, *i.e.*, 124 and 118, of subjects were, respectively, marked as pMCI and sMCI among 403 MCI subjects.

Given the MRI images separated by 93 ROIs, we extracted the HOG features for each ROI. Specifically, we first down-sampled the original MRI images, *i.e.,* from $256 \times 256 \times 256$ to $64 \times 64 \times 64$, followed by partitioning the whole brain into 93 ROIs, which is the same as partitioning the original brain image to extract the ROI features. We dilated each ROI with 3 voxels to achieve a soft boundary among ROIs. Following the method in [6], we set the number of orientation bins to 9, with each bin with 8 orientations to describe a descriptor by a 72-dimensional feature vector. We also set the size (in voxels) of the spatial bins and the size of the blocks, respectively, as 5 and 2, to extract 1728 descriptors from each ROI. Note that descriptor information was divided into overlapping blocks, each of which contained $2 \times 2 \times 2$ 3-dimensional cells. We further clustered descriptors of each ROI of all MRI images to form a 50-dimensional bag-of-words for each ROI.

Finally, we used a 93 dimensional ROI feature vector and a 4650 ($= 93 \times 50$) dimensional HOG feature vector to obtain a multi-view representation of an MRI image.

2.3 Multi-view Learning

A conventional solution of multi-view learning is to search for a common space among different views. For example, Canonical Correlation Analysis (CCA) was designed to search a common space among views in which the diversity among all views was minimized [14]. However, recent studies indicate that such a common space obtained by a symmetric transformation (*i.e.,* the same rotation and scaling to all views) cannot separate classes particularly well [3,14]. To address this, we design a new multi-view learning method to transform HOG features into the ROI feature space by ensuring that the HOG-ROI feature pairs of the same label have high similarity (*i.e.,* high intra-similarity), while those of different labels have low similarity (*i.e.,* low inter-similarity).

Let $\mathbf{X} = \{\mathbf{x}_1, \ldots, \mathbf{x}_i, \ldots, \mathbf{x}_n\}$ and $\mathbf{Y} = \{\mathbf{y}_1, \ldots, \mathbf{y}_i, \ldots, \mathbf{y}_n\}$ denote, respectively, HOG features and ROI features of n samples, where $\mathbf{x}_i \in \mathbb{R}^{d_x}$, $\mathbf{y}_i \in \mathbb{R}^{d_y}$, and d_x and d_y are the dimensionalities of the HOG and ROI features, respectively. We, then, learn a transformation matrix $\mathbf{W} \in \mathbb{R}^{d_x \times d_y}$ from the HOG feature space to the ROI feature space (or equivalently a transformation matrix $\mathbf{W}^T$ from the ROI feature space to the HOG feature space). We first define an inner product similarity function between any sample pair, *i.e.,* $\mathbf{x}_i \in \mathbf{X}$ and $\mathbf{y}_j \in \mathbf{Y}$, as follows

$$sim(\mathbf{x}_i, \mathbf{y}_j) = \mathbf{x}_i^T \mathbf{W} \mathbf{y}_j, \quad i, j = 1, ..., n. \tag{1}$$

In finding a transformation matrix $\mathbf{W}$, we also expect Eq. (1) to have high intra-similarity for samples of the same class, but low inter-similarity for samples of different classes under the supervision of the class labels. In this regard, we formulate the following cost function for a given sample pair $(\mathbf{x}_i, \mathbf{y}_j)$, $i, j = 1, ..., n$:

$$c(\mathbf{x}_i, \mathbf{y}_j) = \begin{cases} max(0, sim(\mathbf{x}_i, \mathbf{y}_j) - \mu), & \text{if } l(i) = l(j) \\ max(0, \nu - sim(\mathbf{x}_i, \mathbf{y}_j)), & \text{otherwise} \end{cases} \tag{2}$$

where $l(i)$ (or $l(j)$) is the label of the HOG features of the i-th sample (or the label of the ROI features of the j-th sample), μ and ν are upper and lower bound parameters to guarantee the constraint, i.e., the largest value of $c(\mathbf{x}_i, \mathbf{y}_j)$, $i, j = 1, ..., n$, for the sample pair $(\mathbf{x}_i, \mathbf{y}_j)$ with the same class label and the smallest value $c(\mathbf{x}_i, \mathbf{y}_j)$ for the sample pair $(\mathbf{x}_i, \mathbf{y}_j)$ with different class labels. Finally, we define a loss function over all sample pairs as follows

$$\mathcal{L}(\mathbf{X}, \mathbf{Y}) = \sum_{i,j=1}^{n} \{c(\mathbf{x}_i, \mathbf{y}_j)\}^2 \tag{3}$$

To avoid over-fitting, we add a Frobenius norm into Eq. (3) to get the final objective function as follows:

$$\min_{\mathbf{W}} \quad \mathcal{L}(\mathbf{X}, \mathbf{Y}) + \lambda \|\mathbf{W}\|_F^2 \tag{4}$$

where $\lambda > 0$ is a tuning parameter. Due to the convexity of both the cost function and the regularization term in Eq. (4), the optimization of Eq. (4) has a global optimum. We employ an alternating projection method based on Bregman's algorithm [1] to optimize Eq. (4). Specifically, the Bregman's method updates the transformation matrix $\mathbf{W}$ with respect to a single constraint in Eq. (2) of a sample pair for each time, which can be easily scaled to large-scale problems and fast convergence in practice.

2.4   AD Classification

After obtaining the transformation matrix $\mathbf{W}$, we concatenate the transformed HOG features $\mathbf{x}_i^T \mathbf{W}$ with the original ROI features $\mathbf{y}_i$ to form a new representation $\mathbf{z}_i = \left[\mathbf{x}_i^T \mathbf{W}, \mathbf{y}_i^T\right]^T \in \mathbb{R}^{2d_y}$. Naturally, we can also directly concatenate the original HOG features with the original ROI features to form another new representation $\mathbf{z}_i = [\mathbf{x}_i^T, \mathbf{y}_i^T]^T \in \mathbb{R}^{(d_x + d_y)}$. We can unify these two kinds of representation as $\mathbf{z}_i = \left[f(\mathbf{x}_i), \mathbf{y}_i^T\right]^T$, where

$$f(\mathbf{x}_i) = \begin{cases} \mathbf{x}_i^T \mathbf{W}, & \text{Linearly mapping HOG to ROI} \\ \mathbf{x}_i^T, & \text{Concatenating HOG with ROI} \end{cases} \tag{5}$$

In this work, we call the former case (i.e., $f(\mathbf{x}_i) = \mathbf{x}_i^T \mathbf{W}$) as the Single-direction Mapping Multi-view Learning (SMML for short) method and the latter case (i.e., $f(\mathbf{x}_i) = \mathbf{x}_i$) as the Directly Concatenating Multi-view Learning (DCML for short) method. Note that SMML transfers HOG features into the space of the ROI features, via a linear transformation matrix (i.e., $\mathbf{W}$), while DCML does that via an identity matrix. We, then, use a linear SVM as a classifier since it has been shown that SVM does not encounter the issue of curse of the dimensionality.

3   Experimental Results and Discussion

We conducted various classification tasks on the ADNI dataset ('www.adni-info.org') to justify the effectiveness of the proposed method.

3.1 Experimental Setting

In our experiments, we considered three binary classification tasks, *i.e.,* AD vs. NC, MCI vs. NC, and pMCI vs. sMCI, to compare our DCML and SMML with the baseline methods (*i.e.,* the SVM classification via the HOG features (HOG for short) and the SVM classification via the ROI features (ROI for short), respectively) and the state-of-the-art methods (*i.e.,* CCA [14] and Multiple Instance Learning method on MRI images (MIL for short) [9]). Among the competing methods, single-view methods include HOG, ROI, and MIL, respectively, while multi-view methods include CCA and the proposed DCML and SSML.

For each binary classification task, we followed the steps of (1) extracting HOG and ROI features; (2) finding a transformation matrix $\mathbf{W}$; (3) conducting SVM learning; and (4) evaluating the performance with classification accuracy.

We used a 10-fold cross-validation method in our experiments. In each fold, we conducted 5-fold inner cross-validation for model parameter selection by a line search method on the parameters with the predefined range, such as $\lambda \in \{10^{-5}, ..., 10^5\}$ in the LIBSVM toolbox. Regarding the upper and lower bounds in Eq. (2), we set them as $\mu = 1$ and $\nu = -1$. The parameters that resulted in the best performance in the inner cross-validation were finally used in testing. We repeated the process 10 times to avoid any possible bias occurring in data partitioning for cross-validation. The final performance was reported by averaging the repeated cross-validation results.

3.2 Performance and Discussion

Table 1 shows the performance of all other competing methods. The proposed SMML achieved the best performances for all three binary classification tasks, followed by CCA, DCML, MIL, ROI and HOG, respectively. For example, SMML achieved improvements of 9.86%, 6.40%, and 6.08%, respectively, on AD vs. NC, MCI vs. NC, and pMCI vs. sMCI, compared to the worst method of all competing methods, *i.e.,* HOG method, and improved by 1.08%, 2.41%, and 2.61%, respectively, on AD vs. NC, MCI vs. NC, and pMCI vs. sMCI, compared to the CCA that achieved the best performance among competing methods.

MIL outperformed all other single-view methods, such as HOG and ROI. MIL is a patch-based method and extracts ROI features within each patch, as it is diverse and also robust, compared to either ROI or HOG. However, our proposed methods outperformed MIL. For example, compared to MIL, our SMML improved by 1.61%, 5.18%, and 8.29%, while our DCML increased by 0.29%, 2.34%, and 4.87%, on AD vs. NC, MCI vs. NC, and pMCI vs. sMCI, respectively. Additionally, HOG outperformed ROI for two out of three classification tasks, such as MCI vs. NC and pMCI vs. sMCI. This indicated that visual feature (*i.e.,* HOG) is useful for AD diagnosis. Besides, multi-view methods (such as CCA, DCML, and SMML) were better than any single-view method (such as HOG, ROI, and MIL). This showed that HOG features and ROI features provide complementary information. However, the proposed SMML still outperformed CCA since our method simultaneously achieved high intra-class similarity and

Table 1. Comparison of the classification accuracy (mean±standard deviation) of all methods at different classification tasks.

Method	AD vs. NC	MCI vs. NC	pMCI vs. sMCI
HOG	0.8145 ± 0.0957	0.7167 ± 0.2088	0.6946 ± 2.5119
ROI	0.8969 ± 0.0951	0.7136 ± 0.1899	0.6638 ± 2.2902
MIL	0.8970 ± 0.0871	0.7289 ± 0.1249	0.6725 ± 1.4298
CCA	0.9023 ± 0.0838	0.7566 ± 0.1152	0.7293 ± 1.3333
DCML	0.8999 ± 0.0987	0.7523 ± 0.0991	0.7212 ± 1.2468
SMML	**0.9131 ± 0.0629**	**0.7807 ± 0.0961**	**0.7554 ± 1.1972**

low inter-class similarity during the estimation of transformation, compared to CCA results.

4   Conclusion

In this paper, we proposed a new multi-view learning method to identify AD using MRI images. The experimental results on the ADNI dataset showed that the proposed method outperformed the state-of-the-art methods for AD diagnosis, as our multi-view representation provides complementary information by extracting both global features (*i.e.,* ROI features) and local features (*i.e.,* HOG features) from MRI images and further imposing high intra-class similarity and low inter-class similarity during feature mapping.

Acknowledgments. This work was supported in part by NIH grants (EB006733, EB008374, EB009634, MH100217, AG041721, AG042599). Xiaofeng Zhu was supported in part by the National Natural Science Foundation of China under grant 61263035. Heung-Il Suk was supported in part by ICT R&D program of MSIP/IITP [B0101-15-0307, Basic Software Research in Human-level Lifelong Machine Learning (Machine Learning Center)].

References

1. Censor, Y.: Parallel Optimization: Theory, Algorithms, and Applications. Oxford University Press (1997)
2. Cuingnet, R., Gerardin, E., Tessieras, J., Auzias, G., Lehéricy, S., Habert, M.O., Chupin, M., Benali, H., Colliot, O.: Automatic classification of patients with Alzheimer's disease from structural MRI: a comparison of ten methods using the ADNI database. NeuroImage **56**(2), 766–781 (2011)
3. Harel, M., Mannor, S.: Learning from multiple outlooks. In: ICML, pp. 401–408 (2011)
4. Jin, Y., Shi, Y., Zhan, L., Gutman, B.A., de Zubicaray, G.I., McMahon, K.L., Wright, M.J., Toga, A.W., Thompson, P.M.: Automatic clustering of white matter fibers in brain diffusion MRI with an application to genetics. NeuroImage **100**, 75–90 (2014)

5. Li, J., Jin, Y., Shi, Y., Dinov, I.D., Wang, D.J., Toga, A.W., Thompson, P.M.: Voxelwise spectral diffusional connectivity and its applications to alzheimer's disease and intelligence prediction. In: Mori, K., Sakuma, I., Sato, Y., Barillot, C., Navab, N. (eds.) MICCAI 2013, Part I. LNCS, vol. 8149, pp. 655–662. Springer, Heidelberg (2013)
6. Sanroma, G., Wu, G., Gao, Y., Shen, D.: Learning to rank atlases for multiple-atlas segmentation. IEEE Transactions Meddical Imaging 33(10), 1939–1953 (2014)
7. Suk, H.I., Lee, S.W., Shen, D.: Latent feature representation with stacked auto-encoder for AD/MCI diagnosis. Brain Structure and Function 220(2), 841–859 (2013)
8. Thung, K., Wee, C., Yap, P., Shen, D.: Neurodegenerative disease diagnosis using incomplete multi-modality data via matrix shrinkage and completion. NeuroImage 91, 386–400 (2014)
9. Tong, T., Wolz, R., Gao, Q., Guerrero, R., Hajnal, J.V., Rueckert, D.: Multiple instance learning for classification of dementia in brain MRI. Medical Image Analysis 18(5), 808–818 (2014)
10. Wan, J., Zhang, Z., Yan, J., Li, T., Rao, B.D., Fang, S., Kim, S., Risacher, S.L., Saykin, A.J., Shen, L.: Sparse bayesian multi-task learning for predicting cognitive outcomes from neuroimaging measures in alzheimer's disease. In: CVPR, pp. 940–947 (2012)
11. Zhan, L., Jahanshad, N., Jin, Y., Toga, A.W., McMahon, K., de Zubicaray, G.I., Martin, N.G., Wright, M.J., Thompson, P.M.: Brain network efficiency and topology depend on the fiber tracking method: 11 tractography algorithms compared in 536 subjects. In: ISBI, pp. 1134–1137 (2013)
12. Zhan, L., Zhou, J., Wang, Y., Jin, Y., Jahanshad, N., Prasad, G., Nir, T.M., Leonardo, C.D., Ye, J., Thompson, P.M.: Comparison of 9 tractography algorithms for detecting abnormal structural brain networks in alzheimers disease. Frontiers in Aging Neuroscience 7(48), 401–408 (2015)
13. Zhang, D., Shen, D.: Multi-modal multi-task learning for joint prediction of multiple regression and classification variables in Alzheimer's disease. NeuroImage 59(2), 895–907 (2012)
14. Zhu, X., Huang, Z., Shen, H.T., Cheng, J., Xu, C.: Dimensionality reduction by mixed kernel canonical correlation analysis. Pattern Recognition 45(8), 3003–3016 (2012)
15. Zhu, X., Li, X., Zhang, S.: Block-row sparse multiview multilabel learning for image classification. IEEE Transactions on Cybernetics (2015)
16. Zhu, X., Suk, H.I., Shen, D.: Matrix-similarity based loss function and feature selection for alzheimer's disease diagnosis. In: CVPR, pp. 3089–3096 (2014)
17. Zhu, X., Suk, H.I., Shen, D.: A novel matrix-similarity based loss function for joint regression and classification in AD diagnosis. NeuroImage 100, 91–105 (2014)
18. Zhu, X., Suk, H.-I., Shen, D.: A novel multi-relation regularization method for regression and classification in AD diagnosis. In: Golland, P., Hata, N., Barillot, C., Hornegger, J., Howe, R. (eds.) MICCAI 2014, Part III. LNCS, vol. 8675, pp. 401–408. Springer, Heidelberg (2014)
19. Zhu, X., Zhang, L., Huang, Z.: A sparse embedding and least variance encoding approach to hashing. IEEE Transactions on Image Processing 23(9), 3737–3750 (2014)

Clustering Analysis for Semi-supervised Learning Improves Classification Performance of Digital Pathology

Mohammad Peikari[1]([✉]), Judit Zubovits[2], Gina Clarke[3], and Anne L. Martel[1,3]

[1] Medical Biophysics, University of Toronto, Toronto, Canada
mpeikari@sri.utoronto.ca
[2] Faculty of Medicine, University of Toronto, Toronto, Canada
[3] Physical Sciences, Sunnybrook Research Institute, Toronto, Canada

Abstract. Purpose: Completely labeled datasets of pathology slides are often difficult and time consuming to obtain. Semi-supervised learning methods are able to learn reliable models from small number of labeled instances and large quantities of unlabeled data. In this paper, we explored the potential of clustering analysis for semi-supervised support vector machine (SVM) classifier. Method: A clustering analysis method was proposed to find regions of high density prior to finding the decision boundary using a supervised SVM and was compared with another state-of-the-art semi-supervised technique. Different percentages of labeled instances were used to train supervised and semi-supervised SVM learners from an image dataset generated from 50 whole-mount images (8 patients) of breast specimen. Their cross-validated classification performances were compared with each other using the area under the ROC curve measure. Result: Our proposed clustering analysis for semi-supervised learning was able to produce a reliable classification model from small amounts of labeled data. Comparing the proposed method in this study with a well-known implementation of semi-supervised SVM, our method performed much faster and produced better results.

1 Introduction

In traditional and state-of-the-art pathology image classification, ground-truth images are manually or semi-manually labeled by a pathologist. A classification function is then trained using the ground-truth images and their labels to find a hyper plane that separates between different image class types. This classification approach belongs to the family of supervised learning in which it is assumed that the labels of all training cases are known. However, labeled instances are often expensive, time consuming, or difficult to obtain. This issue is even more crucial in case of pathology images since they require the effort of experienced human annotators who need to spend much of their time paying attention to highly subjective microscopic details. These details include but are not limited to the texture, morphology, and topology of different tissue components that are present in pathology images. In contrast to supervised learning, which only

© Springer International Publishing Switzerland 2015
L. Zhou et al. (Eds.): MLMI 2015, LNCS 9352, pp. 263–270, 2015.
DOI: 10.1007/978-3-319-24888-2_32

considers labeled data, semi-supervised learning (SSL) methods work with both labeled and unlabeled instances [3]. Unlabeled instances are often easier to obtain and require lesser human effort to generate. Therefore with SSL, it is possible to use large amounts of unlabeled instances together with a few labeled ones to train a classifier. In this paper, we aim to explore the potential of semi-supervised image classification in the context of triaging breast whole slide images. We also propose a new technique that works by analyzing clusters of labeled and unlabeled instance points in the feature space to find areas of high density and guide the learning method to find decision boundaries that passes through the low density regions.

2   Related Works

Semi-supervised learning techniques have previously been integrated with some medical applications to improve classification performances of partially labeled datasets [10,12] but the domain is not yet well explored in the pathology image analysis field. In order to make the most use of the unlabeled data, all semi-supervised methods assume the underlying distribution of data to have some structure [3]. Among the assumptions used in semi-supervised learning, *smoothness* and *cluster assumptions* seem to provide the basis for most of the state-of-the-art techniques [6]. The primary objective of these two assumptions are to ensure that decision boundaries pass through low density rather than high density regions of data instances in the feature space.

Depending on the learning problem in hand, there are many classification functions and methods available. Support vector machine (SVM) classifiers have been shown to be efficient and reliable and to date are one of the most widely used in pathology image classification literature. Semi-supervised SVM on the other hand extends the concept of traditional SVM to include the ability to learn from partially labeled datasets while maintaining accuracy. The idea is to virtually examine all possible label combinations of unlabeled data points along the path that minimizes an objective function and finds low density regions that the decision boundary could potentially pass [4,7,11,13]. There have been many implementations of the objective function optimization which are often lengthy and time inefficient for large datasets for which the reader is invited to see [5] for a review and performance comparison.

Recently, there are attempts to replace the lengthy objective function optimization process of semi-supervised SVMs by cluster analysis [6] [8] . The idea is to first find high density regions (clusters) in feature space through clustering methods and then clusters are passed to standard supervised SVM to find a separating decision boundary that passes through low density regions. In this study, we focus on exploring the potential of semi-supervised learning extension of SVM classifier by proposing a semi-supervised learning method that relies on clustering analysis of instance points in the feature space. To validate the performance of the proposed method with other state-of-the-art techniques, we have applied them to triage (or classify) pathology image patches of breast to clinically relevant or irrelevant.

3   Image Dataset and Data Collection

We used whole-mount H&E stained digital pathology slides ($n = 50$) from breast lumpectomy specimens of 8 patients. They were scanned at 5X (2 μm/pixel) magnification scale by a TissueScope scanner (Huron Technologies International Inc., Waterloo, Canada). Clearly irrelevant regions (fat and background) were removed from image slides using a simple image thresholding. Patches of 512×512 pixels (corresponding to an approximate area of 1 mm^2) were collected from each thresholded slide by overlaying a grid of uniformly spaced boxes on tissue regions (Fig. 1). The locations of overlaid boxes were randomized by their starting point on the tissue area. The horizontal and vertical distances between pairs of grid boxes were 1000 and 500 pixels respectively. A graphical user interface (GUI) was developed in collaboration with a pathologist to capture the biological information within every ROI. The interface allowed the expert pathologist to scroll through the images and evaluate the presence of diagnostically relevant information within every 512×512 pixel patch. In this study, diagnostically relevant regions may include areas of cancers, atypias, microcalcifications and lymphocytic vascular invasion; and irrelevant regions may include the presence of any other structure not included for relevant regions. The collaborating pathologist reviewed more than 2300 image patches (corresponding to 8 patient cases) randomized by their case identification number using the GUI.

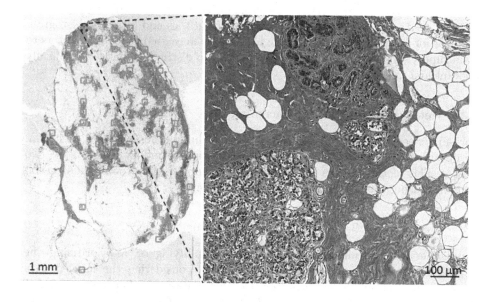

Fig. 1. 512×512 pixel green box patches randomly placed but uniformly spaced on tissue images (left), and a 512×512 pixel image patch at 5X magnification (right).

4   Methodology

The goal in pathology region triaging is to automatically identify diagnostically important (or relevant) regions from digital slides. We do this by finding appropriate texture representations that helps in defining present structures within image patches.

4.1   Texture Feature Extraction from Patches

Image patches were converted from RGB to Lab color space and the luminance channel was kept for texture analysis. The luminance channel was divided into optimum non-overlapping smaller tiles (32×32 pixels) to isolate different tissue components and was normalized (to have zero mean and standard deviation of one). Root filter set (RFS) [9] texture filters with different scales and directions were convolved with normalized tiles to highlight different textures at all scales and directions. The RFS bank used in this study consists of 38 filters of size 4×4 pixels: 2 anisotropic edge and bar filters in 6 directions and 3 scales $((\sigma_x, \sigma_y) = [(1,3), (2,6), (4,12)])$, and 2 rotationally symmetric Gaussian and Laplacian of Gaussian both with $\sigma = 10$ pixels. First order statistical measures were calculated from the maximal filter responses along all filter orientations of individual scales to form a 48 dimensional feature set per tile. Statistical measures used in this study were mean, mode, standard deviation, median, skewness and kurtosis. Bag of words (BoW) technique with an optimum dictionary size of 100 was used to regroup the derived features from tiles and form one histogram of words for every image patch. These histograms were used as feature vectors to train supervised and semi-supervised classifiers to distinguish between clinically relevant and irrelevant patches.

4.2   Method for Supervised Learning

For supervised learning, the standard SVM technique implemented in libsvm [2] library was used to find the separating decision boundary between the two classes. This method works by finding a maximum margin around the decision boundary using the labeled data (regularization).

4.3   Methods for Semi-supervised Learning

Semi-supervised learning methods work by modifying or re-prioritizing the hypothesis (based on unlabeled data) made by considering the labeled data alone. This will be done according to the relationship between unlabeled instances and that of labeled ones. Here, we would like to propose a semi-supervised learning technique that works by cluster analysis based on Ordering Points to Identify the Clustering Structure (OPTICS) [1] clustering algorithm and compare it with a well-known semi-supervised extension of SVM called SVM^{light}:

OPTICS+SVM: This approach works by first identifying areas of high density (in the feature space) through cluster analysis and then passing this information to a standard supervised SVM to find the decision boundary that passes through the low density regions. To find the regions with densely populated points that have any arbitrary shape, we employed the OPTICS clustering technique. This method works by ordering points of a database in such a way that spatially closest points become neighbors (and hence belong to one cluster) in the order set. To order points, this algorithm takes into account the reachability distances of points that are within a radius of ϵ from another point in the database (ϵ-neighborhood). The reachability distance between a point q from a reference point p is defined as the euclidean distance between q and p in such a way that q is within the ϵ-neighborhood of p. Therefore, a point and all its *reachable* neighbors belong to a cluster if they are within the kth reachable distance from each other. This way, points in the database are separated by their spatial distances from each other and therefore it is possible to form clusters of points that have any arbitrary shape. Therefore, OPTICS clustering method finds the regions that match with the previously noted cluster and smoothness assumptions. For a detailed explanation of the OPTICS clustering technique, reader is invited to see [1]. In this study, the value of k was set to one tenth of the size of feature space.

We implemented a semi-supervised version of the original OPTICS technique by forming clusters of points based on calculating reachability distances between labeled points and unlabeled ones. Therefore, clusters were formed by finding unlabeled points that are within reachable distances to labeled ones.

SVM^{light} [11]: this method is based on local combination of different label possibilities for every unlabeled point guided by a label switching mechanism. The label switching mechanism ensures that the balancing constraints between positive and negative classes are maintained and also an objective function is strictly decreased after switching of the labels. Therefore, this algorithm benefits from the standard SVM's regularization process and also gets help from unlabeled points to push the decision boundary away from high density regions.

4.4 Experimental Design

In order to compare the performances of supervised and semi-supervised techniques, we performed an 8 fold subject-wise cross-validation on the 8-patient dataset ($n = 2302$ image patches). For every fold in semi-supervised training methods, some percentage of one patient data were randomly selected to be the labeled set and label of the rest of points were kept hidden (unlabeled set). Similarly, for the supervised method, in every fold some percentage of one patient data were randomly selected to form labeled set and the rest were discarded. The randomly selected labeled points were kept the same for all experimental methods (paired labeled sets). The percentages of labeled points compared in this study were 1, 5, 10, 30, 50, and 70% of one patient data in every fold of the cross-validation scheme.

5 Results and Discussion

Mean of the area under the ROC curve (AUC) of the cross-validated experiments are given in Fig. 2 for each percentage of labeled data. As can be seen from Fig. 2, while performances of SVM^{light} and supervised SVM increased and approached mean AUC=0.78 when 30% or more of data were labeled, OPTICS+SVM had a superior performance and stayed close to the range [0.78, 0.8] at all times even when a portion as low as 1% of data were labeled.

Surprisingly, although no unlabeled points were used to guide the decision boundary for supervised SVM, its performance was better than SVM^{light} semi-supervised technique mainly for 5, and, 10% of labeled data. Thus, for this dataset, making use of unlabeled points made no improvements in the classification performance for the SVM^{light} technique with 5 or 10% labeled instances. This could be because the small amount of labeled points were not enough for SVM^{light} to find an optimum decision boundary and a large amount of unlabeled data might have mis-lead the technique to a sub-optimal solution. This may be a reason to explain its better performance when higher portions of labeled data are provided (Fig. 2).

Table 1 shows the performance comparison for the two semi-supervised techniques at different percentages of paired labeled data. As can be seen, the performance of the OPTICS+SVM is better than SVM^{light} while its training time is significantly lower on a 64-bit Intel(R) Xeon(R) CPU (at 3.50 GHz) machine. The differences reported in Table 1 were not shown to be statistically significant using a two-tailed Wilcoxon signed-rank test. This maybe due to the relatively small sized dataset used in this study.

Table 1. Results comparing the performances of 8 fold subject-wise cross-validated OPTICS+SVM and SVM^{light} at different percentages of labeled data from one patient per fold. OPTICS+SVM is shown to have significantly lower training time while having a better classification performance when compared with SVM^{light}.

	OPTICS+SVM			SVM^{light}		
Labeled Portion (%)	mAUC	95% CI	Train Time (min)	mAUC	95% CI	Train Time (min)
1	0.78	[0.66, 0.90]	25 ± 1.8	0.73	[0.67, 0.80]	2020 ± 1152.7
5	0.80	[0.70, 0.90]	25 ± 1.7	0.72	[0.62, 0.83]	2063 ± 1161.1
10	0.78	[0.68, 0.88]	23 ± 1.6	0.72	[0.61, 0.83]	2055 ± 1145.5
30	0.79	[0.70, 0.88]	24 ± 1.5	0.78	[0.70, 0.86]	1987 ± 1001.3
50	0.80	[0.71, 0.89]	23 ± 1.3	0.80	[0.71, 0.89]	1880 ± 1004.8
70	0.80	[0.70, 0.90]	25 ± 1.8	0.78	[0.68, 0.89]	1865 ± 974.9

CI = Confidence Interval
mAUC = mean AUC

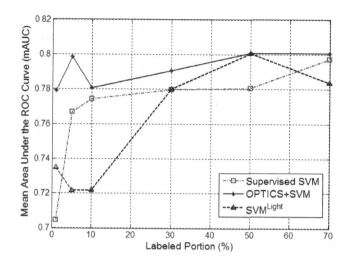

Fig. 2. Mean area under the ROC curve (mAUC) comparison of 8 fold subject-wise cross-validation ($n = 2302$ image patches) for supervised and semi-supervised SVM methods using different percentages of paired labeled data points from one patient data per fold.

5.1   Summary and Conclusion

In summary, getting hold of labeled datasets is usually difficult and expensive. It is particularly difficult for digital pathology slides since experienced human annotators are required to spend much of their time paying attention to highly subjective microscopic details. Therefore, it is beneficial to find ways of using fewer labeled data points in conjunction with many unlabeled data points to train a reliable image classifier. In this study, we compared performances of supervised and semi-supervised SVM methods for the problem of pathology image classification for a partially labeled dataset. We proposed a cluster analysis technique to find high density regions within the feature space prior to finding the decision boundary using standard SVM. We found that our proposed semi-supervised method is much faster than SVM^{light} while its performance is better when the number of labeled points is lower than 30%. On the other hand, comparing the two SSL methods with supervised SVM, we found that the ability to make use of additional unlabeled data did have some improvements on the performance of pathology image classification.

Although SVM^{light} is one of the most successful semi-supervised extension of SVM, its performance have not been shown to be better on synthetic and small sized datasets when compared to the Branch and Bound technique presented in [4]. The Branch and Bound method seems to give the globally optimum result since it searches through all label possibilities in the feature space. However, its performance is reported to be even slower than SVM^{light} and practically not feasible to apply on large datasets such as the one presented in this study.

We believe that the performance of OPTICS+SVM could be further improved by considering a more efficient points selection criteria for clusters. The parameter k (minimum number of points being in a reachable distance to each other) that was used by OPTICS to select candidate points for clusters were set to a constant value of one tenth of the size of feature space. Clusters of points could be found more effectively by considering a more dynamic selection of the value k for each region in the feature space based on local distance averaging. This may help avoiding points from other clusters to be included in each other.

Acknowledgement. This research is funded by Canadian Cancer Society (grant # 703006).

References

1. Ankerst, M., Breunig, M.M., Kriegel, H.P., Sander, J.: OPTICS: ordering points to identify the clustering structure. In: ACM SIGMOD International Conference on Management of Data, pp. 49–60. ACM Press (1999)
2. Chang, C.C., Lin, C.J.: LIBSVM : A Library for Support Vector Machines. ACM Transactions on Intelligent Systems and Technology **2**(3), 27:1–27:27 (2011)
3. Chapelle, O., Schölkopf, B.: Semi-Supervised Learning. The MIT Press, September 2006
4. Chapelle, O., Sindhwani, V., Keerthi, S.: Branch and bound for semi-supervised support vector machines. In: Advances in Neural Information Processing Systems (NIPS) (2006)
5. Chapelle, O., Sindhwani, V., Keerthi, S.: Optimization Techniques for Semi-Supervised Support Vector Machines. Journal of Machine Learning Research **9**, 203–233 (2008)
6. Chapelle, O., Zien, A.: Semi-supervised classification by low density separation. In: Tenth International Workshop on Artificial Intelligence and Statistics (AISTAT 2005) (2005)
7. Chapelle, O., Zien, A.: A continuation method for semi-supervised SVMs. In: International Conference on Machine Learning (2006)
8. Gan, H., Sang, N., Huang, R., Tong, X., Dan, Z.: Using clustering analysis to improve semi-supervised classification. Neurocomputing **101**, 290–298 (2013)
9. Geusebroek, J.M., Smeulders, A.W.M., van de Weijer, J.: Fast anisotropic Gauss filtering. IEEE Transactions on Image Processing: A Publication of the IEEE Signal Processing Society **12**(8), 938–943 (2003)
10. Helmi, H., Teck, D., Lai, C., Garibaldi, J.M.: Semi-supervised techniques in breast cancer classification. In: 12th Annual Workshop on Computational Intelligence (UKCI) (2012)
11. Joachims, T., Dortmund, U., Joachimscsuni-Dortmundde, T.: Advances in kernel methods. In: Support Vector Learning, pp. 169–184 (1999)
12. Shi, M., Zhang, B.: Semi-supervised learning improves gene expression-based prediction of cancer recurrence. Bioinformatics **27**(21), 3017–3023 (2011)
13. Yuille, A.L., Rangarajan, A.: The Concave-Convex Procedure (CCCP). Neural Computation **15**(2), 915–936 (2003)

A Composite of Features for Learning-Based Coronary Artery Segmentation on Cardiac CT Angiography

Yanling Chi[1]([✉]), Weimin Huang[1], Jiayin Zhou[1], Liang Zhong[2], Swee Yaw Tan[2], Keng Yung Jih Felix[2], Low Choon Seng Sheon[3], and Ru San Tan[2]

[1] Institute for Infocomm Research, A*STAR, 1 Fusionopolis Way, #21-01 Connexis, Singapore138632, Singapore
{chiyl,wmhuang,jzhou}@i2r.a-star.edu.sg
[2] National Heart Center Singapore, 5 Hospital Drive, Singapore169609, Singapore
zhong.liang@nhcs.com.sg,
{tan.swee.yaw,felix.keng.y.j,tan.ru.san}@singhealth.com.sg
[3] Department of Diagnostic Radiology, Singapore General Hospital, Singapore169608, Singapore
shoen.low@sgh.com.sg

Abstract. Coronary artery segmentation is important in quantitative coronary angiography. In this work, a novel method is proposed for coronary artery segmentation. It integrates coronary artery features of density, local shape and global structure into the learning framework. The density feature is the vessel's relative density estimated by means of Gaussian mixture models and is able to suppress individual variances. The local tube shape of the vessel is measured with the advantages of the 3-dimensional multi-scale Hessian filter and is able to enhance the small vessels. The global structure feature is predicted from a support vector regression in terms of vessel's spatial position and emphasizes the geometric morphometric attribute of the coronary artery tree running across the surface of the heart. The features are fed into a support vector classifier for vessel segmentation. The proposed methodology was tested on ten 3D cardiac computed tomography angiography datasets. It obtained a sensitivity of 81%, a specificity of 99%, and Dice coefficient of 84%. The performance is good.

1 Introduction

In coronary heart disease (CHD), plaque builds up inside the coronary artery and results in narrowing of artery lumen and limitation of the blood supply to the heart muscle. CHD could lead to a life-threatening heart attack. Cardiac computed tomography angiography (CTA) is a commonly used non-invasive imaging modality for CHD diagnosis. Timely and correct diagnosis requires quantitative approaches to the angiographic evaluation of coronary anatomy, among which coronary artery segmentation is often one of the key elements. Automatic segmentation of coronary artery tree is challenging due to individual variances, vessel abnormalities of stenosis, calcification, and insufficient contrast agent, etc. A robust algorithm is required.

Feature selection is essential in vessel segmentation. On CTA images, the coronary artery appears hyperdense compared with the mayocardium. Thus, the density is a

© Springer International Publishing Switzerland 2015
L. Zhou et al. (Eds.): MLMI 2015, LNCS 9352, pp. 271–279, 2015.
DOI: 10.1007/978-3-319-24888-2_33

straightforward feature for vessel segmentation. Kitslaar et al. [1] proposed to segment the coronary tree using a region growing scheme on the images with the heart and aorta pre-segmented. Wang et al. [2] presented a fuzzy connectedness algorithm for the coronary artery segmentation. Automatic rib cage removal and ascending aorta tracing were included to initialize the segmentation. The density feature works well on large vessels of high contrast, but is not discriminative for tiny vessels of low-contrast. The local shape features, in the form of 3D tubular/cylinder structure or 2D cross-sectional template, are commonly used for vessel enhancement or shape constraints of segmentation. Li et al. [3] proposed to segment vessels using Hessian filters together with Gaussian filter based intensity compensation. Zhou et al. [4] proposed to extract coronary artery tree using multi-scale Hessian filter based vessel enhancement and a 3D dynamic balloon tracking. Yang et al. [5] improved the Frangi's filter by suppressing step-edge responses. The improved filter was employed in a centerline extraction pipeline. Zambal et al. [6] proposed to match two small-scale cylinder-like models via depth-first search to extract the coronary artery tree. Schaap et al. [7] presented a vessel cross sectional segmentation using shape regression. Wong et al. [8] employed non-linear principal curves in vessel centerline detection and the vessels were modelled on cylinders along the polygonal lines. Schneider et al. [9] proposed to segment vessels using multivariate Hough voting and oblique random forests, with local image features extracted by steerable filters. Friman et al. [10] proposed a multiple hypothesis template of the vessels for tracking approach of small arteries. Generally, the local shape features/constraints mentioned in the above methods need an elaborate tracing scheme to complete the segmentation. To simplify the segmentation procedure, a global artery model was built in [11, 12]. Kitamura et al. [11] proposed to build the coronary shape model composed of 30 discrete nodes sampled from three major coronary arteries and two coronary veins. The shape model was then fitted to the detected candidates using a graph matching. Zheng et al. [12] proposed to generate a mean centerline model of the coronary arteries on 108 datasets and the model was employed to constrain the tracing of coronary arteries to detect. The good performance of those two methods indicated the helpfulness from the global structure information of coronary arteries, however, so far, few work has been reported on it.

In this work, we proposed a composite of features for coronary artery segmentation via a supervised learning framework. The composite features describe the coronary arteries' properties of density, local shape, and global structure. A novel relative density feature is estimated using Gaussian mixture models and is able to suppress the individual variances. A local shape feature is measured via the 3D multi-scale Hessian filter to enhance small vessels. A new global structure feature is predicted from a support vector regression (SVR) in terms of vessel position and emphasizes the geometric morphometric attribute of the coronary artery tree running across the surface of the heart. This feature facilitates discriminating the coronary artery tree from other spurious structures. This method is different from the studies in [11, 12], where only the 3 main arteries were separately modelled. Our global structure feature describes the whole coronary tree, which is relatively robust to coronary variants. The composite features are fed into a support vector classifier (SVC) for vessel segmentation. The contributions of our work include (1) a general composite representation of the coronary tree, (2) a novel relative density feature, (3) a new global structure feature, and (4) the integration of composite features into a supervised learning framework.

2   Composite Features

2.1   Relative Density

The imaged vessel density varies due to individual variances or imaging protocols, as observed in the hyper-dense region in Fig. 1(a). An absolute density feature may not work well for all datasets. A relative one is better. On cardiac CTA, the visible tissues are bone, vessel, muscle, skin, fat etc. They form several peaks in the density histogram, which can be modelled by a Gaussian Mixture Model (GMM) [13]. Furthermore, we cropped the CTA images within the field of view of the heart, and the density peaks of the cropped images are similar to that of the original images. As shown in Fig. 1(b), the density centers of those peaks remain same while the counts decrease after cropping. Thus, it is possible for us to achieve a relative density representation consistent in appropriate ROIs, which is defined as the density ratio of vessels to its surrounding tissues, to deal with diverse images.

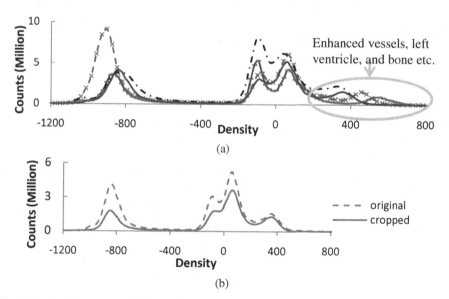

Fig. 1. density histograms of (a) four CTA images, (b) a CTA images cropped around the heart

A GMM is a parametric probability density function represented as a weighted sum of Gaussian component densities: $p(v|\theta) = \sum_{i=1}^{M} w_i \frac{1}{\sqrt{2\pi|\Sigma_i|}} exp\left\{-\frac{1}{2}(v - \mu_i)' \Sigma_i^{-1}(v - \mu_i)\right\}$, where v is the density feature; M is the number of Gaussian components; $\{w_i\}_{i=1}^{M}$ are the mixture weights, satisfying the constraint that $\sum_{i=1}^{M} w_i = 1$; $\{\mu_i\}_{i=1}^{M}$ are the mean vectors and $\{\Sigma_i\}_{i=1}^{M}$ are the covariance matrixes. The complete GMM is parameterized by $\theta = \{w_i, \mu_i, \Sigma_i\}_{i=1}^{M}$. Here, M is empirically set a value of 4, since most of the datasets form four peaks in histogram as shown in Fig. 1. An iterative Expecta-tion-Maximization (EM) algorithm [14] is used to estimate the parameters. If the Gaussian components are ranked in mean density from high to low, the relative densi-ty of a voxel is calculated as the ratio of its image density, v, to the mean density values of the first two components, as shown in (1). The two components are usually the vessel's neighbors which are close to vessels in terms of density or position.

$$F^{RD} = \{v/\mu_1 , \ v/\mu_2 \} \tag{1}$$

2.2   Local Shape Feature

Hessian matrix-based filter has been widely used in coronary artery segmentation [3-5]. A combination of the eigenvalues of the Hessian matrix [15], is adopted here to describe vessel's shape locally. The local shape feature at a voxel is calculated as

$$F^{LS} = \begin{cases} |\lambda_2| - \lambda_1, & if \ \ |\lambda_1| \le |\lambda_2| \le |\lambda_3|, \ and \ \lambda_2, \lambda_3 < 0 \\ 0 & otherwise \end{cases} \tag{2}$$

where $\lambda_1, \lambda_2, \lambda_3$ are the eigenvalues of the Hessian matrix. Multi-scale filtering scheme is also adopted to tackle vessels of various sizes, which is fulfilled by employ-ing Gaussian smoothing with kernel size of δ on the images before Hessian filtering. The upper limit of the coronary lumen diameter is 4.5mm, reported by Dodge et al. [16]. Thus, δ is set as 1, 2, 3, 4 and 5 mm in this study. The maximum value among single scale filter responses is retained as local shape feature at this voxel.

2.3   Global Structure Feature

We proposed to model global spatial structure of the coronary tree using support vec-tor regression (SVR) with radial basis function (RBF) kernel [17].

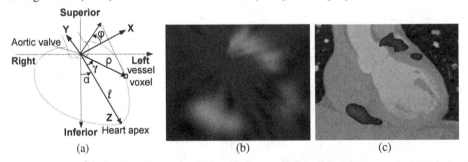

(a)   (b)   (c)

Fig. 2. (a) the polar coordinates of a vessel voxel in a defined coordinate system XYZ, (b) an example of the global feature response map, (c) the artery regions have large responses (red)

Input Vector Preparation. To train a SVR, the input data has to be normalized. The coronary circulation is first introduced. The left and right coronary arteries originate at the root of the aorta, run on the surface of the heart and supply blood to the myo-cardium. The left coronary artery distributes blood to the left side of the heart, the left atrium and ventricle, and the interventricular septum. The right coronary artery proceeds along the coronary sulcus and distributes blood to the right atrium, portions of both ventricles, and the heart conduction system. The apex of the heart is the lowest superficial part of the heart, formed by the left ventricle and directed downward, forward, and to the left [16, 20]. According to the coronary artery anatomy, it can be observed that the aortic root and the heart apex are key points in coronary structure. Thus, the vector from aortic valve to the heart apex is defined as the reference vector to regularize the input data. In our work, the input vectors for SVR training are derived from the vessel's polar coordinates as illustrated in Fig.2 (a). The reference vector's direction is defined as the Z axis or polar axis and its length is written as ℓ. Given an image coordinate system $X'Y'Z'$ with axis X' from right to left, Y' from posterior to anterior, and Z' from superior to inferior; a new coordinate system XYZ is established by rotating $X'Y'Z'$ an angle of α along the axis perpendicular to both Z and Z'. In XYZ, the polar coordinates of a vessel voxel can be calculated as $\{\rho, \gamma, \varphi\}$. Thus, the input vector of a training voxel is

$$x = \{\rho/\ell, \gamma, sin\varphi, cos\varphi\} \tag{3}$$

where the radial coordinate ρ is normalized by ℓ for regularization on size. The angular coordinate γ is directly used, while φ is represented as sin φ and cos φ to retain its periodical and continuous attributes.

Support Vector Regression. Given the input vectors and the corresponding target vectors, SVR is employed to model the global spatial structure using

$$f(x) = \sum_{i=1}^{N} \beta_i \exp\left(-\frac{\|x_i - x\|^2}{2\sigma^2}\right) + b \tag{4}$$

where N is the number of data points, and x_i is the input vectors. The model is trained with the aid of SVM[light] [18]. To select the optimized parameters for SVR, a k-fold cross-validation technique is used. Four training datasets are evenly divided into two groups. One group serves as training set and the other is used to test the model. Then, two groups exchange the roles in training and testing, and the experiments are conducted again. The parameters that minimize the average mean square error are selected. In this work, σ is set as 7.1. Given a voxel with polar coordinates of $\{\rho, \gamma, \varphi\}$, its global structure feature is predicted using the trained SVR as:

$$F^{GS} = f(\{\rho/\ell, \gamma, sin\varphi, cos\varphi\}) \tag{5}$$

The global feature is mainly designed to discriminate coronary arteries from other anatomical structures in terms of spatial position. It will highlight the vessels on the heart surface so as to remove the false positives, which are similar to coronary arteries in density and local shape, e.g. vessels in pulmonary circulation. An example of the global feature map was shown in Fig. 2(b), where voxels around the heart surface has relatively strong responses. When overlaid with the CTA images as shown in Fig. 2 (c), the high response voxels were found covering regions the arteries run through.

3   Supervised Learning-Based Segmentation

To train a supervised-learning based classifier, we first need to decide the training samples. For one CTA dataset, the N^s positive samples are randomly selected from the labelled coronary arteries. The N^{train} training datasets are evenly sampled and we have $N^{train} \times N^s$ positive samples in total. The negative samples are obtained for balance. Here, the negative data refers to image voxels except for the labelled coronary arteries. As described in section 2.1, one dataset was modelled using M Gaussian components with regards to density, which represent various tissues for classifier to discriminate. Therefore, we randomly sample the negative data in the M components respectively. The sample size in each component is the same N^s/M. In this work, N^s is set as 100 empirically. The composite features of the samples, $F = \{F^{RD}, F^{LS}, F^{GS}\}$, can be calculated using (1), (2), and (5). The aortic valve and the heart apex, for F^{GS} computation, are manually located on the images by the user.

With the samples and their composite features obtained, a support vector classifier (SVC) is trained for coronary artery segmentation. In the classification problem using SVC, the objective is to find a hyperplane that separate the classes with a maximized separation margin. In this work, a linear unbiased hyperplane was sought to separate the coronary arteries from other tissues.

To extract a connected coronary artery tree, a region growing scheme is employed on the output images from SVC, which starts growing from the aorta. The aorta appears hyperdense on cardic CT angiography and can be segmented by an appropriate threshold. Here, the threshold is set as $\mu_1 - \Sigma_1$, where μ_1 and Σ_1 are defined in Section 2.1. The upper limit of ascending aortic diameter is 42.6 mm reported by Mao et al. [19]. The angle of aortic insertion on the left ventricle is from 30 to 60 degrees [20]. Based on these statistics, a separation disc of 5cm in diameter is placed on the aortic valve to isolate the aorta from the left ventricle. The separation disc's normal direction is along the polar axis Z defined in Section 2.3. The segmented aorta is superposed on the output images of the classifier to start the region growing.

4   Experimental Results and Discussion

Experimental Results. After approval by the Institutional Review Board, ten anonymized cardiac CTA datasets, from ten CHD patients, were evaluated in this work. The CTA scans were acquired on a 320-row scanner (Aquilion ONE, Toshiba Medical System) in the National Heart Centre Singapore (NHCS) between May and July 2014. Diastolic reconstructions were used and the voxel size of the datasets was $(0.39 \pm 0.05) \times (0.39 \pm 0.05) \times 0.5mm^3$. Six datasets were randomly selected for training and the other four were used for testing. With the supervision from a cardiologist, an engineer manually labelled the aortic valve, the heart apex, and the coronary arteries on the images using an interactive image analysis tool. The labelling results were used as the ground truth for system's training and evaluation.

The common performance measurements of sensitivity, specificity and Dice coefficient were used for the evaluation. The larger the measurements, the more similar the result and the ground-truth are. To focus on the segmented coronary artery, the aorta was manually removed from each segmentation result. The method was trained on the six training datasets and tested on the four testing datasets. It obtained a sensitivity of 0.81 ± 0.05 , a specificity of 0.99 ± 0.005 , and Dice coefficient of

0.84 ± 0.03. One example is shown in Fig. 3. It can be observed that our method performed well on most of the vessels and had limitations with tiny vessels.

Discussion. Schaap el al. [21] proposed a standard methodology to evaluate coronary artery centerline extraction algorithms with a public Rotterdam database. The database consists of two parts. The first part includes 8 CTA datasets and the corresponding reference centerlines. The second part includes 24 CTA datasets. Even though the Rotterdam evaluation framework focuses on the centerlines of four major coronary arteries while our method aims to segment the full coronary artery tree, it is still interesting to evaluate our pre-trained classifier on the public database for data diversity.

Our results on the first part were evaluated under the framework using the provided reference centerlines and software. To tailor our results to be comparable to the reference centerlines, we extracted the segmentation's skeletons using a thinning algorithm [22]. Before skeletonization, morphological operations of dilation and erosion were employed for hole-filling. The average performance was: 95.2% of *overlap* (OV), 70.4% of *overlap until first error* (OF), 98.1% of *overlap with the clinically relevant part of the vessel* (OT) and 0.41 mm of *average inside* (AI). The results were encouraging. The AI was about one voxel. It was probably because the hole-filling and skeletonization were conducted on the original images and the minimal magnitude of error was one voxel. Since extra work has been involved to adapt our results for evaluation under the Rotterdam's framework, the evaluation was viewed as an indirect assessment of our method, thus, was included in the discussion section.

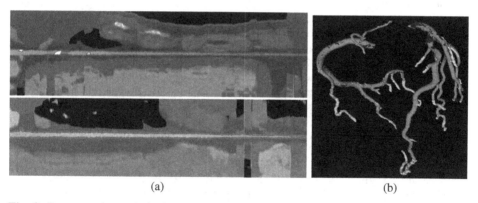

(a)   (b)

Fig. 3. One example result for illustration (a) segmented left anterior descending artery (top) and right coronary artery (bottom) overlaid with CTA images using curved multi-planar reformation (b) a segmented complete coronary artery tree compared with the ground truth (green: true positives, blue: false positives, yellow: false negatives)

5   Conclusions and Future works

In this paper, we proposed a new representation of coronary arteries. The relative density feature is able to supress individual variances, and the global feature is helpful in excluding the spurious structures. The composite of features was integrated into the supervised-learning framework to develop a classifier for coronary artery segmentation. The classifier is applicable to diverse images, and has achieved good performance on both our data and public data. Future work will include algorithm improvement on accuracy for the comprehensive evaluation of CHD.

Acknowledgement. This work was supported by a research grant (1321480008) from the Biomedical Engineering Programme, Agency for Science, Technology and Research (A*STAR), Singapore.

References

1. Kitslaar, P., Frenay, M., Oost, E., Dijkstra, J., Stoel, B., Reiber, J.: Connected component and morphology based extraction of arterial centerlines of the heart (CocomoBeach). In: MICCAI Workshop S4 (2008)
2. Wang, C., Smedby, O.: An automatic seeding method for coronary artery segmentation and skeletonization in CTA. In: MICCAI Workshop S4 (2008)
3. Li, Z., Zhang, Y., Liu, G., Shao, H., Li, W.: A robust coronary artery identification and centerline extraction method in angiographies. Biomed. Signal Proce. 16, 1–8 (2015)
4. Zhou, C., Chan, H., Chughtai, C., Patel, S., Hadijiiski, L., Wei, J., Kazerooni, E.: Automated coronary artery tree extraction in coronary CT angiography using a multi-scale enhancement and dynamic balloon tracking (MSCAR-DBT) method. Comput. Med. Imag. Grap. 36, 1–10 (2012)
5. Yang, G., Kitslaar, P., Frenay, M., Broersen, A., Boogers, M., Bax, J., Reiber, J., Dijkstra, J.: Automatic centerline extraction of coronary arteries in coronary computed tomographic angiography. Int. J. Card. Imaging 28(4), 921–933 (2012)
6. Zambal, S., Hladuvka, J., Kanitsar, A., Buhler, K.: Shape and appearance models for automatic coronary artery tracking. In: MICCAI Workshop S4 (2008)
7. Schaap, M., Walum, T., Neefjes, L., Metz, C., Capuano, E., Bruijne, M., Niessen, W.: Robust shape regression for supervised vessel segmentation and its application to coronary segmentation in CTA. IEEE Trans. Med. Imaging 30(11), 1974–1986 (2011)
8. Wong, W., So, R., Chung, A.: Principal curves for lumen center extraction and flow channel width estimation in 3-D arterial networks: theory, algorithm, and validation. IEEE Trans. Image Process. 21(4), 1847–1862 (2012)
9. Schneider, M., Hirsch, S., Weber, B., Szekely, G., Menze, B.: Joint 3-D vessel segmentation and centerline extraction using oblique Hough forests with steerable filters. Med Image Anal 19, 220–249 (2015)
10. Friman, O., Hindennach, M., Kuhnel, C., Peitgen, H.: Multiple hypothesis template tracking of small 3D vessel structures. Med. Image Anal. 14, 160–171 (2010)
11. Kitamura Y., Li Y., and Ito W.: Automatic coronary extraction by supervised detection and shape matching. In: Proc. of ISBI, pp. 234-237 (2012)
12. Zheng, Y., Tek, H., Funka-Lea, G.: Robust and accurate coronary artery centerline extraction in CTA by combining model-driven and data-driven approaches. In: Mori, K., Sakuma, I., Sato, Y., Barillot, C., Navab, N. (eds.) MICCAI 2013, Part III. LNCS, vol. 8151, pp. 74–81. Springer, Heidelberg (2013)
13. Bishop, C.: Pattern Recognition and Machine Learning, pp. 78–124. Springer Science Business Media, Heidelberg (2006)
14. Dempster, A.P., Laird, N.M., Rubin, D.B.: Maximum-likelihood from incomplete data via the EM algorithm. J. Royal Statist. Soc. Ser. B. 39(1), 1–38 (1977)

15. Sato, Y., Nakajima, S., Shiraga, N., Atsumi, H., Yoshida, S., Koller, T., Gerig, G., Kikinis, R.: Three-dimensional multi-scale line filter for segmentation and visualization of curvilinear structures in medical images. Med. Image Anal. **2**(2), 143–168 (1998)

16. Dodge, J., Brown, B., Bolson, E., Dodge, H.: Lumen diameter of normal human coronary arteries. Influence of age, sex, anatomic variation, and left ventricular hypertrophy or dilation. Circulation **86**, 232–246 (1992)

17. Smola, A., Scholkopf, B.: A tutorial on support vector regression. Stat. Comp. **14**, 199–222 (2004)

18. Joachims T.: Estimating the generalization performance of an SVM efficiently. In: Proc. ICML, pp. 431-438 (2000)

19. Mao, S., Ahmadi, N., Shah, B., Beckmann, D., Chen, A., Ngo, L., Flores, F., Gao, Y., Budoff, M.: Normal thoracic aorta diameter on cardiac computed tomography in healthy asymptomatic adult; impact of age and gender. Acad Radiol **15**(7), 827–834 (2008)

20. Hazel, R., Pollack, S., Reichek, N.: Investigation of the relationship between age and the angle of aortic insertion on the left ventricle using 3D MRI. J. Cardiov. Magn. Resonance **14**, 77–78 (2012)

21. Schaap, M., Metz, C., Walsum, T., Giessen, A., et al.: Standardized evaluation methodology and reference database for evaluating coronary artery centerline extraction algorithms. Med. Image Anal. **13**, 701–714 (2009)

22. Lee, T., Kashyap, R., Chu, C.: Building skeleton models via 3-D medical surface/axis thinning algorithms. Graph. Model and Im. Proc. **56**(6), 462–478 (1994)

Ensemble Prostate Tumor Classification in H&E Whole Slide Imaging via Stain Normalization and Cell Density Estimation

Michaela Weingant[1], Hayley M. Reynolds[2,3], Annette Haworth[2,3], Catherine Mitchell[4], Scott Williams[5], and Matthew D. DiFranco[6]([✉])

[1] Vienna University of Technology, Vienna, Austria
[2] Department of Physical Sciences, Peter MacCallum Cancer Centre, Melbourne, Australia
[3] Sir Peter MacCallum Department of Oncology, University of Melbourne, Melbourne, Australia
[4] Department of Pathology, Peter MacCallum Cancer Centre, Melbourne, Australia
[5] Division of Radiation Oncology and Cancer Imaging, Peter MacCallum Cancer Centre, Melbourne, Australia
[6] Center for Medical Physics and Biomedical Engineering, Medical University Vienna, Vienna, Austria
matthew.difranco@meduniwien.ac.at

Abstract. Classification of prostate tumor regions in digital histology images requires comparable features across datasets. Here we introduce adaptive cell density estimation and apply H&E stain normalization into a supervised classification framework to improve inter-cohort classifier robustness. The framework uses Random Forest feature selection, class-balanced training example subsampling and support vector machine (SVM) classification to predict the presence of high- and low-grade prostate cancer (HG-PCa and LG-PCa) on image tiles. Using annotated whole-slide prostate digital pathology images to train and test on two separate patient cohorts, classification performance, as measured with area under the ROC curve (AUC), was 0.703 for HG-PCa and 0.705 for LG-PCa. These results improve upon previous work and demonstrate the effectiveness of cell-density and stain normalization on classification of prostate digital slides across cohorts.

Keywords: Machine learning · Digital pathology · Tumor prediction · Prostate · Cell counting

1 Introduction

A variety of clinical and research applications would benefit from computer aided methods for accurate and reliable tumor classification in whole mount

H.M. Reynolds—Funded by a Movember Young Investigator Grant awarded through Prostate Cancer Foundation of Australia Research Program.

A. Haworth—Supported by PdCCRS grant 628592 with funding partners: Prostate Cancer Foundation of Australia; Radiation Oncology Section of the Australian Government of Health and Ageing; Cancer Australia.

© Springer International Publishing Switzerland 2015
L. Zhou et al. (Eds.): MLMI 2015, LNCS 9352, pp. 280–287, 2015.
DOI: 10.1007/978-3-319-24888-2_34

histology images. Current fields of research include computer aided methods to classify tumor location [3] and correlation studies assessing histology ground-truth data with multi-parametric MRI (mpMRI) [1,5].

Computer-aided interpretation of prostate H&E histopathology images relies heavily on color information. However, the chromatic appearance of digital whole-slide imagery is subject to many sources of variability, such as manufacturer-dependent staining agents for dying the tissue, institute-dependent staining protocols and hardware-dependent scanning conditions [8]. Stain normalization using color deconvolution, in which RGB pixel data is transformed into stain-specific color channels, helps overcome this obstacle. Fixed stain vector values have been determined for a range of histology stains, including H&E [10], more recent publications proposed image-specific stain vectors [2,6,7].

The use of color and texture-based features for predicting LG-PCa and HG-PCa on whole slide images is desired due to the efficiency and simplicity of feature extraction on such large images. However, a recent study [4] reported unsatisfactory results (AUC=0.632 for HG-PCa, 0.486 for LG-PCa) when training a classifier on cohort and testing on another, suggesting the need for stain-normalized color and texture features, as well as more descriptive measures such as cell density [9].

In this work we aimed to improve on the cross-cohort classifier performance from [4] by (1) including a cell density feature into the classification framework and (2) by applying stain normalization as proposed in [7] prior to color and texture feature extraction in order to account for variations in H&E staining (Fig. 1).

2 Methods

Datasets. Three H&E-stained datasets were used in this work. The first, available as a supplement to [11], has nuclei annotations and served as the ground-truth for developing and quantifying the optimized cell density estimation. It consisted of 36 H&E image-tiles of 600x600 pixels from multiple human tissue sites with a resolution of 0.23 m per Pixel (MPP).

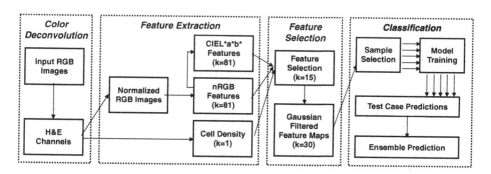

Fig. 1. Flowchart of normalization and cell density within classification framework

Table 1. Number of tiles from annotated regions for each image, with number of annotated detailed ROIs in parentheses.

Sample	Non-Cancer	LG-PCa	HG-PCa	Sample	Non-Cancer	LG-PCa	HG-PCa
A01	14939 (17)	924 (5)	1444 (10)	B01	855 (6)	646 (9)	11 (4)
A02	14770 (14)	63 (3)	668 (18)	B02	2073 (49)	1 (1)	36 (11)
A03	25673 (8)	0 (0)	319 (3)	B03	0 (0)	4516 (2)	0 (0)
A04	6499 (7)	900 (4)	866 (16)	B05	6337 (15)	95 (12)	80 (10)
A05	9668 (6)	445 (4)	221 (4)	B06	16569 (18)	159 (18)	458 (20)
A06	1898 (7)	951 (4)	290 (3)	B07	1026 (15)	411 (15)	14 (3)
A07	0 (0)	775 (9)	453 (3)	B08	14167 (20)	114 (24)	0 (0)
A08	2462 (13)	845 (7)	719 (3)	B09	2335 (13)	174 (10)	34 (5)
A09	8969 (9)	800 (3)	0 (0)	B10	12525 (23)	286 (15)	106 (13)
A10	11159 (7)	39 (1)	914 (4)				
A11	10684 (5)	450 (1)	2190 (12)				
A12	5622 (16)	1273 (2)	1087 (2)				
A13	1310 (1)	800 (8)	94 (3)				
A14	3613 (7)	608 (2)	0 (0)				
Cohort A	117266 (117)	8873 (53)	9265 (81)	Cohort B	55887 (159)	6402 (106)	739 (66)

The second and third dataset, called *Cohort A* and *Cohort B* and previously described in [4], consisted of post-resection prostate H&E digital slides. Cohort A consisted of 14 H&E prostate histopathology whole slide images from one pathology center, taken at 400x magnification and stored with 0.238 MPP. Cohort B was composed of 9 H&E prostate histopathology whole slide images taken at 200x magnification and stored with 0.504 MPP from a different pathology center. Each cohort was annotated by a different expert pathologist.

These two datasets included annotated ROIs, refered to as *detailed* in the results, of homogeneous high-grade, low-grade and benign tissue patterns used here to define training and testing data for various supervised classification scenarios. Tile and region counts for these detailed ROIs are shown in Table 1. For Cohort B, we also have clinical ROIs from the original glass slides which delineate tumor and non-tumor regions more generally, and we refer to these in the results as *clinical* ROIs.

H&E Color Deconvolution and Stain Normalization. In order to mitigate the effects of H&E stain variation between our datasets we included a color normalization method based on [7]. The normalization process involves identification of image-specific stain-vectors, stain deconvolution, and finally normalization to a target appearance in RGB space.

For the stain vector identification, the RGB values of the image in question were first converted to optical density (OD) [10]. The transformation is calculated as $OD = -log_{10}(I)$ where I holds the RGB intensity values of each pixel, normalized to [0 1]. After identifying the image-specific stain vectors V according to [7], the deconvolution was realized using the equation $C = V^{-1}OD$ on

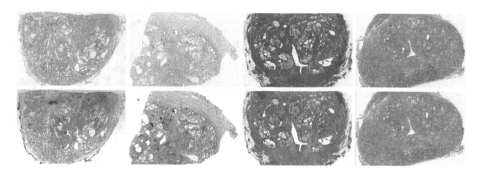

Fig. 2. Two images from Cohort A (left, middle left) and two images from Cohort B (middle right, right). Top row shows original staining, bottom row shows normalized staining.

all OD-tuples, where the three-channel matrix C contains the intensity in every pixel for each of the stains (i.e. H, E and a vector orthogonal to H and E). The results of color deconvolution were used in the cell density algorithm.

Finally, the normalized images I_{norm} were computed using $I_{norm} = e^{-V_{target}*C}$, where V_{target} denotes the stain-matrix containing the desired appearance. The effect of the normalization can be seen in Fig. 2. The previously heterogeneous appearances of different images are transformed to a commonly used uniform appearance, applying a standard H&E vector V_{target} from [10]. Normalized images were used for subsequent color and texture feature extraction (Fig. 1).

Cell Density Estimation. The parameters used in [9] had been empirically tuned to images from Cohort B using a subset of representative benign and tumor tiles. Here, we aimed to determine the parameters more objectively to ensure they were suitable for application across data from multiple centers rather than biased towards one particular center. The optimization was conducted via a grid-search of the parameter space, using the multiple-site dataset from [11] with per-nucleus annotations to quantify the respective outcome. The five parameters were: (1) the radius r_1 of an object to be accepted as a nucleus candidate in the radial symmetry transform (2) the roundness constraint α, which lies between 0, allowing an arbitrary shape and 4, allowing only strictly round shapes (3) the minimum intensity gradient threshold γ for pixels contributing to the symmetry measurement (4) the region radius r_2 of the non-maxima suppression (NMS) and (5) a threshold t below which local maxima are ignored as a maximum candidate for the NMS.

The final parameters were chosen considering two metrics: (1) an adjusted recall measure ($Recall + \frac{FalsePositives}{TruePositives + FalseNegatives}$) of close to 1.5, and (2) a high F_2-scores (similar to the F-score, but weighting recall twice as important as precision).

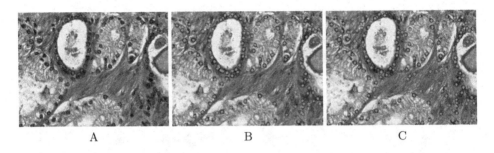

A   B   C

Fig. 3. Nuclei identification on a sample image from Cohort B: (A) original ROI (B) using fixed value deconvolution and empirically determined parameters according to [9] (C) using the proposed adaptive deconvolution and optimized parameters.

Classification Framework. Our approach to whole-slide classification comes from [3], and our training scenarios are the same as [4]. Here we use stain normalization prior to calculating color channel histogram and gray level co-occurrence texture features for each tile, and we also include cell density in the feature vector. Images were divided into non-overlapping tiles of approximately 127 m, and for each tile cell density ($k_{cd} = 1$) co-occurence texture features ($k_{co} = 21$) as well as histogram-based features ($k_{hist} = 6$) for each of the six channels of the RGB and $CIEL^*a^*b^*$ colorspaces were calculated, for a total of ($k = 163$) features per tile. Expert annotations were used to assign a class label to each training tile based on the underlying tissue class. For each classification scenario, a Random Forest based feature selection was performed, and the 15 highest ranking features based on Gini-importance were chosen to build a training model. After feature selection, 2-D Gaussian filters ($\sigma = 2.4, 2.8$) were applied to generate smoothed feature maps for inclusion into training models.

For each classification model, up to 3000 tiles were randomly sampled, with the constraint that each ROI from the training images was represented in the training set. Classifiers were trained using radial basis function support vector machines (RBF-SVMs) with $C = 2^{-2}$ and $\gamma = 2^{-9}$. For each training scenario, multiple models were generated and used as an ensemble for pooling predictions on the test sets. For each query image, predictions always based on training models that did not include that image. In total, we ran 5 training scenarios: 01 and 02 used only data from Cohort A, 04 and 05 used only data from Cohort B, and 03 used data from both cohorts. Classifier performance is reported as area under the ROC curve (AUC) for each cohort of images.

3   Results

The optimized parameters and the updated metrics for the proposed cell density method in comparison to [9] are summarized in Table 2. An illustration of the nuclei detection on a sample image before and after optimization is shown in Fig. 3.

Classification results are shown in Table 3. Scenario 03 includes data from both cohorts, and we see comparable AUC values for LG-PCa classification between detailed annotations from cohorts A and B (0.854 and 0.870, respectively). For HG-PCa, we note that scenario 03 performs better on Cohort B than Cohort A (0.952 vs. 0.875). For classification of Cohort B using Cohort A for training (Runs 01 and 02), an AUC of 0.705 and 0.657 for LG-PCa and 0.686 and 0.703 for HG-PCa is achieved. Classification of Cohort A using Cohort B as training data (Runs 04 and 05) produces AUC values of 0.563 and 0.568 for LG-PCa and 0.484 and 0.487 for HG-PCa.

Fig. 4(A) shows an example heat map using our ensemble results for image B05 which was clinically annotated with a large, heterogeneous lesion (blue outline) which was given a score of Gleason 3+4. Fig.s 4(B) and (D) show results for LG-PCa (yellow) and HG-PCa (blue) from scenario 02, while figures 4(C) and (E) are from scenario 03. Scenario 02 detected regions of low-grade tumor within the larger tumor, but completely failed to detect high-grade tumor. Scenario 03 was able to detect both low-grade and high-grade tumor regions.

4   Discussion

In this study, we have adapted the cell density algorithm of [9] by introducing adaptive color deconvolution and by optimizing the parameters for cell detection (see Table 2) based on a validation dataset from [11]. Our method improved the F2-score and moved our adjusted recall metric to a desired median detection rate of 1.5. Fig. 3 illustrates that the parameters in [9] led to a detection-bias for nuclei near ducts, compared to the presented parameter setting, which detects nuclei more homogeneously across multiple tissue sites. The latter promises a more stable and reliable cell density estimation across whole slides, seeing as the presence of ducts will not distort the local density in a ROI.

Although the cell density measure overestimates the true cell count per tile, it presents a meaningful estimation for comparison between different tiles of a whole-slide image. A true quantitative verification of the nuclei detection on

Table 2. Update of the parameters and quantifying metrics (MAD = Median absolute deviation) based on the dataset from [7] with 0.23 m per pixel.

	Reynolds et al. [9]	proposed
Parameters		
r_1, radius of the object in question in px	5:8	5:8
α, roundness constraint	4	3
γ, minimum intensity gradient threshold	15	15
r_2, region radius for NMS	1	2
t, minimum threshold for being a NMS candidate	1.5	1.6
Metric		
Adj. Recall (Median / MAD)	1.13 / 0.20	1.55 / 0.19
F2-score (Median / MAD)	0.63 / 0.11	0.68 / 0.06

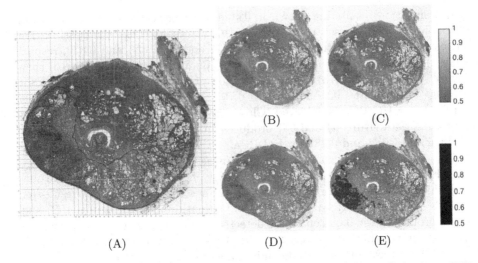

Fig. 4. Prediction maps of LG-PCa (B and C) and HG-PCa (D and E) for imageB05 in Cohort B, along with original annotations (A). Note that for the large tumor region (blue ROI in A), the classification has separated the tumor into regions of HG tumor (E, bottom left) and LG tumor (B,C). The failure to detect tumor in D indicates the inability of the model built using Cohort A data to detect HG-tumor in Cohort B.

prostate images such as those from Cohort A and B would be beneficial, but would require tedious manual cell counting.

Classifier performance using mixed cohorts (scenario 03) was comparable to that from [4]. However, training with Cohort A and testing with Cohort B shows an improvement of 21% for LG-PCa and 8% for HG-PCa, demonstrating the impact of including stain normalization prior to texture and histogram feature extraction.

Results for training with Cohort B and testing with Cohort A only achieved 56% and 48% AUC, respectively. This discrepancy likely arises from the differences in annotation detail levels between the two cohorts, since ROIs were drawn by two different pathologists. Furthermore, smaller, more specific ROIs

Table 3. Area under the ROC curve (AUC) for classification of both LG-PCa and HG-PCa for images from Cohort A and B using both clinical and detailed ground truth annotations.

	Low-grade (LG-PCa)			High-grade (HG-PCa)		
Run	Detailed A	Detailed B	Clinical B	Detailed A	Detailed B	Clinical B
01	0.910	0.705	0.642	0.834	0.686	0.760
02	0.893	0.657	0.682	0.882	0.703	0.674
03	0.854	0.870	0.711	0.875	0.952	0.847
04	0.563	0.968	0.756	0.484	0.978	0.842
05	0.568	0.961	0.748	0.487	0.961	0.808

were drawn from cohort B in comparison to cohort A. The difference in magnification may also play a role here.

5   Conclusions

Improving the reliability of whole-slide image classification is of critical importance for the adoption of this technology into pathology workflows. The results presented here show a promising improvement in classification of LG- and HG-PCa in whole slide H&E images when training and testing on separate cohorts. This improvement can be attributed to the inclusion of stain normalization for texture-based features, as well as the introduction of a cell-density feature. Future work to perform more rigorous parameter tuning, feature extraction and feature selection should lead to further improvements in performance.

References

1. Borren, A., Groenendaal, G., Moman, M.R., Boeken Kruger, A.E., van Diest, P.J., van Vulpen, M., Philippens, M.E.P., van der Heide, U.A.: Accurate prostate tumour detection with multiparametric magnetic resonance imaging: Dependence on histological properties. Acta Oncol. **53**(1), 88–95 (2014)
2. Cosatto, E., Mille, M., Grad, H.P., Meyer, J.S.: Grading nuclear pleomorphism on histological micrographs. In: 19th Int. Conf. Pattern Recogn. (2008)
3. DiFranco, M.D., O'Hurley, G., Kay, E.W., Watson, W.G., Cunningham, P.: Ensemble based system for whole-slide prostate cancer probability mapping using color texture features. Comput. Med. Imaging Graph. **35**, 629–645 (2011)
4. DiFranco, M.D., Reynolds, H.M., Mitchell, C., Williams, S., Allan, P., Haworth, A.: Performance assessment of automated tissue characterization for prostate H and E stained histopathology. In: SPIE Medical Imaging, p. 94200M (2015)
5. Gibbs, P., Liney, G.P., Pickles, M.D.: Correlation of ADC and T2 measurements with cell density in prostate cancer at 3.0 Tesla. Invest. Radiol. **44**(9), 572–576 (2009)
6. Khan, A.M., Rajpoot, N., Treanor, D., Magee, D.: A nonlinear mapping approach to stain normalization in digital histopathology images using image-specific color deconvolution. IEEE Trans. Biomed. Eng. **61**(6), 1729–1738 (2014)
7. Macenko, M., Niethammer, M., Marron, J.S., Borland, D., Woosley, J.T., Guan, X., Schmitt, C., Thomas, C.: A method for normalizing histology slides for quantitative analysis. In: Proceedings of IEEE ISBI 2009, pp. 1107–1110 (2009)
8. McCann, M.T., Ozolek, J.A., Castro, C.A., Parvin, B., Kovacevic, J.: Automated histology analysis: Opportunities for signal processing. IEEE Signal Process. Mag. **32**(1), 78–87 (2015)
9. Reynolds, H.M., Williams, S., Zhang, A.M., Ong, C.S., Rawlinson, D., Chakravorty, R., Mitchell, C., Haworth, A.: Cell density in prostate histopathology images as a measure of tumor distribution. In: SPIE Medical Imaging, p. 90410S (2014)
10. Ruifrok, A.C., Johnston, D.A.: Quantification of histochemical staining by color deconvolution. Analyt. Quant. Cytol. Histol. **23**, 291–299 (2001)
11. Wienert, S., Heim, D., Saeger, K., Stenzinger, A., Beil, M., Hufnagl, P., Dietel, M., Denkert, C., Klauschen, F.: Detection and segmentation of cell nuclei in virtual microscopy images: A minimum-model approach. Scientific Reports **2**, 503 (2012)

Computer-Assisted Diagnosis of Lung Cancer Using Quantitative Topology Features

Jiawen Yao[1], Dheeraj Ganti[1], Xin Luo[2], Guanghua Xiao[2], Yang Xie[2], Shirley Yan[3], and Junzhou Huang[1]([⊠])

[1] Department of Computer Science and Engineering,
University of Texas at Arlington, Arlington, TX 76019, USA
jzhuang@uta.edu
[2] Department of Clinical Science, The University of Texas Southwestern Medical Center, Dallas, TX 75390, USA
[3] Department of Pathology, The University of Texas Southwestern Medical Center, Dallas, TX 75390, USA

Abstract. In this paper, we proposed a computer-aided diagnosis and analysis for a challenging and important clinical case in lung cancer, i.e., differentiation of two subtypes of Non-small cell lung cancer (NSCLC). The proposed framework utilized both local and topological features from histopathology images. To extract local features, a robust cell detection and segmentation method is first adopted to segment each individual cell in images. Then a set of extensive local features is extracted using efficient geometry and texture descriptors based on cell detection results. To investigate the effectiveness of topological features, we calculated architectural properties from labeled nuclei centroids. Experimental results from four popular classifiers suggest that the cellular structure is very important and the topological descriptors are representative markers to distinguish between two subtypes of NSCLC.

1   Introduction

Lung cancer is one of serious diseases causing death for humans. Disease progression and response to treatment in lung cancer varies widely among patients. Therefore, it has clinical importance to be able to classify tumor type and predict patient clinical outcomes. In lung cancer, non-small cell lung cancer (NSCLC) accounts for the majority (84%) type and two major subtypes of NSCLC are adenocarcinoma (ADC) (40%) and squamous cell carcinoma (SCC) (25-30%) [1]. Therefore, how to classify NSCLC patients as ADC and SCC has become a very important topic in lung cancer pathology. However, most of lung cancer pathology diagnosis is still based on subjective opinions of pathologists. This process could result in large interpretation errors or bias. Therefore, in order to avoid subjectivity, it is necessary to design a quantitative analysis framework in lung cancer diagnosis.

J. Huang—This work was partially supported by U.S. NSF IIS-1423056, CMMI-1434401, CNS-1405985.

L. Zhou et al. (Eds.): MLMI 2015, LNCS 9352, pp. 288–295, 2015.
DOI: 10.1007/978-3-319-24888-2_35

Since the diagnosis of most disease grades highly depends on the cell-level information, researchers proposed to analyze individual cells for accurate diagnosis [2,3]. In [2], Wang et al. proposed three kinds of local features for quantitative analysis. They are geometry features, pixel intensity statistics and texture features. Geometry features consider all segmented lung cancer cells and capture geometric properties such as area and contour perimeter. Pixel intensity statistics calculate values like mean, standard deviation in *Lab* color space. Texture features measure properties derived from gray-level intensity profiles and Haralick gray-level co-occurrence matrix [4] to quantify image sharpness, contrast and changes in intensity. Zhang et al. [3] designed a framework to automatically detect and segment all cells from thousands of lung cancer images, resulting in half million of cell images. Then texture features are extracted from cell images and the system performs large-scale cell image retrieval for each segmented cell to classify its category. The final classification result of testing image is decided by the majority voting from all cells' classification. The most recent work [2,3] only focus on individual cells and ignore the internal connection and organization of cells. In fact, the arrangement of nuclei has been demonstrated to be very important markers in breast cancer histopathology [5,13]. To describe such cellular structures, graph-based topological features are proposed based on nuclei centroids. Compared to local features in [2], topological or architecture features describe the organization of cells and contain higher level information. However, to best of our knowledge, there are few works to discuss the performance of topological features in Lung cancer pathology.

In this paper, we investigated topological features in NSCLC images and proposed a computer-assisted diagnosis which could alleviate the subjectivity in NSCLC pathology. We extracted both local and topological features and then employed different classification schemes. Experiments were conducted using the adenocarcinoma and squamous cell carcinoma lung cancer images from the NLST (National Lung Screening Trial) Data Portal[1]. Experimental results demonstrated that topological features are representative to differentiate two subtypes of NSCLC.

2   Methodology

2.1   Overview

An overview of our method is presented in Fig.1. Slides of Hematoxylin and Eosin stained lung biopsy tissue are scanned at 40x magnification. Since the extreme high resolution of the original slide, an expert pathologist labeled regions of tissues and several image tiles will be extracted from the interested regions. When image tiles are prepared, we extract local and topological features from images. These features cover both local and holistic information and benefit the diagnostic accuracy of histopathological images.

---

[1] https://biometry.nci.nih.gov/cdas/

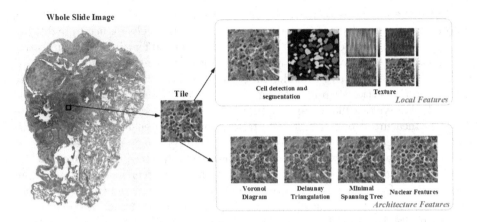

Fig. 1. Overview of the proposed framework. Both local appearance and holistic topological features are extracted from the tile of whole slide image.

2.2 Local Features

Local features include texture and cell-level information (e.g. appearance and shapes) of individual cells. To measure texture, we calculate Haralick features [4] and Gabor "wavelet" texture [6]. To capture cell-level information, it requires a successful cell detection and segmentation method to extract nuclei regions. Motivated by [7], we adopt a contour-based "minimum-model" cell detection and segmentation approach to detect cells in virtual microscopy images.

The minimum-model approach [7] uses a minimal priori information and detects contours independent of their shape. It avoids segmentation bias with respect to shape features and allows for an accurate cell segmentation. Fig.2 shows segmentation results of a randomly selected patch by comparing the minimum-model with Otsu [8] and isoperimetric (ISO) method [9]. It can be clearly seen that the minimum-model can accurately detect robust boundaries of cells.

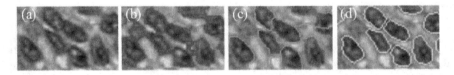

Fig. 2. Segmentation results of three methods on a randomly picked patch. From left to right: a. Original image, b. Otsu, c. ISO, d. Minimum-model

Based on the segmented cell boundaries, we will extract geometry and textural features from cells. Geometry properties include area, compactness, eccentricity and other 12 properties (can be found in Table 1), and 30 Zernike shape features. Then we extract texture features from each cell. A cell without much texture has a smooth appearance else it will appear rough and show a wide variety of pixel intensities. Haralick [4] and Gabor "wavelet" features [6] will be measured as texture properties of objects.

2.3 Topological Features

Within a histological image region, the arrangement of nuclei is related to the cancer type and this architecture can be described by graph-based techniques such as Voronoi Diagram, Delaunay Triangulation and Minimum Spanning Tree [5]. First, we define the undirected and complete graph as $\mathcal{G} = (\mathcal{O}, E, W)$ where $\mathcal{O}$ is the set of nuclear centroids, E is the set of edges connecting the nuclear centroids, and W is the set of weights of each E.

Voronoi Diagram - The Voronoi Diagram $\mathcal{G}_V$ includes a set of polygons $\mathbf{P} = \{P_1, P_2, ..., P_m\}$ surrounding all nuclear centroids $\mathcal{O}$. Each pixel is linked with the nearest centroid and added to the associated polygon P. After the graph construction, the mean, standard deviation, minimum/maximum (min/max) ratio, and disorder (standard deviation divided by the mean) are calculated for the area, perimeter length, and chord length over all polygons.

Delaunay Triangulation - The Delaunay graph $\mathcal{G}_D$ is a spanning subgraph of $\mathcal{G}$ and the dual graph of $\mathcal{G}_V$. Here we show how it is constructed: if $P_i, P_j \in \mathbf{P}$ share a side $(i, j \in 1, 2, ..., L)$ and then their nuclear centroids $o_i, o_j \in \mathcal{O}$ will be connected by an edge (o_i, o_j). Following the same calculation, we compute the mean, standard deviation, min/max ratio and disorder for the side length and area of all triangles in $\mathcal{G}_D$.

Minimum Spanning Tree - A spanning tree $\mathcal{G}_S$ refers to any spanning subgraph of $\mathcal{G}$. The total weight for each subgraph is calculated by summing up all individual weights. The minimum spanning tree $\mathcal{G}_{MST}$ is the spanning tree with the lowest total weight. The same calculation of the branch lengths in $\mathcal{G}_{MST}$ can be found in Table 1.

Nuclear Features - For any nuclear centroid $o_i \in \mathcal{O}$, a corresponding nuclear neighborhood is defined as $\eta^\zeta(o_i) = \{o_j : \|o_i - o_j\|_2 < \zeta, o_j \in \mathcal{O}, o_j \neq o_i\}$, where $\zeta \in \{10, 20, ..., 50\}$. Moreover, we estimate the minimum radius ζ^* such that $|\eta^{\zeta^*}(o_i)| \in 3, 5, 7$, and also calculate the mean, standard deviation, and disorder over all centroids.

2.4 Summary of Features

Table. 1 lists both local and topological features used in this paper. In summary, 155 local features include geometry and texture properties of individual cells and the whole image tile. 48 topological features are calculated based on three kinds of graph and nuclear neighborhoods.

3 Experiments

To prepare the data, 100 histopathological image slides from NLST were gathered which contain 50 adenocarcinoma (ADC) and 50 squamous cell carci-

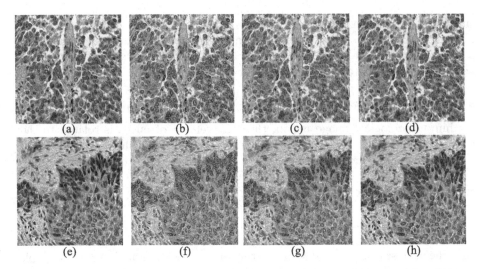

Fig. 3. Graph-based architecture features on image from adenocarcinoma (a) and squamous cell carcinoma (e). Voronoi Diagram (b-f), Delaunay Triangulation (c-g) and Minimum Spanning Tree (d-h)

Table 1. The total features used for analysis

Feature Set	Description	Number
f_G	Area, Perimeter, Compactness, FormFactor, Solidity, Extent EulerNumber, Eccentricity, Axis Length (Major, Minor) Radius (Max, Mean, Median), Feret diameter (Max, Min) Zernike features	45
f_T	Gabor and Haralick Features (Nuclei, Intensity)	106
f_S	Area, Perimeter, Number (Nuclei), Stain area	4
f_L	Local features	155
f_V	Polygon area, perimeter and chord length (mean, std dev., min/max ratio, disorder)	12
f_D	Triangle side length and triangle area (mean, std dev., min/max ratio, disorder)	8
f_{MST}	Edge length (mean, std dev., min/max ratio, disorder)	4
f_{NF}	Distance to {3,5,7} nearest nuclei: mean, std dev., disorder Nuclei in {10, 20,...,50} pixel radius: mean, std dev., disorder	24
f_{Arch}	Topological Features	48
f	Local and Topological Features	203

noma (SCC) tissues. Local features are calculated by Cellprofiler[2]. It is a free open-source software designed to enable researchers to quantitatively measure phenotypes from thousands of images automatically [10]. All experiments are conducted using RStudio (Ver. 0.98.1103) and MATLAB 2013b on a desktop with 3.4GHz Intel core i7 4770 3.4GHz CPU and 16.0 GB RAM.

---

[2] http://www.cellprofiler.org/

Table 2. Evaluation of the classification accuracy. From left to right: local features, architecture features, both local and architecture features

	Mean	STD	Mean	STD	Mean	STD
kNN	0.4938	0.0411	**0.7969**	0.0397	0.7625	0.0493
RF	0.5250	0.0655	0.8031	0.0467	**0.8187**	0.0384
SVM	0.5094	0.0860	0.7969	0.0630	**0.8094**	0.0311
PLR	0.6531	0.0498	0.8125	0.0607	**0.8375**	0.0527

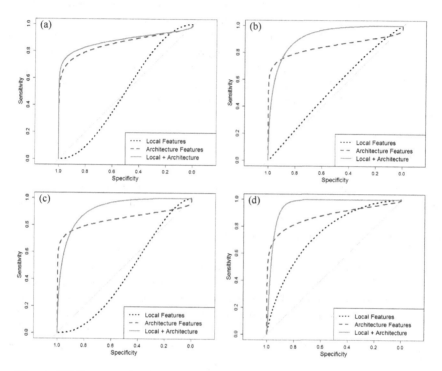

Fig. 4. ROC curves showing the performance of a. kNN b. RF c. SVM d. PLR

We compare our scheme with several effective classifiers employed for NSCLC image analysis. k-nearest neighbor (kNN) method is first used as the baseline classification because of its simplicity and efficacy [11]. As an ensemble learning method, Random Forest (RF) can generate a permutation score to rank the importance of features in classification [12]. A supervised method Support Vector Machine (SVM) has been widely used for breast and prostate cancer diagnosis [13]. Here we choose an RBF kernel with optimized gamma value for SVM. Penalized Logistic Regression (PLR) is an efficient lasso regularization path for logistic regression and enables feature selection for high dimensional data [14].

To conduct the comparison, we randomly select 1/3 samples as testing data and use the remaining as training. The random procedure is repeated ten times to obtain the mean and standard deviation and training process is completed by 10-fold cross-validation. For fair comparison, model parameters and kernel selections are optimized by cross-validation. Table 2 shows quantitative results of classification accuracy. First, it fails to produce reasonable results by using only local features. This means that the local information is not differentiated to subtypes of NSCLC. The classification accuracy is significantly improved (around 80%) when adding topological features and incorporate with holistic structure properties. When compared with performances of four classifiers using both local and topological features, it can be shown that kNN cannot achieve satisfactory results, that may be due to the large variance and noise in features. Since Random Forest (RF) and Penalized Logistic Regression (PLR) can rank the importance of variables and enable feature shrinkage, they can handle with high dimensional data and provide the best results. Fig. 4 shows Receiver Operating Characteristic (ROC) curves from four models. The results indicate that combining both local and architecture features performs better accuracy than other two cases.

4   Conclusion

In this paper, we investigated the performance of topological features in lung cancer pathology and proposed a quantitative image analysis framework. Since few efforts have been put on the classification of NSCLC, the main contribution of this paper is to enable cell-level analysis by using local and holistic features. Experimental results demonstrated that architecture features are very useful to differentiate two types of lung cancer as adenocarcinoma and squamous carcinoma. Although architecture features provide important information for classification, they highly depend on the detection accuracy of nuclei centroids. In our future work, we plan to investigate performances when nuclei centroids are provided by automated methods. Also, inspired by recent structure sparse learning techniques [15–17], we will use feature selection methods based on structured sparsity to select important features and further improve the accuracy.

Acknowledgments. The authors thank the National Cancer Institute for access to NCI's data collected by the National Lung Screening Trial. The statements contained herein are solely those of the authors and do not represent or imply concurrence or endorsement by NCI.

References

1. Anagnostou, V.K., Dimou, A.T., Botsis, T., Killiam, E.J., Gustavson, M.D., Homer, R.J., Boffa, D., Zolota, V., Dougenis, D., Tanoue, L., et al.: Molecular classification of nonsmall cell lung cancer using a 4-protein quantitative assay. Cancer **118**(6), 1607–1618 (2012)
2. Wang, H., Xing, F., Su, H., Stromberg, A., Yang, L.: Novel image markers for non-small cell lung cancer classification and survival prediction. BMC Bioinformatics **15**(1), 310 (2014)

3. Zhang, X., Su, H., Yang, L., Zhang, S.: Fine-grained histopathological image analysis via robust segmentation and large-scale retrieval. In: Proceedings of the IEEE Conference on Computer Vision and Pattern Recognition, pp. 5361–5368 (2015)
4. Haralick, R.M., Shanmugam, K., Dinstein, I.H.: Textural features for image classification. IEEE Transactions on Systems, Man and Cybernetics 6, 610–621 (1973)
5. Basavanhally, A.N., Ganesan, S., Agner, S., Monaco, J.P., Feldman, M.D., Tomaszewski, J.E., Bhanot, G., Madabhushi, A.: Computerized image-based detection and grading of lymphocytic infiltration in HER2+ breast cancer histopathology. IEEE Transactions on Biomedical Engineering 57(3), 642–653 (2010)
6. Gabor, D.: Theory of communication. part 1: The analysis of information. Journal of the Institution of Electrical Engineers-Part III: Radio and Communication Engineering 93(26), 429–441 (1946)
7. Wienert, S., Heim, D., Saeger, K., Stenzinger, A., Beil, M., Hufnagl, P., Dietel, M., Denkert, C., Klauschen, F.: Detection and segmentation of cell nuclei in virtual microscopy images: a minimum-model approach. Scientific reports 2 (2012)
8. Otsu, N.: A threshold selection method from gray-level histograms. IEEE Transactions on Systems, Man and Cybernetics 9(1), 62–66 (1979)
9. Grady, L., Schwartz, E.L.: Isoperimetric graph partitioning for image segmentation. IEEE Transactions on Pattern Analysis and Machine Intelligence 28(3), 469–475 (2006)
10. Carpenter, A.E., Jones, T.R., Lamprecht, M.R., Clarke, C., Kang, I.H., Friman, O., Guertin, D.A., Chang, J.H., Lindquist, R.A., Moffat, J., et al.: Cellprofiler: image analysis software for identifying and quantifying cell phenotypes. Genome Biology 7(10), R100 (2006)
11. Tabesh, A., Teverovskiy, M., Pang, H.Y., Kumar, V.P., Verbel, D., Kotsianti, A., Saidi, O.: Multifeature prostate cancer diagnosis and gleason grading of histological images. IEEE Transactions on Medical Imaging 26(10), 1366–1378 (2007)
12. Breiman, L.: Random forests. Machine Learning 45(1), 5–32 (2001)
13. Doyle, S., Agner, S., Madabhushi, A., Feldman, M., Tomaszewski, J.: Automated grading of breast cancer histopathology using spectral clustering with textural and architectural image features. In: IEEE International Symposium on Biomedical Imaging, pp. 496–499. IEEE (2008)
14. Friedman, J., Hastie, T., Tibshirani, R.: Regularization paths for generalized linear models via coordinate descent. Journal of statistical software 33(1), 1 (2010)
15. Huang, J., Zhang, S., Metaxas, D.: Efficient MR image reconstruction for compressed MR imaging. Medical Image Analysis 15(5), 670–679 (2011)
16. Huang, J., Zhang, T., Metaxas, D.: Learning with structured sparsity. The Journal of Machine Learning Research 12, 3371–3412 (2011)
17. Liu, X., Zhao, G., Yao, J., Qi, C.: Background subtraction based on low-rank and structured sparse decomposition. IEEE Transactions on Image Processing 24(8), 2502–2514 (2015)

Inherent Structure-Guided Multi-view Learning for Alzheimer's Disease and Mild Cognitive Impairment Classification

Mingxia Liu[1,2], Daoqiang Zhang[2], and Dinggang Shen[1(✉)]

[1] Department of Radiology and BRIC, University of North Carolina at Chapel Hill,
Chapel Hill, NC 27599, USA
dgshen@med.unc.edu
[2] School of Computer Science and Technology, Nanjing University of Aeronautics
and Astronautics, Nanjing 210016, China

Abstract. Multi-atlas based morphometric pattern analysis has been recently proposed for the automatic diagnosis of Alzheimer's disease (AD) and its early stage, i.e., mild cognitive impairment (MCI), where multi-view feature representations for subjects are generated by using multiple atlases. However, existing multi-atlas based methods usually assume that each class is represented by a specific type of data distribution (i.e., a single cluster), while the underlying distribution of data is actually a prior unknown. In this paper, we propose an inherent structure-guided multi-view leaning (ISML) method for AD/MCI classification. Specifically, we first extract multi-view features for subjects using multiple selected atlases, and then cluster subjects in the original classes into several sub-classes (i.e., clusters) in each atlas space. Then, we encode each subject with a new label vector, by considering both the original class labels and the coding vectors for those sub-classes, followed by a multi-task feature selection model in each of multi-atlas spaces. Finally, we learn multiple SVM classifiers based on the selected features, and fuse them together by an ensemble classification method. Experimental results on the Alzheimer's Disease Neuroimaging Initiative (ADNI) database demonstrate that our method achieves better performance than several state-of-the-art methods in AD/MCI classification.

1 Introduction

Multi-atlas based morphometric pattern analysis using magnetic resonance imaging (MRI) data are recently proposed for automatic diagnosis of Alzheimer's disease (AD) and its early stage, i.e., mild cognitive impairment (MCI) [1,2,3,4]. Generally, multi-atlas based methods mainly focus on the direct morphometric measurement of spatial brain atrophy of subjects, by non-linearly registering a brain image onto multiple atlases. Thus, multi-view feature representations can be generated from those multi-atlas spaces for each subject, where each atlas is regarded as a specific view. Compared with single-atlas based methods, multi-atlas based methods can reduce registration errors by using multiple atlases, which is helpful in improving subsequent learning performance [1,2,5].

© Springer International Publishing Switzerland 2015
L. Zhou et al. (Eds.): MLMI 2015, LNCS 9352, pp. 296–303, 2015.
DOI: 10.1007/978-3-319-24888-2_36

In the literature, most of existing multi-atlas based methods simply assume that each class is represented by a specific type of data distribution (i.e., a single cluster). Although such assumption may simplify the problem at hand, it will definitely degrade the learning performance because the underlying distribution structure of data is actually a prior unknown. In practice, the potentially complicated distribution structure of neuroimaging data within a specific class could result from several facts [6], e.g., 1) different sub-types of a specific disease, and 2) an inaccurate clinical diagnosis. Intuitively, modeling such inherent structure of data distribution can bring more prior information to the learning process. However, no previous methods employ such information in their learning models.

In this paper, we propose an inherent structure-guided multi-view learning (ISML) method for AD/MCI classification. Specifically, we first non-linearly register each brain image onto multiple selected atlases, through which multi-view feature representations for each subject can be obtained from different atlases. To uncover the inherent distribution structure of data, we partition subjects in original classes into several sub-classes (i.e., clusters) by using a clustering algorithm. Then, we encode each of sub-classes with a unique coding vector, and regard these coding vectors as new class labels for corresponding subjects. Next, we adopt a multi-task feature selection method to select the most informative features in each atlas space. Based on these selected features, we then learn multiple SVM classifiers, with each SVM corresponding to a specific atlas space. Finally, we fuse these classifiers by an ensemble classification method. Experiments on the ADNI database demonstrate that our method outperforms several state-of-the-art methods in AD/MCI classification.

2   Proposed Method

Figure 1 illustrates the overview of our inherent structure-guided multi-atlas learning (ISML) method, which includes three main steps, i.e., 1) feature extraction, 2) inherent structure-guided sparse feature selection and 3) ensemble classification. Specifically, we first non-linearly register the brain images of those subjects onto multiple selected atlases, and then extract volumetric features from the gray matter (GM) tissue density map within each of multi-atlas spaces. Afterwards, we perform feature selection using the proposed inherent structure-guided sparse feature selection method, where we cluster the original classes into several sub-classes and perform sparse feature selection using a multi-task feature selection method. With the selected features, we then learn a support vector machine (SVM) classifier in each of multi-atlas spaces, followed by an ensemble classification approach to combine those SVMs for making a final decision. In what follows, we will introduce each step in detail.

2.1   Feature Extraction

In this study, we apply a standard image pre-processing procedure to the T1-weighted MR brain images for all studied subjects. Specifically, we first perform

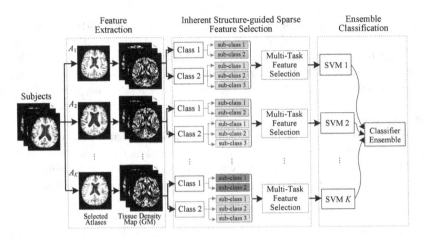

Fig. 1. The overview of our proposed ISML method.

a non-parametric non-uniform bias correction [7] on the MR images to correct intensity in-homogeneity. Then, we perform a skull stripping [8] procedure, followed by a manual review or correction to ensure that the skull and the dura have been removed cleanly. Next, we remove the cerebellum by warping a labeled atlas to each skull-stripping image. Afterwards, we use the FAST method proposed in [9] to segment each brain image into three tissues, i.e., gray matter (GM), white matter (WM) and cerebrospinal fluid (CSF). Finally, all brain images are affine-aligned by the FLIRT method [10].

To select appropriate atlases, we adopt a clustering method to select multiple atlases from all studied subjects. Specifically, we first partition the whole population of AD and NC brain images into K ($K = 10$ in this study) non-overlapping clusters by using the Affinity Propagation (AP) clustering algorithm [11], through which an exemplar image can be automatically determined for each cluster. We then regard these exemplar images as selected atlases (i.e., $A_1, \cdots, A_K$), which is shown in Fig. 1. By performing feature extraction as described in [12] in each atlas space, we can obtain D-dimensional ($D = 1500$ in this study) features from the GM tissue density map for each subject. Given K atlases, we now have K sets of feature representations for each subject.

2.2 Inherent Structure-Guided Sparse Feature Selection

To utilize the structure information of data, we first divide subjects in original classes into several sub-classes, and then encode these sub-classes with a popular one-versus-all (OVA) encoding strategy [13], followed by a multi-task feature selection model to select the most informative features in each atlas space.

Sub-class Clustering and Encoding. For a specific class, we exploit the affinity propagation (AP) algorithm [11] to automatically partition the subjects within this class into several sub-classes (i.e., clusters) in each atlas space, where

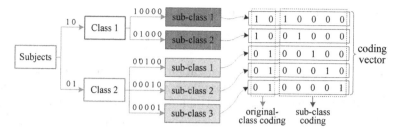

Fig. 2. Illustration of the sub-class clustering and encoding method.

the cluster number can be determined by cross validation on training data. As shown in Fig. 2, subjects belong to two original classes, i.e., Class 1 and Class 2. Using the AP algorithm, we partition the subjects in Class 1 into two sub-classes, and divide subjects in Class 2 into three sub-classes (see Fig. 2).

Then, we label all subjects with new class labels by encoding the original classes and those sub-classes using the OVA encoding strategy. For the original classes (see Fig. 2), each class is represented by a unique OVA coding vector, i.e., [1 0] for Class 1 and [0 1] for Class 2. For those sub-classes in Class 1 and Class 2, they are encoded in a combined encoding manner, by concatenating the coding vectors of their original classes and their own OVA coding vectors. For example, the coding vector for sub-class 1 in Class 1 is set as [1 0 1 0 0 0 0], where the first two bits denote the OVA coding for Class 1, and the last five bits represent its unique OVA coding among five sub-classes (2 sub-classes in Class 1 and 3 sub-classes in Class 2). Afterwards, we regard these 7-bit coding vectors as the new class labels for corresponding subjects. In this way, the original binary classification problem is transformed into a multi-task (e.g., 7 tasks in Fig. 2) learning problem, through which the structure information of the original classes can be incorporated into the learning process.

Multi-task Feature Selection. As high-dimensional features could be redundant or noisy that has attracted research attention in many fields (e.g.,image retrieval [14] and classification [15]), feature selection remains a popular research topic for dealing with high-dimensional features. Here, we exploit a multi-task feature selection model to perform feature selection in each atlas space. We denote matrices as boldface uppercase letters, vectors as boldface lowercase letters, and scalars as normal italic letters, respectively. Denote $\mathbf{a}_i$ and $\mathbf{a}^j$ as the ith row and the jth column of a matrix $\mathbf{A}$, respectively. We further denote the Frobenius norm and the $\ell_{2,1}$ norm of $\mathbf{A}$ as $\|\mathbf{A}\|_F = \sqrt{\sum_i \|\mathbf{a}_i\|^2}$ and $\|\mathbf{A}\|_{2,1} = \sum_i \|\mathbf{a}_i\|$, respectively. Denote $\mathbf{X} \in \mathbb{R}^{N \times D}$ as the data matrix with N subjects of D-dimensional features. Let $\mathbf{Y} \in \mathbb{R}^{N \times C}$ denote the new class label matrix for N subjects, where each subject is labeled with a C-bit row vector. Here, C is the sum of the number of original classes and the number of sub-classes of all original classes. Denote $\mathbf{W} = [\mathbf{w}^1, \mathbf{w}^2, \cdots, \mathbf{w}^c, \cdots, \mathbf{w}^C] \in \mathbb{R}^{D \times C}$ as the weight matrix for C learning tasks, where $\mathbf{w}^c$ is the column weight vector for the cth learning task. To jointly select common features among different tasks, the multi-task feature selection (MTFS) model is defined as follows:

$$\min_{\mathbf{W}} \|\mathbf{Y} - \mathbf{XW}\|_F^2 + \lambda \|\mathbf{W}\|_{2,1} \tag{1}$$

where $\|\mathbf{W}\|_{2,1}$ is a group sparsity regularization, and λ is a parameter to trade off the balance between the empirical loss on the training data and the regularization term. Due to the group sparsity nature of $\ell_{2,1}$ norm, the estimated optimal coefficient matrix $\widehat{\mathbf{W}}$ will have some zero-value row vectors, implying that the corresponding features are not useful in predicting the new class labels of training data. With the MTFS model defined in (1), we can select the most informative features in each atlas space, where the distribution structure of the original classes are used to guide the feature selection process.

2.3 Ensemble Classification

Then, we further propose an ensemble classification approach. To be specific, after feature selection in each atlas space, we can obtain K feature subsets using K atlases. Based on those selected features, we then learn K SVM classifiers, with each SVM corresponding to a specific atlas space. Finally, we combine these classifiers together by a majority voting strategy that is a simple and effective classifier fusion method. Given a new test sample, its class label can be determined by majority voting for the outputs of those SVMs.

3 Experiments

3.1 Data and Experimental Settings

To demonstrate the efficacy of our proposed method, we perform experiments on part of subjects in the ADNI database with T1-weighted MR images. There are totally 459 subjects randomly selected from those scanned with 1.5T scanners, including 97 AD, 117 progressive MCI (pMCI), 117 stable MCI (sMCI) and 128 normal controls (NC). In this study, we perform four groups of experiments, including 1) AD vs. NC classification, 2) pMCI vs. sMCI classification, 3) pMCI vs. NC classification, and 4) sMCI vs. NC classification. We employ a 10-fold cross-validation strategy to evaluate the performance of different methods. Specifically, all samples are partitioned into 10 subsets (each subset with a roughly equal size), and each time samples in one sub-set are successively selected as the test data, while those in the other nine subsets are used as the training data to perform feature selection and classifier construction. Finally, we report the average values of classification results among those 10 folds.

We demonstrate the advantages of our proposed ISML method from two aspects. First, we compare ISML with three feature selection algorithms using the proposed ensemble classification strategy, including 1) Pearson Correlation (PC), 2) COMPARE proposed in [12], and 3) LASSO. Second, we compare our ensemble classification method with conventional feature concatenation methods (i.e., PC_con, COMPARE_con, LASSO_con, and ISML_con). That is, we

Table 1. Comparison of ISML with different methods in four classification tasks

Method	AD vs. NC			pMCI vs. sMCI			pMCI vs. NC			sMCI vs. NC		
	ACC (%)	SEN (%)	SPE (%)	ACC (%)	SEN (%)	SPE (%)	ACC (%)	SEN (%)	SPE (%)	ACC (%)	SEN (%)	SPE (%)
PC_con	84.01	81.56	89.23	72.78	74.62	70.91	75.42	65.17	88.41	61.53	62.35	66.32
PC	85.59	82.44	89.93	73.92	73.38	72.32	78.09	70.15	89.17	65.93	64.92	72.63
COMPARE_con	84.93	80.11	87.03	73.35	75.76	70.83	76.71	68.22	85.26	62.75	55.68	69.68
COMPARE	86.61	85.44	89.23	75.56	75.75	73.48	80.63	73.18	89.55	67.81	65.90	**76.97**
LASSO_con	86.62	84.78	89.80	71.49	76.06	66.67	84.96	79.54	89.74	62.02	68.86	56.54
LASSO	87.27	84.78	89.23	75.32	81.36	69.17	85.35	82.48	87.15	68.38	70.69	54.80
ISML_con(ours)	88.06	88.78	87.50	76.13	78.63	73.33	86.99	85.38	88.02	69.29	71.17	71.03
ISML(ours)	**93.83**	**92.78**	**95.69**	**80.90**	**85.95**	**78.41**	**89.09**	**87.66**	**90.25**	**71.20**	**72.42**	70.91

first concatenate those multi-view feature representations as a long vector, and then use a specific feature selection method (e.g., PC, COMPARE, LASSO, and ISML) to select the most informative features, followed by a SVM classifier. For fair comparison, all compared methods share the same multi-view feature representations generated from K atlases.

The regularization parameter (i.e., λ) in equation 1 and that in LASSO are chosen from the range $\{2^{-10}, 2^{-9}, \cdots, 2^0\}$ through inner cross-validation on the training data. There are K ($K = 10$ in this study) atlases selected from AD and NC subjects. Using these selected atlases, we extract D-dimensional ($D = 1500$ in this study) features from each of K atlas spaces. Here, we use the linear SVM with default parameters as the benchmark classifier. In addition, we evaluate the performance of different methods via three criteria, including classification accuracy (ACC), sensitivity (SEN), and specificity (SPE).

3.2 Results and Discussion

We first record the averaged number of sub-classes (i.e., clusters) identified by our ISML method in the cross-validation process, i.e., 2.1/2.9 for AD/NC, 3.2/3.8 for pMCI/sMCI, 3.1/2.5 for pMCI/NC, and 3.2/2.3 for sMCI/NC. These results validate our intuition that there exists heterogeneity within a specific class.

Then, we report the results achieved by different methods in four classification tasks in Table 1, where the best results are shown in boldface. We further plot the ROC curves achieved by four ensemble-based methods in Fig. 3. From Table 1 and Fig. 3, one can observe two main points. First, in four classification tasks, our proposed ISML method generally outperforms the compared methods in terms of accuracy, sensitivity and specificity. For example, the accuracy achieved by ISML in AD vs. NC classification is 93.83%, which is much higher than the second best accuracy achieved by ISML_con (i.e., 88.06%). Although the COMPARE method obtains the best specificity in sMCI vs. NC classification, its accuracy and sensitivity are much lower than those achieved by ISML. Second, methods using the ensemble classification strategy (i.e., PC, COMPARE, LASSO, and ISML) generally outperform their conventional counterparts that adopt the feature concatenation strategy (i.e., PC_con, COPARE_con, LASSO_con, and ISML_con).

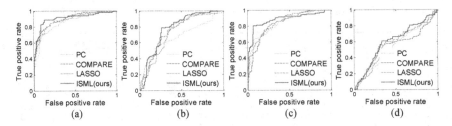

Fig. 3. ROC curves achieved by four ensemble-based methods in (a) AD vs. NC, (b) pMCI vs. sMCI, (c) pMCI vs. NC, and (d) sMCI vs. NC classification.

Table 2. Comparison with the state-of-the-art methods using MRI data of ADNI.

Method	AD vs. NC			pMCI vs. sMCI			pMCI vs. NC		
	ACC (%)	SEN (%)	SPE (%)	ACC (%)	SEN (%)	SPE (%)	ACC (%)	SEN (%)	SPE (%)
Cuingnet et al. [16]	88.58	81.00	95.00	70.40	57.00	78.00	81.17	73.00	85.00
Wolz et al. [1]	89.00	85.00	93.00	68.00	67.00	69.00	84.00	82.00	86.00
Koikkalainen et al. [2]	86.00	81.00	91.00	72.10	77.00	71.00	-	-	-
Min et al. [3]	91.64	88.56	93.85	72.41	72.12	72.58	-	-	-
Liu et al. [5]	92.51	**92.89**	88.33	78.88	85.45	76.06	88.26	86.43	89.94
ISML(ours)	**93.83**	92.78	**95.69**	**80.90**	**85.95**	**78.41**	**89.09**	**87.66**	**90.25**

Furthermore, we compare our ISML method with several state-of-the-art methods using MRI data of ADNI, with results given in Table 2. Since very few works reports the results of sMCI vs. NC classification, we only show the results of three classification tasks (i.e., AD vs. NC, pMCI vs. sMCI, and pMCI vs. NC classification) in Table 2. It is worth noting that the method proposed in [16] employs single-atlas feature representation extracted from one single atlas, while the others use multi-atlas based feature representations. It can be seen from Table 2 that, in three classification tasks, our ISML method yields the best classification results in terms of both accuracy and specificity, and comparable sensitivity with the work in [5].

4   Conclusion

In this paper, we propose an inherent structure-guided multi-view learning (ISML) method for AD/MCI classification. Specifically, we first extract multi-view features for subjects, and then cluster subjects in original classes into several sub-classes, followed by a multi-task feature selection algorithm. Finally, we develop an ensemble classification method by fusing multiple classifiers constructed in multi-atlas spaces. Experimental results on the ADNI database demonstrate the efficacy of our ISML method.

Acknowledgments. This study was supported by NIH grants (EB006733, EB008374, EB009634, MH100217, AG041721, and AG042599), the National Natural Science Foundation of China (Nos. 61422204, 61473149), the Jiangsu Natural Science Foundation for Distinguished Young Scholar (No. BK20130034).

References

1. Wolz, R., Julkunen, V., Koikkalainen, J., Niskanen, E., Zhang, D.P., Rueckert, D., Soininen, H., Lötjönen, J., Initiative, A.D.N., et al.: Multi-method analysis of MRI images in early diagnostics of Alzheimer's disease. PloS One **6**(10), e25446 (2011)
2. Koikkalainen, J., Lötjönen, J., Thurfjell, L., Rueckert, D., Waldemar, G., Soininen, H., Initiative, A.D.N., et al.: Multi-template tensor-based morphometry: Application to analysis of Alzheimer's disease. NeuroImage **56**(3), 1134–1144 (2011)
3. Min, R., Wu, G., Cheng, J., Wang, Q., Shen, D.: Multi-atlas based representations for alzheimer's disease diagnosis. Human Brain Mapping **35**(10), 5052–5070 (2014)
4. Jin, Y., Shi, Y., Zhan, L., Gutman, B.A., de Zubicaray, G.I., McMahon, K.L., Wright, M.J., Toga, A.W., Thompson, P.M.: Automatic clustering of white matter fibers in brain diffusion mri with an application to genetics. Neuroimage **100**, 75–90 (2014)
5. Liu, M., Zhang, D., Shen, D.: View-centralized multi-atlas classification for alzheimer's disease diagnosis. Human Brain Mapping **36**(5), 1847–1865 (2015)
6. Noppeney, U., Penny, W.D., Price, C.J., Flandin, G., Friston, K.J.: Identification of degenerate neuronal systems based on intersubject variability. NeuroImage **30**(3), 885–890 (2006)
7. Sled, J.G., Zijdenbos, A.P., Evans, A.C.: A nonparametric method for automatic correction of intensity nonuniformity in MRI data. IEEE Transactions on Medical Imaging **17**(1), 87–97 (1998)
8. Wang, Y., Nie, J., Yap, P.T., Li, G., Shi, F., Geng, X., Guo, L., Shen, D., Initiative, A.D.N., et al.: Knowledge-guided robust MRI brain extraction for diverse large-scale neuroimaging studies on humans and non-human primates. PloS One **9**(1), e77810 (2014)
9. Zhang, Y., Brady, M., Smith, S.: Segmentation of brain MR images through a hidden markov random field model and the expectation-maximization algorithm. IEEE Transactions on Medical Imaging **20**(1), 45–57 (2001)
10. Jenkinson, M., Smith, S.: A global optimisation method for robust affine registration of brain images. Medical Image Analysis **5**(2), 143–156 (2001)
11. Frey, B.J., Dueck, D.: Clustering by passing messages between data points. Science **315**(5814), 972–976 (2007)
12. Fan, Y., Shen, D., Gur, R.C., Gur, R.E., Davatzikos, C.: COMPARE: Classification of morphological patterns using adaptive regional elements. IEEE Transactions on Medical Imaging **26**(1), 93–105 (2007)
13. Liu, M., Zhang, D., Chen, S., Xue, H.: Joint binary classifier learning for ecoc-based multi-class classification. IEEE Transactions on Pattern Analysis and Machine Intelligence (2015)
14. Gao, Y., Wang, M., Tao, D., Ji, R., Dai, Q.: 3-d object retrieval and recognition with hypergraph analysis. IEEE Transactions on Image Processing **21**(9), 4290–4303 (2012)
15. Ji, R., Gao, Y., Hong, R., Liu, Q., Tao, D., Li, X.: Spectral-spatial constraint hyperspectral image classification. IEEE Transactions on Geoscience and Remote Sensing **52**(3), 1811–1824 (2014)
16. Cuingnet, R., Gerardin, E., Tessieras, J., Auzias, G., Lehéricy, S., Habert, M.O., Chupin, M., Benali, H., Colliot, O., Initiative, A.D.N., et al.: Automatic classification of patients with Alzheimer's disease from structural MRI: A comparison of ten methods using the ADNI database. NeuroImage **56**(2), 766–781 (2011)

Nonlinear Feature Transformation and Deep Fusion for Alzheimer's Disease Staging Analysis

Yani Chen[1], Bibo Shi[1], Charles D. Smith[2], and Jundong Liu[1(✉)]

[1] School of Electrical Engineering and Computer Science,
Ohio University, Athens, USA
liu@cs.ohio.edu
[2] Department of Neurology, University of Kentucky, Lexington, USA

Abstract. In this study, we develop a novel nonlinear metric learning method to improve biomarker identification for Alzheimer's Disease (AD) and Mild Cognitive Impairment (MCI). Formulated under a constrained optimization framework, the proposed method learns a smooth nonlinear feature space transformation that makes the input data points more linearly separable in SVMs. The thin-plate spline (TPS) is chosen as the geometric model due to its remarkable versatility and representation power in accounting for sophisticated deformations. In addition, a deep network based feature fusion strategy through stacked denoising sparse autoencoder (DSAE) is adopted to integrate cross-sectional and longitudinal features estimated from MR brain images. Using the ADNI dataset, we evaluate the effectiveness of the proposed feature transformation and feature fusion strategies and demonstrate the improvements over the state-of-the-art solutions within the same category.

1 Introduction

The Alzheimer's Disease Neuroimaging Initiative (ADNI) [1] has provided a wealth of new data including structural and functional MR images to support the research on intervention, prevention and treatments of AD. Significant research efforts have been conducted using ADNI data to identify neuroimage biomarkers for the diagnoses of AD/MCI and various mixed pathologies. There is a pressing need to refine the solutions for patient classification as well as feature extraction, selection and fusion.

Many pattern classification algorithms rely on Euclidean metrics to compute pairwise dissimilarities, with equal weights assigned to the feature components. Replacing Euclidean with a metric learned from the inputs, which is equivalent to learn a feature transformation [2], can often improve the algorithm's performance significantly [2,3]. Depending on the feature space transformation to be sought, metric learning (ML) can be divided into linear and nonlinear groups [3]. Linear models commonly try to estimate a "best" affine transformation to deform the feature space, such that the resulted Mahalanobis distance would well agree with the supervisory information brought by training samples. While easy to use and convenient to optimize, linear models show inherently

© Springer International Publishing Switzerland 2015
L. Zhou et al. (Eds.): MLMI 2015, LNCS 9352, pp. 304–312, 2015.
DOI: 10.1007/978-3-319-24888-2_37

limited expressive power and separation capability in handling data with non-linear structures. Nonlinear models are usually designed through kernelization or localization of certain linear models. The idea of localization is to build a overall nonlinear metric through combination of multiple piecewise linear metrics that are learned based on either local neighborhoods or class memberships. Although the multi-metric strategies are more powerful in accommodating non-linear structures, generalizing these methods to fit other classifiers than kNN is not trivial. To avoid non-symmetric metrics, extra cares are commonly needed to ensure the smoothness of the transformed feature space.

Other than learning distance metrics, feature extraction and fusion from the ADNI database is also in great need of further exploration. For structural features extracted from brain MRIs, cortical thickness [4], volumetry of brain strucrures [5,6] and voxel tissue probability maps [7,8] across the whole brain or around certain regions of interest (ROI), are among the popular choices. Most of them are either cross-sectional features obtained at one point in time, or "static" longitudinal volumetric information acquired at two or multiple time points but only through structural segmentation. In part due to the unavailability of defor-mation data in ADNI, "dynamic" longitudinal information such as the atrophies at various gray matter (GM) areas, which is a major hallmark in the progression of AD, has not been fully utilized in the literature.

In this paper, we propose to improve the quality of AD/MCI neuroimage biomarker identification along two directions: 1) feature space transformation through a novel nonlinear ML technique, and 2) extraction and integration of dynamic longitudinal atrophy features into the classification framework. The proposed ML solution is a generalization of linear ML through the application of a deformable geometric model — the thin-plate spline (TPS) - to transform the feature space in SVMs. Toward the integration of longitudinal information, we adopt a deep network model – multi-modal stacked denoising sparse autoencoder (DSAE), with both cross-sectional (baseline) and longitudinal atrophy features extracted from MR brain images.

2   TPS Metric Learning for Support Vector Machines (TML-SVM)

Since learning a metric is equivalent to learn a feature transformation [2], metric learning can be applied to SVM models [9,10]. However, the existing SVM-based ML models employ only linear transformations, limiting their capabilities in dealing with complex data. In this study, we propose a new nonlinear ML solution for SVMs, which is a direct generalization of linear metric learning through the application of deformable geometric models to transform the entire input space. We choose thin-plate splines (TPS) as the transformation model, as TPS are well-known for their remarkable versatility and representation power in accounting for high-order deformations. To our best knowledge, this is the first work that utilizes nonlinear dense transformations, or spatially varying deformation models in metric learning. Next, we will briefly describe the theoretical background of the TPS in the general context of transformations, followed by the presentation of our proposed ML model.

TPS When utilized to align a set of n corresponding point-pairs $\mathbf{u}_i$ and $\mathbf{v}_i$, $(i = 1, \ldots, n)$, a TPS transformation is a mapping function $f(\mathbf{x}) : \mathbb{R}^d \to \mathbb{R}^d$ within a suitable Hilbert space $\mathcal{H}$, that matches $\mathbf{u}_i$ and $\mathbf{v}_i$, as well as minimizes a smoothness TPS penalty functional:

$$J_m^d(f) = \int ||\mathcal{D}^m f||^2 dX = \sum_{a_1 + \cdots + a_d = m} \frac{m!}{a_1! \ldots a_d!} \int \cdots \int (\frac{\partial^m f}{\partial x_1^{a_1} \ldots \partial x_d^{a_d}})^2 \prod_{j=1}^d dx_j \quad (1)$$

where $\mathcal{D}^m f$ is the matrix of m-th order partial derivatives of f, with a_k being positive, and $dX = \prod_{j=1}^d dx_j$, where x_j are the components of $\mathbf{x}$. The classic solution of Eqn. (1) has a representation in terms of a radial basis function (TPS interpolation function),

$$f_k(\mathbf{x}) = \sum_{i=1}^n \psi_i G(||\mathbf{x} - \mathbf{x}_i||) + \boldsymbol{\ell}^T \mathbf{x} + c, \quad (2)$$

where $||.||$ denotes the Euclidean norm and $\{\psi_i\}$ are a set of weights for the nonlinear part; ℓ and c are the weights for the linear part. The corresponding radial distance kernel of TPS, which is the Green's function to solve Eqn. (1), is as follows:

$$G(\mathbf{x}, \mathbf{x}_i) = G(||\mathbf{x} - \mathbf{x}_i||) \propto \begin{cases} ||\mathbf{x} - \mathbf{x}_i||^{2m-d} \ln ||\mathbf{x} - \mathbf{x}_i||, & \text{if } 2m - d \text{ is even;} \\ ||\mathbf{x} - \mathbf{x}_i||^{2m-d}, & \text{otherwise.} \end{cases} \quad (3)$$

The TPS transformation for point interpolation, as specified in Eqn. (2), can be employed as the geometric model to deform the input space for nonlinear metric learning. Such a transformation would ensure certain desired smoothness as it minimizes the bending energy $J_m^d(f)$ in Eqn. (1). Within the metric learning setting, let $\mathbf{x}$ be one of the training samples in the original feature space $\mathcal{X}$ of d dimensions, and $f(\mathbf{x})$ be the transformed destination of $\mathbf{x}$, also of d dimensions. Through a straightforward mathematical manipulations [11], we can get $f(\mathbf{x})$ in matrix format:

$$f(\mathbf{x}) = L\mathbf{x} + \Psi \begin{pmatrix} G(\mathbf{x}, \mathbf{x}_1) \\ \cdots \\ G(\mathbf{x}, \mathbf{x}_p) \end{pmatrix} = L\mathbf{x} + \Psi \boldsymbol{G}(\mathbf{x}), \quad (4)$$

where L (size $d \times d$) is a linear transformation matrix, Ψ (size $d \times p$) is the weight matrix for the nonlinear parts, and p is the number of anchor points $(\mathbf{x}_1, \ldots, \mathbf{x}_p)$ to compute the TPS kernel. We can use all the training data points as the anchor points. However, in practice, p anchor points are extracted through k-medoids method under the consideration of reducing computational cost.

TML-SVM By utilizing the nonlinear TPS transformation, we formulate our model under the *Margin-Radius-Ratio* bounded SVM paradigm, similarly as in [10]. Given training dataset $\mathcal{X} = \{\mathbf{x}_i | \mathbf{x}_i \in \mathbb{R}^d, i = 1, \cdots, n\}$ together with the class label information $y_i \in \{-1, +1\}$, our proposed TML-SVM aims to simultaneously learn the nonlinear transformation f as described in Eqn. (4) and a SVM classifier, which can be formulated as follows:

$$\min_{L, \Psi, \mathbf{w}, b} \quad J = \frac{1}{2}\|\mathbf{w}\|^2 + C_1 \sum_{i=1}^{n} \xi_i + C_2 \|\Psi\|_F^2$$

$$\text{s.t.} \quad y_i(\mathbf{w}^T f(\mathbf{x}_i) + b) \geq 1 - \xi_i, \quad \xi_i \geq 0, \quad \forall i = 1 \ldots n; \text{ (I \& II)}$$

$$\|f(\mathbf{x}_i) - \mathbf{x}_c\|^2 \leq 1, \quad \forall i = 1 \ldots n; \text{ (III)} \tag{5}$$

$$\sum_{i=1}^{p} \Psi_i^k = 0, \quad \sum_{i=1}^{p} \Psi_i^k \mathbf{x}_i^k = 0, \forall k = 1 \ldots d. \text{ (IV)}$$

f is in the form of Eqn. (4); Ψ^k is the kth column of Ψ; $\mathbf{x}^k$ is the kth component of $\mathbf{x}$. Besides the components for the traditional soft margin SVMs, another component $\|\Psi\|_F^2$, the squared Frobenius norm of Ψ, is added to the objective function as a regularizer to prevent overfitting. C_1 and C_2 are two trade-off hyper-parameters. The first two nonequivalent constraints (I and II) are the same as used in traditional SVMs. The third nonequivalent constraint (III) is a unit-enclosing-ball constraint, which forces the radius of minimum-enclosing-ball to be unit in the transformed space and avoids trivial solutions. $\mathbf{x}_c$ is the center of all samples. The last two equivalent constraints (IV) are used to maintain the properties for TPS transformation at infinity.

To solve this optimization problem, we propose an efficient EM-like iterative minimization algorithm by updating $\{\mathbf{w}, b\}$ and $\{L, \Psi\}$ alternatively. The details of this algorithm can be found in the supplementary material (http://media.cs.ohio.edu/mlmi2015_supplementary.pdf).

3   Neuroimage Data and Feature Extraction

The neuroimage data used in this work were obtained from the ADNI database [1]. We consider only the subjects for whom the baseline (M0) visits and 12-month follow-up (M12) T1-weighted MRIs, together with their *MIDAS Whole Brain Masks*, are all available. As a result, 338 subjects were selected : 94 patients with AD, 121 with MCI and 123 normal controls (NC).

Recently, patch-level neuroimage features extraction and fusion [8,12] have been used in producing excellent performance for AD/MCI/NC classifications. The features utilized in their work are cross-sectional, extracted from the baseline MRIs and Positron emission tomography images (PETs). Different from the existing work, we propose a strategy that utilizes patch extraction and deep network based feature fusion with longitudinal brain atrophy, which is one of the pathological hallmarks of AD, as an addition information source. Our proposed framework consists of two main steps: The first step is the extraction of class-discriminative patches from both baseline and longitudinal MRIs; the second step is a deep network based feature fusion step to learn a fused feature representation from the extracted patch pools.

Patch Extraction: After spatially normalized into an International Consortium for Brain Mapping template (with the dimensions reduced to $79 \times 79 \times 95$ and the voxel sizes to $2 \times 2 \times 2$ mm^3), each baseline M0-MRI was segmented into three brain tissues: gray matter (GM), white matter (WM), and cerebrospinal fluid (CSF). We choose the spatially normalized GM tissue densities from the baseline MRIs as the cross-sectional information source in our work. A voxel-wise t-test is first performed based on the group labels, i.e., AD vs. NC and MCI vs. NC. Voxels with statistically significant group difference (with the p-value smaller than 0.05) are identified as the seeds for patch extraction. The mean p values in the seed voxels' enclosing patches of size $5 \times 5 \times 5$ are then used to sort the patch seeds. Based on their ascending order, we select the first 100 class-discriminative patches in a greedy manner with the condition that no candidate patch pair should have more than 50% overlapping volume. The corresponding patch-wise average GM densities consist a cross-sectional feature vector.

Our longitudinal features are obtained based on the estimated voxel deformations matching the baseline and follow-up MRIs for each subject. A diffeomorphic registration method provided via ANTs package [13] is utilized to generate the deformation vector fields. We then calculate the magnitude (or length) of the deformation vector at each voxel, and a 3D scalar field of deformation magnitudes (DM) is obtained. Based on the DM fields, which show the longitudinal atrophy, we conduct the same patch extraction as for the cross-sectional GM features, resulting in a set of 3D local patches along with the local average DM of each patch.

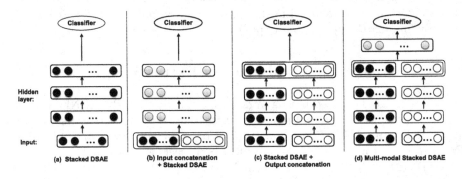

Fig. 1. Deep network structures of stacked DSAE, and three fusion strategies.

Feature Fusion: In our experiments, the above patch extraction steps return 100 discriminative patches for GM and DM respectively. Ideally, the two types of features should be fused with a reduced dimensionality. To this end, deep neural networks [4] provide very powerful solutions. Deep networks have been utilized in several recent AD/MCI works [6,12,14], with the same goal to learn a latent and compressed representation of the input feature vectors. Stacked Auto-encoder [6], Restricted Boltzman machine [12] and convolutional networks [14] are among the choices that have been examined. In this paper, we adopt a different model — stacked denoising sparse auto-encoder (DSAE), a direct combination of both denoising and sparse auto-encoder [15,16]. This choice is based on the nature of the GM/DM features in our model. While easy to obtain, the GM/DM vectors contain many non-discriminative components, or in other words, high noise level.

On top of the stacked DSAE, several strategies are available to fuse different types of features, as shown in Fig. 1.(b)∼ (d): (b) shows the most intuitive way that concatenates different types of feature in the input layer, and learns a single deep neural network, as used in [6]; (c) learns separate deep neural networks for each feature type, and concatenates the output layers; (d) adds one more fully connected fusion layer on top of (c). In this paper, we choose the last strategy, the so-called multi-modal stacked DSAE as the solution to learn a discriminative fused feature representation.

4   Experiments and Results

In this section, we evaluate the proposed nonlinear feature transformation introduced by TML-SVM, as well as the integrated feature representation obtained via multi-modal stacked DSAE, through two binary classification problems: AD vs. NC, and MCI vs. NC. The performance of various classification solutions is compared based on three measures: classification accuracy (ACC), sensitivity (SEN), and specificity (SPE).

4.1   Comparisons of Different Features

The first set of experiments is to investigate the efficacy of different features in distinguishing AD and MCI from normal controls. Specifically, the three types of features, i.e., "GM only"– features learned using stacked DSAE from only GM patches, "DM only"–features learned using stacked DSAE from only DM patches, and "Fused GM & DM"– features learned using multi-modal stacked DSAE from both GM and DM patches, are evaluated based on three performance measures, ACC, SEN, and SPE. To reduce the potential bias introduced by any particular classifier, here we utilize softmax regression model as the classifier, which is also regarded as "the classifier for stacked auto-encoder" [6]. Unlike other classifiers, softmax regression model makes "fine-tuning" deep networks for stacked DSAE and multi-modal stacked DSAE straightforward.

To better compare the classification performance, we run each experiment 10 times with different random 5-fold splits (three folds for training, one fold for validation, and one fold for testing). Similarly as in [6], we use three hidden layers for DSAE, with the numbers for the three layer's hidden nodes selected from $[100, 300, 500, 1000] - [50, 100] - [10, 20, 30]$ (bottom to up); the hyper-parameters for sparsity control and denoising corruption are both set to 0.2. For the fusion layer in multi-modal DSAE, the number of hidden nodes is selected from $[3, 5, 10, 20]$. The classification results based on the three different features, averaging over the 10 runs, are summarized in Table 1. It is evident that the idea of combining longitudinal and baseline features paid off – "Fused GM &

DM" feature has generally improved the classification performance over the two single feature types, "GM only" and "DM only", with the highest ACC, SEN and SPE for both AD vs. NC and MCI vs. NC.

Table 1. Comparisons of the three different features for AD vs. NC and MCI vs. NC classifications. Boldface denotes the best performance for each measure.

Classifier	Feature	AD versus NC			MCI versus NC		
		ACC(%)	SEN(%)	SPE(%)	ACC(%)	SEN(%)	SPE(%)
	GM only	81.80	75.32	86.75	74.71	72.63	76.75
Softmax	DM only	80.49	75.13	84.56	70.21	68.46	71.93
	Fused GM & DM	**86.55**	**85.88**	**87.05**	**77.78**	**76.71**	**78.85**

4.2 Comparisons of Different Feature Fusion Strategies

The second set of experiments is to test the effectiveness of our adopted multi-modal stacked DSAE in improving AD/MCI versus NC classifications, with three other feature fusion strategies compared: 1) traditional "PCA based" strategy – concatenate the feature from GM and DM patches, and use Principle Component Analysis (PCA) to reduce the dimension with 99% variances kept; 2) "Input concatenation + Stacked DSAE", as shown in Fig. 1.(b); 3) "Stacked DSAE + Output concatenation", as shown in Fig. 1.(c); 4) our adopted multi-modal Stacked DSAE. We adopt the same performance measures (ACC, SEN, SPE), experimental setting (5-fold splits with 10 runs), and softmax regression classifier as in Section 5.1. The classification results of each strategy for AD/MCI versus NC are summarized in Table 2. As we can see from the results, the adopted multi-modal stacked DSAE has the best overall classification performance with the highest ACC, SEN for both AD vs. NC and MCI vs. NC. Although the 'Stacked DSAE + Output concatenation" strategy results in a slightly higher SPE values than multi-modal stacked DSAE, it is at the cost of sacrificing SEN values.

Table 2. Four feature fusion strategies for AD vs. NC and MCI vs. NC classifications.

Classifier	Fusion strategy	AD versus NC			MCI versus NC		
		ACC(%)	SEN(%)	SPE(%)	ACC(%)	SEN(%)	SPE(%)
	PCA based	79.77	73.30	84.72	53.71	53.96	53.46
Softmax	Input concat. + Stacked DSAE	80.82	76.42	84.12	75.26	72.89	77.57
	Stacked DSAE + Output concat.	85.58	81.32	**88.83**	75.46	71.82	**79.01**
	Multi-modal Stacked DSAE	**86.55**	**85.88**	87.05	**78.20**	**77.77**	78.60

4.3 Comparisons of TML-SVM with Other Classifiers

The last set of experiments is to test the effectiveness of the nonlinear feature transformation introduced by our proposed TML-SVM classifier in improving AD/MCI versus NC classifications. We compare TML-SVM against two other classifiers without feature transformation: the softmax regression and the traditional SVM. For all the three classifiers, the same multi-modal Stacked DSAE are used to obtain the fused feature representation. It is worth noting that only the deep network in softmax regression model is fine-tuned. For SVM, the slackness coefficient C is selected from $\{2^{-5} \sim 2^{15}\}$. TML-SVM has three hyperparameters to be tuned: the number of anchor points p and the tradeoff coefficients C_1 and C_2. For p, we empirically set it to 30% of the training samples; for C_1 and C_2, we select them from $\{2^{-5} \sim 2^{15}\}$ and $\{5^{-5} \sim 5^{25}\}$ respectively. We still adopt the same experimental setting and performance measures, and report the results averaged from 10 runs in Table 3.

Table 3. Comparisons of three different classifiers for AD vs. NC and MCI vs. NC classifications.

Classifier	AD versus NC			MCI versus NC		
	ACC(%)	SEN(%)	SPE(%)	ACC(%)	SEN(%)	SPE(%)
Softmax regression	86.55	85.88	87.05	78.20	77.77	78.60
SVM	85.76	82.11	88.54	76.83	74.60	79.04
Our proposed TML-SVM	**88.98**	**87.42**	**90.17**	**81.66**	**78.09**	**85.16**

As evident, our proposed TML-SVM has the best classification performance with the highest ACC, SEN, SPE for both AD vs. NC and MCI vs. NC. Especially, the improvements made by TML-SVM over the baseline classifier SVM is significant, which means adding the nonlinear feature transformation is effective in leading to a more separable feature space. Also, it is worth pointing out that the deep networks used in SVM and TML-SVM are not fine-tuned as in softmax regression model, and we believe the performance of our TML-SVM can be further improved if fine-tuning is utilized.

5   Conclusions

Our proposed AD/MCI vs. NC diagnosis solution consists of two major components: feature transformation through TML-SVM and feature fusion based on multi-modal stacked DSAE. TML-SVM learns a globally smooth deformation for the input space, and it is the first work that utilizes nonlinear dense transformations, or spatially varying deformation models in metric learning. Multi-modal stacked DSAE integrates longitudinal atrophy with baseline cross-sectional information, and it can be easily generalized to fuse other types of features. For AD/MCI vs. NC classification, some recent works [6,8,12] reported rather high classification rates through extracting features from different types of medical images (mainly MRIs and PETs) and sophisticated multi-classifier decision fusion schemes. To explore features from other data modalities and to enhance our TML-SVM with multi-kernelization are the directions of our ongoing efforts.

References

1. Jack, C.R., et al.: The alzheimer's disease neuroimaging initiative (adni): Mri methods. Journal of Magnetic Resonance Imaging 27(4), 685–691 (2008)
2. Bellet, A., Habrard, A., Sebban, M.: A survey on metric learning for feature vectors and structured data (2013). arXiv preprint arXiv:1306.6709
3. Yang, L., Jin, R.: Distance metric learning: A comprehensive survey, vol. 2. Michigan State Universiy (2006)
4. Klöppel, S., et al.: Automatic classification of mr scans in alzheimer's disease. Brain 131(3), 681–689 (2008)
5. Chupin, M., et al.: Automatic segmentation of the hippocampus and the amygdala driven by hybrid constraints: method and validation. Neuroimage 46(3), 749–761 (2009)
6. Suk, H.-I., et al.: Latent feature representation with stacked auto-encoder for ad/mci diagnosis. Brain Structure and Function 220(2), 841–859 (2013)
7. Fan, Y., et al.: Compare: classification of morphological patterns using adaptive regional elements. IEEE Transactions on Medical Imaging 26(1), 93–105 (2007)
8. Liu, M., Zhang, D., Shen, D.: Hierarchical fusion of features and classifier decisions for alzheimer's disease diagnosis. Human brain mapping 35(4), 1305–1319 (2014)
9. Xu, Z., et al.: Distance metric learning for kernel machines (2012). arXiv:1208.3422
10. Zhu, X., et al.: Learning similarity metric with svm. In: IJCNN (2012)
11. Chui, H., Rangarajan, A.: A new point matching algorithm for non-rigid registration 89(2–3), 114–141 (2003)
12. Suk, H.-I., et al.: Hierarchical feature representation and multimodal fusion with deep learning for ad/mci diagnosis. NeuroImage 101, 569–582 (2014)
13. Avants, B.B., et al.: Advanced normalization tools (ants). Insight J., 1–35 (2009)
14. Gupta, A., Ayhan, M., Maida, A.: Natural image bases to represent neuroimaging data. In: Proceedings of the 30th ICML, pp. 987–994 (2013)
15. Vincent, P., et al.: Extracting and composing robust features with denoising autoencoders. In: Proceedings of the 25th ICML, pp. 1096–1103. ACM (2008)
16. Bengio, Y.: Learning deep architectures for ai. Foundations and trends® in Machine Learning 2(1), 1–127 (2009)

Tumor Classification by Deep Polynomial Network and Multiple Kernel Learning on Small Ultrasound Image Dataset

Xiao Liu, Jun Shi[✉], and Qi Zhang

School of Communication and Information Engineering, Shanghai University, Shanghai, China
junshi@staff.shu.edu.cn

Abstract. Ultrasound imaging is a most common modality for tumor detection and diagnosis. Deep learning (DL) algorithms generally suffer from the small sample problem. The traditional texture feature extraction methods are still commonly used for small ultrasound image dataset. Deep polynomial network (DPN) is a newly proposed DL algorithm with excellent feature representation, which has the potential for small dataset. However, the simple concatenation of the learned hierarchical features from different layers in DPN limits its performance. Since the features from different layers in DPN can be regarded as heterogeneous features, they then can be effectively integrated by multiple kernel learning (MKL) methods. In this work, we propose a DPN and MKL based feature learning and classification framework (DPN-MKL) for tumor classification on small ultrasound image dataset. The experimental results show that DPN-MKL algorithm outperforms the commonly used DL algorithms for ultrasound image based tumor classification on small dataset.

1 Introduction

The ultrasound-based computer-aided diagnosis (CAD) for tumors provides an excellent decision support and second opinion tool for radiologists. Feature extraction and representation plays an essential role in CAD.

Deep learning (DL) has achieved great success in the field of medical image analysis [1-4]. DL algorithms can effectively learn data representation from patch-level samples. However, in ultrasound image, the local patch-level features don't always work as well as in other medical imaging modality. For example, the breast tumor in B-mode ultrasound images reflects lower level of echoes and appears relatively darker than surrounding tissues [5]. In this case, local patch usually only provides less or even poor information. DL algorithms usually suffer from the small sample problem. Therefore, the traditional texture feature extraction methods are still very commonly used instead of DL in ultrasound image, especially for small dataset.

Recently, a new DL algorithm, deep polynomial network (DPN), is proposed, in which the output of each node is a quadratic function of its inputs with an efficient layer-by-layer learning algorithm [6]. DPN has achieved competitive or even better performance on large scale image datasets compared with deep belief network (DBN)

© Springer International Publishing Switzerland 2015
L. Zhou et al. (Eds.): MLMI 2015, LNCS 9352, pp. 313–320, 2015.
DOI: 10.1007/978-3-319-24888-2_38

and stacked autoencoder (SAE) [6]. Moreover, the way of building the deep networks makes DPN feasible to compactly learn data representation on finite sample dataset.

In the current DPN, the final output features are built by concatenating the learned hierarchical features in DPN networks, which depress the representative performance of the features in different layers. In fact, the hierarchical features with different dimensions can be regarded as the heterogeneous features. Instead of the feature-level fusion methods, such as feature concatenation, another way to properly integrate these features is classifier- or decision-level fusion. Multiple kernel learning (MKL) is originally developed to combines multiple sub-kernels to seek better results for single view data. MKL has been successfully extended to combine heterogenous features or multi-modal features, whose kernels can naturally correspond to features of different views [7]. Therefore, MKL can be applied to fuse these hierarchical features in DPN.

In this study, we propose a DPN and MKL based texture feature re-learning and classification framework (DPN-MKL) for tumor classification on small ultrasound image dataset. The main contributions are twofold: 1) we employ DPN as a feature learning method for small ultrasound image dataset to generate more representative features for tumor classification task; 2) we propose to use MKL to fuse the learned hierarchical features in different layers instead of the simple feature concatenation in original DPN, which can further improve the classification performance.

2   DPN-MKL Framework

The DPN and DPN-MKL based classification frameworks are shown in Fig. 1. The network architecture of original DPN is also given in Fig. 1(a) with polynomials of degree 4 as an example. The DPN-MKL is introduced in following sections.

2.1   Deep Polynomial Network Algorithm

For DPN algorithm [6], let $X=\{x_1, x_2, \ldots, x_m\} \in \mathbb{R}^{m \times d}$ be a set of m training samples. When building the 1st-layer network, the set of values obtained by degree-1 polynomials (linear) function over the training samples is given by

$$\{(<w, [1\ x_1]>, \ldots, <w, [1\ x_m]>): w \in R^{d+1}\} \tag{1}$$

which is the $(d+1)$-dimensional linear subspace of $\mathbb{R}^m$. To conduct a basis for it, it only need to find $d+1$ vector $(w_1, \ldots, w_{d+1})$ by such as singular value decomposition. A linear transformation (specified by a matrix W) is used to maps $[1\ X]$ into the constructed basis. The columns of W specify the $d+1$ linear functions forming the 1st-layer in DPN : For all $j=1, \ldots, d+1$, the j'th node of first layer is the function

$$n_j^1(x) = <W_j, [1\ X]> \tag{2}$$

The $\{(n_j^1(x_1), \ldots, n_j^1(x_m))\}_{j=1}^{d+1}$ is a basis for all value obtained by degree-1 polynomials over training samples. Let F^1 denotes the $m \times (d+1)$ matrix, its columns are the vectors of this set, namely, $F_{i,j}^1 = n_j^1(x_i)$. So far, a one-layer network is finished.

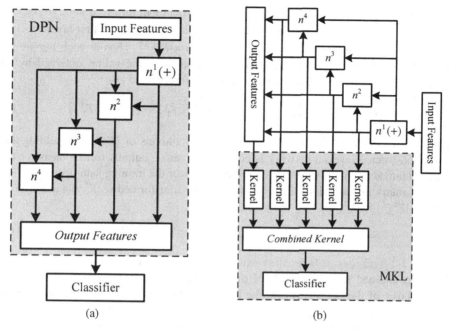

Fig. 1. Flowchart of DPN-based classification framework with a 4-degree polynomial DPN. (a) the original DPN classification framework; (b) the proposed DPN-MKL framework

It has been proved that any degree t polynomial can be written as

$$\Sigma_i \, g_i(x) \, h_i(x) + k(x) \tag{3}$$

where $g_i(x)$ is the degree-1 polynomial, $h_i(x)$ is degree-$(t-1)$ polynomial, and $k(x)$ is a polynomial of degree at most $(t-1)$ [6]. Since the nodes at the first layer network span all degree-1 polynomials, they in particular span the polynomials g_i, h_i and k. Therefore, any degree-2 polynomial can be written as

$$\Sigma_i \left(\Sigma_j \, \alpha_i^{(g_i)} n_j^1(x) \right) \left(\Sigma_j \, \alpha_s^{(h_i)} n_s^1(x) \right) + \left(\Sigma_j \, \alpha_j^{(k)} n_j^1(x) \right) =$$
$$\Sigma_{j,i} \, n_j^1(x) n_s^1(x) \left(\Sigma_i \, \alpha_j^{(g_i)} \alpha_s^{(h_i)} \right) + \Sigma_j \, n_j^1(x) \left(\alpha_j^{(k)} \right) \tag{4}$$

where all the α are scales. Eq. (4) indicates that the vector of values obtained by any degree-2 polynomial is in the span of the vector of values achieved by nodes in the first layer, and products of the outputs of every two nodes in the first layer.

Let $\tilde{F}^2$ be defined as following:

$$\tilde{F}^2 = \left[\left(F_1^1 \circ F_1^1 \right) \cdots \left(F_1^1 \circ F_{|F_1|}^1 \right) \cdots \left(F_{|F_1|}^1 \circ F_1^1 \right) \cdots \left(F_{|F_1|}^1 \circ F_{|F_1|}^1 \right) \right] \tag{5}$$

where $\circ$ denotes the Hadamard product. Then, the concatenated new matrix $[F \, \tilde{F}^2]$ spans all possible values attainable by degree-2 polynomials, leading to that $[F \, F^2]$'s columns are a linearly independent basis for $[F \, \tilde{F}^2]$'s columns. The columns of F^2 (which are a subset of the columns of $\tilde{F}^2$) specify the 2nd layer network: each such column, which corresponds to $F_i^1 \circ F_j^1$, corresponds in turn to a node in the 2nd layer, which computes the product of nodes $n_i^1(\cdot)$ and $n_j^1(\cdot)$ in the first layer.

Now Let F be redefined as the augmented matrix $[F \ F^2]$. Then at each iteration t, matrix F is maintained, whose columns form a basis for the values obtained by all polynomials of degree $\leq (t-1)$. The new matrix is represented as

$$\tilde{F}^t = \left[\left(F_1^{t-1} \circ F_1^1\right) \cdots \left(F_1^{t-1} \circ F_{|F_1|}^1\right) \cdots \left(F_{|F_1|}^{t-1} \circ F_1^1\right) \cdots \left(F_{|F^{t-1}|}^{t-1} \circ F_1^1\right) \right] \tag{6}$$

where the columns of $[F \ F^t]$ form a basis for the columns of $[F \ \tilde{F}^t]$. By adding this newly constructed layer, a network is constructed whose outputs form a basis for the values obtained by all polynomials of degree $\leq t$ over the training samples.

To maintain numerical stability, $\tilde{F}_t$ then can be transformed to F^t via a matrix W of size $|F^{t-1}| \times |F^1|$ by

$$F_s^t := W_{i(s),j(s)} F_{i(s)}^{t-1} \circ F_{j(j)}^1 \qquad s = 1, 2, \dots, |F^t| \tag{7}$$

After T-1 iterations, it is finished with a matrix F, whose columns form a basis for all values attained by polynomials of degree $\leq (T-1)$ over the training samples. On the top layer of the deep network, the learned features are concatenated into a new feature vector. The resulting network architecture of DPN is shown in Fig. 1(a).

This DPN algorithm can only be used for small datasets presently, because the larger the training samples, the wider the network width (i.e. the number of nodes created in each layer), which results in huge networks and high computational complexion. To solve this problem, a simple solution is to explicitly constrain the network width in each iteration [6]. Therefore, DPN can be applied to both large and small datasets. More detailed information about DPN is referred to [6].

2.2   Multiple Kernel Learning

As shown in Fig. 1(b), the hierarchical learned features from different layers are then fed to MKL algorithm to further improve the feature representation.

For kernel algorithms, such as support vector machines (SVM), the solution of the learning problem can be formed as

$$f(x) = \sum_{i=0}^{l} \alpha_i k(x, x_i) + b \tag{8}$$

where x_i is training sample, α_i and b are the coefficients to be learned from training samples, while $k(x, x_i)$ is a given positive definite kernel associated with a reproducing kernel Hilbert space (RKHS).

MKL aims to learn an optimal combination of multiple kernels usually given by

$$k(x, x_i) = \sum_{i=0}^{m} \beta_i k(x, x^{'}) \tag{9}$$

where m is the total number of kernels, and β_i is the weight for each basis kernel.

MKL should learn both coefficients and weights in a single optimization problem. Various optimization methods have been proposed to solve the kernel combination problem. In this work, the commonly used simple MKL (SimpleMKL) algorithm and a recently proposed soft margin MKL (SMMKL) algorithm are used due to their effectiveness [8, 9]. More detailed introduction about SimpleMKL and SMMKL is referred to [8] and [9].

3   Experiments and Results

The performance of DPN-MKL algorithms for ultrasound-based tumor classification is evaluated on two small datasets, namely breast B-mode ultrasound image dataset and prostate ultrasound elastography image dataset. For comparison, the original texture features are also further learned by two commonly used DL algorithms, namely SAE and DBN, and the widely used principal SAE component analysis (PCA) algorithm. The parameters of SAE, DBN and DPN are given in Table 1 and 2 for two datasets.

Two kinds of classifiers are adopted to more comprehensively evaluate the performance of different features. For fair comparison, the most commonly used support vector machine (SVM) algorithm is used for the original features and the features generated by DPN, SAE, DBN and PCA, due to its well performance for classification. Moreover, for DPN, S-DPN, SAE and DBN, the corresponding embedded classifiers are also used for classification, which have been proved their effectiveness.

Table 1. Parameters of Different DL Algorithms for Breast Ultrasound Image Dataset

	SAE	DBN	DPN
Hidden node	50	60	/
Layer	3	2 RBMs	3
Batch size	5	5	/
Epoch	3000	2000/2000	/

Table 2. Parameters of Different DL Algorithm for Prostate Ultrasound Image Dataset

	SAE	DBN	DPN
Hidden node	50	80	/
Layer	3	2 RBMs	3
Batch size	2	2	/
epoch	2500	2500/3000	/

3.1   Breast Ultrasound Image Dataset

A total of 200 pathology-proved B-mode breast ultrasound images, which include 100 benign mass cases and 100 malignant tumor cases, were tested. The lesion region was cropped to the size of 128×128. Figure 2 shows the examples of the benign breast mass and malignant tumor images.

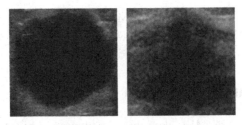

Fig. 2. Example images of benign breast mass and malignant breast tumor from left to right

The shearlet transform was applied to extract texture feature due to its superior performance to wavelet transform [10]. Totally 148 statistical descriptors, such as entropy, correlation, mean, variance and energy, were extracted based a 3-layer shearlet. The dataset was randomly split into half for training set and testing set. This procedure was repeated five times, and the classification result was averaged over five runs.

Table 3 shows the classification results of different methods. It can be found that all the DPN-based algorithms significantly outperform other compared algorithms, while two DPN-MKL algorithms are superior to DPN. The best performance is achieved by DPN-SMMKL with the mean classification accuracy of 92.40±1.67%, sensitivity of 93.84±0.89% and specificity of 90.84±3.15%. It is also clear from Table 1 that DBN and SAE are even worse than the original features for this dataset, which indicates that they can't work well on such small dataset.

Table 3. Classification Results on Breast Ultrasound Image Dataset (Unit: %)

	Accuracy	Sensitivity	Specificity
148-features-SVM	88.40±1.82	90.41±4.48	86.45±6.23
PCA-SVM	88.80±0.45	89.11±4.21	89.34±4.13
DBN-E-Classifier	85.40±3.05	84.25±6.42	86.41±4.14
SAE-E-Classifier	87.20±2.17	83.95±5.31	89.96±3.83
DPN-E-Classifier	89.20±1.10	90.78±3.28	86.07±3.77
DBN-SVM	87.20±2.17	84.49±4.65	89.54±3.40
SAE-SVM	85.20±3.27	82.32±6.43	88.04±3.53
DPN-SVM	89.20±1.30	90.32±2.41	88.02±4.99
DPN-SimpleMKL	90.80±1.10	91.01±1.93	90.50±3.15
DPN-SMMKL	**92.40±1.67**	**93.84±0.89**	**90.84±3.15**

3.2   Prostate Ultrasound Elastography Image Dataset

The second experiment was conducted on 70 pathology-proved prostate ultrasound elastography images (42 benign masses and 28 malignant tumors) with the examples shown in Fig. 3. The region for feature extraction was cropped to include the lesion. Totally 35 statistical feature desciptors, such as means, deviation, entropy, skewness, kurtness, coefficient variance and their variants from all pixel values, were extracted to represent the texture properties. The 4-fold cross-validation strategy was performed.

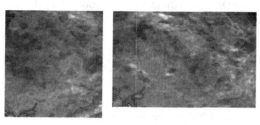

Fig. 3. Example images of benign prostate mass and malignant prostate tumor from left to right

As shown in Table 4, DPN-MKL algorithms are again superior to other non-DPN algorithms. The best classification accuracy and sensitivity are 77.78±4.54% and 70.15±7.51%, respectively, achieved by DPN-SMMKL with significant improvements. DPN-SimpleMKL has the second-best performance. It indicates that MKL algorithm is crucial for heterogeneous feature fusion.

It is worth noting that standard deviation for all the algorithms are relative large, because this ultrasound image dataset is very small with unbalance samples. When performing 4-fold cross-validation strategy, there are only about 16 testing samples, resulting in the large standard deviation. However, the results of DPN-SMMKL are still relative stable, which indicates that MKL algorithm itself is very important for hierarchical DPN features on very small dataset.

Table 4. Classification Results on Prostate Ultrasound Elastography Image Dataset (Unit: %)

	Accuracy	Sensitivity	Specificity
35-features-SVM	59.72±2.78	33.42±9.76	74.08±5.77
PCA-SVM	68.06±2.78	54.29±5.08	74.91±4.43
DBN-E-Classifier	61.12±6.41	49.88±11.95	67.64±13.74
SAE- E-Classifier	55.56±4.54	67.02±12.62	50.17±3.43
DPN- E-Classifier	72.22±0.00	65.15±5.01	76.16±3.08
DBN-SVM	62.50±2.78	33.60±19.73	81.51±13.36
SAE-SVM	58.33±5.56	31.73±6.49	74.47±11.35
DPN-SVM	68.06±2.78	65.15±5.01	69.47±4.65
DPN-SimpleMKL	73.61±5.32	38.04±18.29	**93.37±8.65**
DPN-SMMKL	**77.78±4.54**	**70.15±7.51**	83.44±11.41

4   Conclusion

In this study, we propose a DPN-MKL based feature learning and classification framework for tumor classification on small ultrasound image dataset. The results indicate three conclusions: 1) DPN works well as a feature re-representation method to further improve the performance of hand-designed texture features; 2) DPN outperforms other compared DL algorithms for ultrasound-based tumor classification on small sample dataset; 3) the hierarchical learned features in DPN are well integrated by MKL to further improve DPN's feature representation instead of the concatenation fusion in original DPN for small sample dataset.

Even for small training samples, the network architectures of commonly used DL algorithms are still complex with huge nodes. Consequently, small samples seriously limit the effectiveness of deep network training, which finally depresses the feature representation. While DPN builds the networks with small nodes for small training samples, which guarantee a well trained deep network with small samples. Therefore, the algorithm structure of DPN makes it suitable for both large and small datasets.

Acknowledgments. This work is supported by the National Natural Science Foundation of China (61471231, 61401267) and the Innovation Program of Shanghai Municipal Education Commission (13YZ016).

Reference

1. Prasoon, A., Petersen, K., Igel, C., Lauze, F., Dam, E., Nielsen, M.: Deep feature learning for knee cartilage segmentation using a triplanar convolutional neural network. In: Mori, K., Sakuma, I., Sato, Y., Barillot, C., Navab, N. (eds.) MICCAI 2013, Part II. LNCS, vol. 8150, pp. 246–253. Springer, Heidelberg (2013)
2. Shin, H.C., Orton, M.R., Collins, D.J., Doran, S.J., Leach, M.O.: Stacked autoencoders for unsupervised feature learning and multiple organ detection in a pilot study using 4D patient data. IEEE Trans. Pattern Anal. Mach. Intell. **35**(8), 1930–1943 (2013)
3. Roth, H.R., Lu, L., Seff, A., Cherry, K.M., Hoffman, J., Wang, S., Liu, J., Turkbey, E., Summers, R.M.: A new 2.5D representation for lymph node detection using random sets of deep convolutional neural network observations. In: Golland, P., Hata, N., Barillot, C., Hornegger, J., Howe, R. (eds.) MICCAI 2014, Part I. LNCS, vol. 8673, pp. 520–527. Springer, Heidelberg (2014)
4. Carneiro, G., Nascimento, J.C.: Combining multiple dynamic models and deep learning architectures for tracking the left ventricle endocardium in ultrasound data. IEEE Trans. Pattern Anal. Mach. Intell. **35**(11), 2592–2607 (2013)
5. Sehgal, C.M., Weinstein, S.P., Arger, P.H., Conant, E.F.: A review of breast ultrasound. J. Mammary Gland Biol. **11**(2), 113–123 (2006)
6. Livni, R., Shalev-Shwartz, S., Shamir, O.: An algorithm for training polynomial networks. arXiv: 1304.7045 (2014)
7. Xu, C., Tao, D., Xu, C.: A aurvey on multi-view learning. arXiv: 1304.5634 (2013)
8. Rakotomamonjy, A., Bach, F.R., Canu, S., Grandvalet, Y.: SimpleMKL. J. Mach. Learn. Res. **9**, 2491–2521 (2008)
9. Xu, X.X., Tsang, I.W., Xu, D.: Soft Margin Multiple Kernel Learning. IEEE Trans. Neural Network Learn. Sys. **24**(5), 749–761 (2013)
10. Easley, G., Labate, D., Lim, W.Q.: Sparse directional image representations using the discrete shearlet transform. Appl. Comput. Harmon. Anal. **25**, 25–46 (2008)
11. Bengio, Y., Courville, A., Vincent, P.: Representation learning: a review and new rerspectives. IEEE Trans. Pattern Anal. Mach. Intell. **35**(8), 1798–1828 (2013)

Multi-source Information Gain for Random Forest: An Application to CT Image Prediction from MRI Data

Tri Huynh[1], Yaozong Gao[1,2], Jiayin Kang[1], Li Wang[1], Pei Zhang[1],
Dinggang Shen[1,2(✉)], and Alzheimer's Disease Neuroimaging Initiative (ADNI)

[1] IDEA Lab, Department of Radiology and BRIC,
University of North Carolina at Chapel Hill, Chapel Hill, NC, USA
dgshen@med.unc.edu
[2] Department of Computer Science,
University of North Carolina at Chapel Hill, Chapel Hill, NC, USA

Abstract. Random forest has been widely recognized as one of the most powerful learning-based predictors in literature, with a broad range of applications in medical imaging. Notable efforts have been focused on enhancing the algorithm in multiple facets. In this paper, we present an original concept of *multi-source information gain* that escapes from the conventional notion inherent to random forest. We propose the idea of characterizing information gain in the training process by utilizing *multiple beneficial sources of information*, instead of the *sole governing of prediction targets* as conventionally known. We suggest the use of location and input image patches as the secondary sources of information for guiding the splitting process in random forest, and experiment on the challenging task of predicting CT images from MRI data. The experimentation is thoroughly analyzed in two datasets, i.e., human brain and prostate, with its performance further validated with the integration of auto-context model. Results prove that the *multi-source information gain* concept effectively helps better guide the training process with consistent improvement in prediction accuracy.

1 Introduction

Since introduced by Breiman [1] in 2001, random forest has become one of the most powerful learning-based predictors with state-of-the-art performance on a broad range of applications, ranging from detection, classification, to segmentation, etc.

With its increasing success, random forest has attracted growing efforts in improving the method from various facets. Menze et al. [2] proposed a supervised approach to define the optimal *"oblique"* split direction on the features, instead of the popular *orthogonal* split in the training process. This approach adapts more effectively to the nature of data and dramatically reduces the complexity of decision trees. Marin [3] et al. also adopted this idea with the use of Support Vector Machine in learning the splitting direction. While in [4], Robnik-Šikonja provided insight that using multiple attribute evaluation measures in different trees for split selection would improve the performance by decreasing the correlation among the trees. The author also showed significant improvement in deriving final prediction result by weighting the trees based on their per-

© Springer International Publishing Switzerland 2015
L. Zhou et al. (Eds.): MLMI 2015, LNCS 9352, pp. 321–329, 2015.
DOI: 10.1007/978-3-319-24888-2_39

formance on similar inputs. Recently, the most notable advancement of random forest is the introduction of structured random forest, which extends random forest from predicting scalar outputs to directly predicting structured outputs. Structured random forest can better preserve the neighborhood information in the structured outputs as a whole, which has shown preeminent performance [5][6].

Although many enhancements have been proposed for random forest, all of the methods follow the same strategy in growing trees based solely on minimizing the variety of the prediction targets in each child node. The purity of prediction targets or labels is unarguably the most important factor in choosing the splits on data. However, prediction targets are not the only source of information that is beneficial to guide the process. In this paper, we, for the first time, explore the use of *multiple sources of information* as the splitting criteria in random forest. Specifically, we devise the general model for multi-source information gain, and suggest the use of location and input image patches (built upon the success of structured random forest) as other secondary sources of information to guide the splitting process. The method is then analyzed through the challenging problem of predicting computed tomography (CT) image from magnetic resonance (MR) image in two datasets, human brain and prostate region. The performance is also further thoroughly examined and validated with the integration of auto-context model. Results provide insights into the method as well as show that significant improvement could be gained by the proposed approach.

2   Random Forest

We first review the *classic* random forest, followed by *structured* random forest. They are the foundation for extending to *multi-source information gain* in Section 3.

2.1   Classic Random Forest

Random forest comprises of multiple decision trees. At each internal node of a tree, a feature is chosen to split the incoming training samples to maximize the information gain. A training sample consists of an *input* feature vector and its *output* target. Let $u \in U \subset \mathbb{R}^q$ be an input feature vector, and $v \in V \subset \mathbb{Z}$ be its corresponding prediction target in the classification problem. For a set of samples $S_j \subset U \times V$ arriving at node j, the information gain achieved by choosing the k-th feature is computed by:

$$I_j^k = H(S_j) - \frac{|S_{j,\mathrm{L}}^k|}{|S_j|} H(S_{j,\mathrm{L}}^k) - \frac{|S_{j,\mathrm{R}}^k|}{|S_j|} H(S_{j,\mathrm{R}}^k), \tag{1}$$

$$H(S) = -\sum_v p_v \log(p_v), \tag{2}$$

where L and R denote the left and right child nodes, $S_{j,\mathrm{L}}^k = \{(u, v) \in S_j \mid u^k < \theta_j^k\}$, $S_{j,\mathrm{R}}^k = S_j \backslash S_{j,\mathrm{L}}^k$, u^k is the k-th feature in u, θ_j^k is the splitting threshold chosen to maximize the information gain I_j^k, and $|\cdot|$ is the cardinality of the set. $H(S)$ denotes the entropy of target values in S, with p_v the fraction of elements in S having value v. For regression problem ($V \subset \mathbb{R}$), the entropy is replaced by variance as follows:

$$H(S) = \sum_v p_v(v - \bar{v})^2, \tag{3}$$
$$\bar{v} = \sum_v p_v v, \tag{4}$$

2.2   Structured Random Forest

In the classic random forest, the output space is *either* a class label for the case of classification, *or* a real value for the case of regression. Recently, a few pioneering works [5][6] advanced random forest into structured random forest, which directly predicts a structured patch instead of a single value, and achieved preeminent performance. The difference between *structured* random forest and *classic* random forest is illustrated in Fig. 1, using an example of predicting CT image from MRI data. *Structured* random forest helps preserve the neighborhood information in the predicted structured patch and further reduce the expected number of decision trees since a voxel now receives information from multiple neighboring patches.

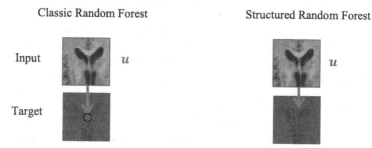

Fig. 1. Illustration of *classic* random forest and *structured* random forest. In the classic random forest, the input feature vector $\boldsymbol{u}$ derived from MR image patch is used to predict a target value v for a voxel (red point) in the CT image, while, in the structured random forest, the same feature vector $\boldsymbol{u}$ is used to predict all values $\boldsymbol{v}$ in a target CT patch (red rectangle).

When extending to *structured* random forest, the main issue is how to characterize the entropy of the structured patches. That is, how to efficiently capture the similarity of different target patches. One naïve way is formulating the similarity based on individual voxels inside the patches. However, the computation is highly expensive and the method is too sensitive to individual voxel changes rather than high-level patch structure. A more effective way is to find a mapping that can effectively capture the information from each image patch. In this paper, we characterize the image patches by principal component analysis (PCA), i.e., the mapped coefficients of $\boldsymbol{v}$ represent its first d PCA coefficients. This mapping has the advantage of being computationally efficient while effectively deriving the most significant information in each target patch. Suppose the prediction targets now are $\boldsymbol{v} \in \boldsymbol{V} \subset \mathbb{R}^g$, and $\boldsymbol{w} = \Pi(\boldsymbol{v})$ denotes the mapped coefficients of $\boldsymbol{v}$, where $\boldsymbol{w} \in \mathbb{C} \subset \mathbb{R}^d$, $d < g$. Then, the entropy $H(S)$ from Eqs. (3) and (4) can be computed as:

$$H(S) = \sum_w p_w \|w - \bar{w}\|_2^2 \tag{5}$$

$$\bar{w} = \sum_w p_w w \tag{6}$$

By using *structured* random forest, the predicted neighboring patches can be fused, i.e., by averaging, to reconstruct a final predicted image.

3   Multi-source Information Gain

In random forest, the splitting maximizes the information gain by minimizing the variety of prediction targets in each child node (Eqs. 1-6). The rationale of this process is to find the best feature and threshold that have the highest discriminative power to categorize the samples. That discriminative power is measured solely by the convergence of prediction targets, which is intuitive and the prediction targets are unarguably the most important information to guide the learning procedure. However, they are not the only source of information that is helpful to guide the splitting process. For example, many applications hold the spatial constraint, in which certain output patterns usually appear in certain locations. In these cases, a split results in the grouping of similar output patterns and is more informative and robust in nearby locations, which should also carry higher information gain compared to the case of having those output patterns in highly scattered locations. In this case, location is another source of information that could contribute to the information gain obtained at each split. Therefore, we propose to include multiple indicators in guiding the splitting process, and devise the notion of multi-source information gain for this purpose.

Suppose we have N sources of information that we would like to integrate to the final information gain. The sources can be of various forms, from discrete labels, real values, or structured patches, with their individual entropies to be computed as in Eqs. 2, 3-4, and 5-6, respectively. Since the information gain from different sources could have very different ranges, we define the information gain ratio for one source as a variant of the information gain in Eq. 1 to normalize the gain from different sources:

$$R_j^k = \frac{I_j^k}{H(S_j)} \tag{7}$$

where R_j^k denotes the information gain ratio obtained from one source by choosing the k-th feature to split the samples at node j, I_j^k is the information gain as defined in Eq. 1, and $H(S_j)$ is the entropy of set S_j. Letting $R_j^k(n)$ denote the information gain ratio obtained from source $n \in \{1, \ldots, N\}$, we define the multi-source information gain as the weighted combination of the information gain ratios from all sources as follows:

$$M_j^k = \sum_{n=1}^{N} \alpha(n) G_j^k(n) \tag{8}$$

$$G_j^k(n) = \begin{cases} R_j^k(n) & R_j^k(n) \geq 0 \\ 0 & R_j^k(n) < 0 \end{cases} \tag{9}$$

where M_j^k denotes the multi-source information gain when choosing the k-th feature to split the samples at node j, and $\alpha(n)$ is the weighting factor which indicates the relative importance of different sources.

In this paper, we suggest and analyze the use of three different sources of information gain: 1) the prediction target patches, 2) the location of the samples, and 3) the corresponding input image patches. The contribution of location information has been previously discussed, while input image patches also can potentially provide helpful information to better guide the splitting process. In many problems where there are strong correlations between the input and output structures, we could expect that a similarity in input structures should also correspond to the similarity in output structures. Thus, information gain from input structures could potentially further enhance the confidence of similarity of output structures. This is especially helpful with the introduction of *structured* random forest, where the information gain from both input and output can be measured in the corresponding structured patches, thus better exploiting their correlation.

4   Experimental Analysis

4.1   Predicting CT Image from MR image

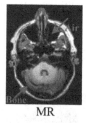
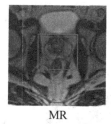
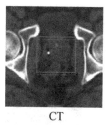

MR	CT

| MR | CT |

Fig. 2. A pair of MR image and corresponding CT image from the same human brain. Example of "one-to-multiple" relationship: both air and bone have very low response in MR images, but can be highly differentiated in CT images.

Fig. 3. A pair of an MR image and its corresponding CT image around the prostate area. Example of "multiple-to-one" relationship: there are many intensity levels in MR image corresponding to the same intensity level in CT image (red rectangle).

We apply the proposed method to the problem of predicting CT image from corresponding MR image. We choose to perform analysis on this problem because it is a challenging problem, with complex relationship between CT and MR images, and also location information could be exploited. These conditions allow us to best demonstrate the proposed multi-source information gain model. This task is highly important in performing attenuation correction (AC) for Positron emission tomography (PET) images in the PET/MRI system. AC is required to make PET images readily applicable for clinical diagnosis, which relies on the attenuation map obtained from CT images. Therefore, predicting CT image from MR image is crucial in PET/MRI system. Examples of the MR and CT image pairs are shown in Figs. 2-3. As can be seen in the figures, predicting CT image from MR image is very challenging, with the complex relationship between two modalities. The same range of MR intensity values can correspond to different ranges of CT values (Fig. 2), while multiple ranges of MR values can also correspond to the same CT value range (Fig. 3).

4.1.1   Datasets

We experiment on two datasets: 1) The brain data were acquired from 16 subjects with both MR and CT scans in the Alzheimer's Disease Neuroimaging Initiative database (adni.loni.usc.edu). 2) The prostate dataset is our in-house data, which has 22 subjects, each with the corresponding MR and CT scans.

4.1.2   Training Procedure

Pre-alignment. In order to learn the relationship between MR and CT images, we first need to perform the intra-alignment for the MR and CT image pair of each subject [8]. Afterwards, in order to utilize the spatial information, we perform inter-subject registration [7] to roughly bring all the subjects onto a common space.

Training. We utilize structured random forest to predict CT image from corresponding MR image, as discussed in Section 2.2. Different combinations from three sources of information gain are experimented: MR patches, target CT patches, and location. The following parameters were used - MR input patch size: 15x15x15; CT target patch size: 3x3x3; Number of PCA coefficients used in structured random forest: 10; Weighing factors for CT patches, MR patches, and locations in the multi-source information gain model are 1, 0.2, and 0.2, respectively.

4.1.3   Results

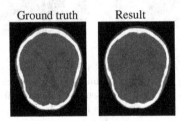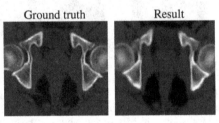

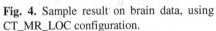

Fig. 4. Sample result on brain data, using CT_MR_LOC configuration.

Fig. 5. Sample result on prostate data, using CT_LOC configuration.

To provide thorough evaluation of the performance using different sources of information gain, we experiment on **four** different configurations: **1)** information gain from target CT patches alone (CT), **2)** from CT and MR patches (CT_MR), **3)** from CT patches and Locations of the patches (CT_LOC), and **4)** from MR, CT patches, and Locations of the patches (CT_MR_LOC). Leave-one-out cross validation was performed on both datasets using two popular metrics: Peak signal-to-noise ratio (PSNR) and normalized mean square error (NMSE). Results are provided in Figs. 6-7, with qualitative samples in Figs. 4-5. Following conclusions could be drawn:

- The information gain from **location** always notably improves the performance in both brain and prostate data (CT_LOC versus CT, and CT_MR_LOC versus CT_MR).

The location information gain helps favoring the grouping of similar image patches in nearby locations, making the grouping more robust.

- The information gain from **MR patches** slightly improves the prediction performance in brain dataset, but degrades the prediction in prostate dataset (CT_MR versus CT, and CT_MR_LOC versus CT_LOC). One possible reason is due to the nature of datasets. In brain data, we have more one-to-multiple mappings from MR to CT images, where similar intensities from MR (e.g., air and bone) correspond to highly different CT intensities. Thus, the added refinement from MR patches helps better differentiate the CT patches. On the other hand, in prostate data, there are more multiple-to-one mappings from MR to CT images. Thus, the further information gain from MR patches does not help, and actually makes the grouping overfitting and leads to more wrong predictions.

To validate the confidence in improvement of the multi-source model, we also performed statistical tests with the obtained p-values well below 0.05 for both datasets.

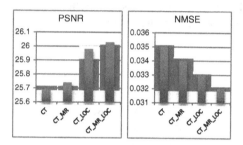 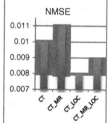

Fig. 6. Prediction results on brain data.   **Fig. 7.** Prediction results on prostate data.

4.2   Integration to Auto-context Model

To perform in-depth analysis of the method, we further experiment the multi-source information gain in the second layer of auto-context model (ACM) [9]. ACM utilizes the prediction result from the previously learned model as the added contextual information, and uses features extracted from this result together with features from the original input image to train a new refining model.

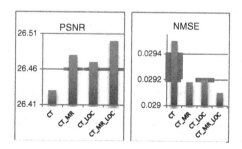 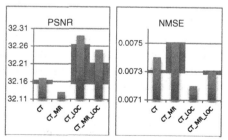

Fig. 8. Prediction results of second layer ACM on brain data.

Fig. 9. Prediction results of second layer ACM on prostate data.

We use the *best predicted results* from the first layer (CT_MR_LOC for brain, CT_LOC for prostate data) as the context features to train the second layer random forest. The prediction performance of different sources of information gain is provided in Figs. 8-9. We can see that although the improvement has been more saturated in the second layer, adding more sources of information gain still has the same effect as in the first layer. Specifically, location information gain always improves the performance in both datasets, while information gain from MR image patches helps advance the prediction in brain dataset, but degrades in prostate dataset.

To further provide a complete comparison, we also show the performance of auto-context model using the *traditional* random forest (information gain based solely on CT patches) and our *multi-source information gain* based random forest (CT_MR_LOC for brain, and CT_LOC for prostate data). In this experiment, each method uses *its own predicted results* as context features. Results are presented in Figs. 10-11. From this experiment, we can clearly see the improvement of the proposed method compared to the traditional one. In both datasets, the performance of the multi-source model in the first layer almost reaches the result of the traditional model in the second layer.

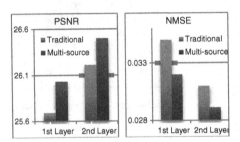

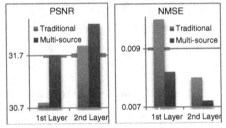

Fig. 10. Prediction results on brain data, in different layers of ACM.

Fig. 11. Prediction results on prostate data, in different layers of ACM.

5   Discussion and Conclusion

In this paper, we proposed the use of multiple sources of information in characterizing the information gain in random forest. A general model was proposed and the experimentation was carried out for the challenging task of predicting CT images from MRI data. Results clearly show that, when using appropriately, the information gain from other contributive sources besides the prediction targets consistently improves the prediction performance. This is the first time a multi-source information gain concept is proposed with promising results, which could open potentials for future shifts into this line of research. In the future, we would like to investigate the use of other sources of information gain that could also be taken into consideration.

References

1. Breiman, L.: Random Forests. Machine Learning **45**, 5–32 (2001)
2. Menze, B.H., Kelm, B., Splitthoff, D.N., Koethe, U., Hamprecht, F.A.: On oblique random forests. In: Gunopulos, D., Hofmann, T., Malerba, D., Vazirgiannis, M. (eds.) ECML PKDD 2011, Part II. LNCS, vol. 6912, pp. 453–469. Springer, Heidelberg (2011)
3. Marin, J., Vazquez, D., Lopez, A. M., Amores, J., Leibe, B.: Random forests of local experts for pedestrian detection. In: IEEE International Conference on Computer Vision (ICCV), pp. 2592–2599 (2013)
4. Robnik-Šikonja, M.: Improving random forests. In: Boulicaut, J.-F., Esposito, F., Giannotti, F., Pedreschi, D. (eds.) ECML 2004. LNCS (LNAI), vol. 3201, pp. 359–370. Springer, Heidelberg (2004)
5. Kontschieder, P., Bulò, S.R., Bischof, H., Pelillo, M.: Structured class-labels in random forests for semantic image labeling. In: ICCV, pp. 2190–2197 (2011)
6. Dollar, P., Zitnick, C.L.: Structured forests for fast edge detection. In: ICCV, pp. 1841–1848 (2013)
7. Jenkinson, M., Smith, S.M.: A global optimisation method for robust affine registration of brain images. Medical Image Analysis **5**(2), 143–156 (2011)
8. Klein, S., Staring, M., Murphy, K., Viergever, M.A., Pluim, J.P.W.: Elastix: a toolbox for intensity based medical image registration. IEEE Transactions on Medical Imaging **29**(1), 196–205 (2010)
9. Tu, Z.: Auto-context and its application to high-level vision tasks. In: IEEE Conference on Computer Vision and Pattern Recognition, pp. 1–8 (2008)

Joint Learning of Multiple Longitudinal Prediction Models by Exploring Internal Relations

Baiying Lei, Dong Ni$^{(\boxtimes)}$, and Tianfu Wang$^{(\boxtimes)}$

Department of Biomedical Engineering, School of Medicine, Shenzhen University,
National-Regional Key Technology Engineering Laboratory for Medical Ultrasound,
Guangdong Key Laboratory for Biomedical Measurements and Ultrasound Imaging,
Shenzhen, China
{nidong,tfwang}@szu.edu.cn

Abstract. Longitudinal prediction of the brain disorder such as Alzheimer's disease (AD) is important for possible early detection and early intervention. Given the baseline imaging and clinical data, it will be interesting to predict the progress of disease for an individual subject, such as predicting the conversion of Mild Cognitive Impairment (MCI) to AD, in the future years. Most existing methods predicted different clinical scores using different models, or predicted multiple scores at different future time points separately. This often misses the chance of coordinated learning of multiple prediction models for jointly predicting multiple clinical scores at multiple future time points. In this paper, we propose a novel method for joint learning of multiple longitudinal prediction models for multiple clinical scores at multiple future time points. First, for each longitudinal prediction model, we explore three important relationships among training samples, features, and clinical scores, respectively, for enhancing its learning. Then, we further introduce additional relation among different longitudinal prediction models for allowing them to select a common set of features from the baseline imaging and clinical data, with $l_{2,1}$ sparsity constraint, for their joint training. We evaluate the performance of our joint prediction models with the data from the Alzheimer's Disease Neuroimaging Initiative (ADNI) database, showing much better performance than the state-of-the-art methods in predicting multiple clinical scores at multiple future time points.

1 Introduction

In the recent decades, neuroimaging-based longitudinal studies prove to be an important research direction in characterizing the neurodegenerative process of many brain diseases such as Alzheimer's disease (AD) [1], in which data from multiple time points are used [2-4]. The temporal change of the neurodegenerative cognitive measures, e.g., the Alzheimer's Disease Assessment Scale Cognitive Subscale (ADAS-Cog) and the Mini Mental State Examination (MMSE), can partly reveal the AD progression. But, due to the complicated characteristics of the disease development, the accurate prediction of AD progression still remains an important topic.

© Springer International Publishing Switzerland 2015
L. Zhou et al. (Eds.): MLMI 2015, LNCS 9352, pp. 330–337, 2015.
DOI: 10.1007/978-3-319-24888-2_40

In longitudinal studies for AD diagnosis and prognosis, the dimensionality of the data has long been a problem (i.e., small number of samples with large feature size). To address this problem, researchers developed various models with different clinical scores (e.g., ADAS-Cog and MMSE) to identify disease-related biomarkers among multiple time points [5-7]. Although many existing longitudinal studies have shown promising predictive power, the underlying relations among features, subjects, and clinical scores at different time points are seldom considered simultaneously. These relationships could serve as inherent high-level information in the observations. Intuitively, we observe that modeling and utilizing such relationship information can further enhance the learning performance for AD progression prediction. This high-level relational information could be considered, with the intuition that the learned model shall preserve the relationships present in the training data.

To model the disease progression, we need to observe the behavior of changes in condition of the patients through time. On the other hand, the huge amount of information in the data, especially from multiple time-points, leads to a challenging problem when with quite a lot of irrelevant information. Therefore, we should utilize the aforementioned relational constraints to build a more robust regression model by selecting the best and most relevant features for predicting the individual patient's clinical behavior in multiple future time points.

In this paper, we propose a joint learning procedure for multiple longitudinal predictions by exploiting their inherent relations and applying for AD progression prediction. Particularly, we propose three novel regularization terms, each modeling a set of crucial relationship at different time points. We incorporate these terms into a multi-task sparse feature selection model. We also introduce a loss function specifically designed to jointly predict the patients' clinical scores at multiple future time points. This enables us to condense the common information shared by data from different time points and then select the most meaningful features for multiple prediction tasks. We evaluate our method on the ADNI database, and achieve promising results on estimating multiple clinical scores at multiple future time points, using only baseline data.

2   Method

2.1   Notation and Problem Statement

In this work, capital bold letters represent matrices, small bold letters denote vectors, and non-bold letters denote regular variables. Let $\mathbf{X} \in \mathbf{R}^{S \times F}$ be the data of S different subjects, each with F-dimensional feature sets from the baseline MR image. We denote $\mathbf{x}_{u,:}$ and $\mathbf{x}_{:,v}$ as the u-th row vector and the v-th column vector of $\mathbf{X}$. Let $\mathbb{Y} = \left\{ \mathbf{Y}^{(t)} \in \mathbf{R}^{S \times C}, t = 1, ..., T \right\}$ represent C types of clinical cognitive scores (e.g., ADAS-Cog and MMSE) for S subjects at T time points, where $\mathbf{Y}^{(t)} \in \mathbf{R}^{S \times C}$ is the corresponding clinical scores at the t-th time point for S subjects. Denote $\mathbb{W} = \left\{ \mathbf{W}^{(t)} \in \mathbf{R}^{F \times C}, t = 1, ..., T \right\}$ as the set of weight matrices map the original features to the clinical scores, where $\mathbf{W}^{(t)}$ represents the weight matrix for the t-th time point.

Our goal is to learn a linear regression model to reveal the longitudinal associations between the original features and the cognitive trajectories, through time, and predict the clinical scores at multiple future time points from the baseline data ($t = 1$). This is illustrated in Fig. 1. Each subject's features are put as a row in the matrix $\mathbf{X}$. By learning the weight vectors in each $\mathbf{W}^{(t)}$, we can reconstruct the corresponding clinical scores in each $\mathbf{Y}^{(t)}$. The details are explained in the following subsections.

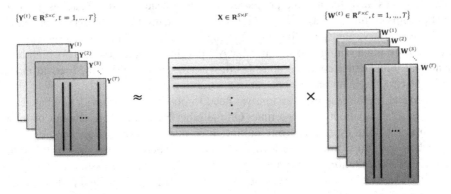

Fig. 1. An illustration of the proposed regression model using longitudinal data.

2.2   Proposed Method

A key advantage in longitudinal studies is that we could observe the patient changes through time, and can effectively utilize the shared common information in different time points. This enables us to select the best set of features for monitoring the progression of MCI patients and thereafter predict their future scores. This shared common information in different time points could be captured efficiently for better predicting the patient scores. There are three different aspects that this common information could be leveraged, among features, subjects and their clinical scores, respectively. These relations can be measured through similarities between any pair of columns and between any pair of rows in matrices. Intuitively, we propose that the pairwise similarities between features, subjects and clinical scores should be preserved in the predictions by the regression model. In this section, we introduce a method to incorporate this information in a multi-task learning framework and jointly learn a model from multiple longitudinal data. We define a linear regression model for each time point using the baseline data as a single task, and then formulate the global regression model in a multi-task learning formulation with an $l_{2,1}$ sparsity constraint, where the above three relational aspects are incorporated as regularization terms.

Some previous studies (e.g., [5]) reveal the associations among imaging features and cognitive scores at each time point separately, with the assumption that each task at each time point is independent. However, this assumption does not hold due to the ignorance of the temporal correlation of clinical scores. In fact, the correlation among different time points can potentially help predict the clinical cognitive scores. This motivates us to jointly learn a regression model across all time points, which would help identify the most relevant imaging markers for prediction of cognitive scores. Specifically, we seek to learn the weight coefficient matrices to uncover the temporal change of clinical scores, through which the information from each learning task and the common structures among multiple time points can be jointly discovered.

In order to select the most relevant and discriminant features for each time point, we propose a correlation-induced sparsity model, along with a least-squares loss function. The loss function would control the prediction error, while the sparsity assumption leads to the least number of contributing features. As a result, for each time point, we would select the features that are most correlated with the actual clinical scores. A general form of the objective function would be as follows:

$$\min_{\{W^{(t)}, t=1,\dots,T\}} \sum_{t=1}^{T} \left\| Y^{(t)} - XW^{(t)} \right\|_F^2 + \lambda_1 \sum_{t=1}^{T} \Phi\left(W^{(t)}\right) + \lambda_2 \left\| \widehat{W} \right\|_{2,1}, \qquad (1)$$

where $\|\cdot\|_F^2$ is the Frobenius norm of a matrix, $\widehat{W}$ is the coefficient weight matrix, defined by concatenating all $W^{(t)}$s as $\widehat{W} = [W^{(1)}, W^{(2)}, \cdots, W^{(t)}, \cdots, W^{(T)}] \in \mathbf{R}^{F \times CT}$, and λ_1 and λ_2 are the regularization parameters. The second term, $\Phi(W^{(t)})$, is our regularizer, which is comprised of multiple parts, corresponding to three relationships among features, subjects and clinical scores, respectively. In the rest of this section, we will explain it in details and discuss all its characteristics. The last term in Eq. (1) is a group regularizer to uncover the correlation among different features and jointly select features for multiple tasks, which is defined as $\left\| \widehat{W} \right\|_{2,1} = \sum_{i=1}^{F} \left\| \widehat{w}_{i,:} \right\|_2$, where $\widehat{w}_{i,:}$ is the i-th row vector of $\widehat{W}$, and $\|\cdot\|_{2,1}$ is $l_{2,1}$-norm. It is worth noting that $l_{2,1}$-norm computes the sum of the l_2-norm of each row of $\widehat{W}$, which enforces many rows to be zero, and hence it is suitable for feature selection. Then, features corresponding to those non-zero rows in $\widehat{W}$ are regarded as the most discriminative features in subsequent learning models.

To define the proposed regularization term, $\Phi(W^{(t)})$, the 'feature-feature', 'subject-subject' and 'clinical score-clinical score' relations at each different time point are incorporated. We use the idea of Laplacian matrices and graphs to obtain the similarity in the local structures [8, 10].

The 'feature-feature' relational information is imposed as the relationship between columns of the input matrix X, and is reflected in the relation between the corresponding rows in the coefficients weight matrix $W^{(t)}$. Hence, the widely used graph Laplacian is leveraged. To measure the similarity between the u-th feature and v-th feature of X in the original feature space, we use a heat kernel defined as below:

$$f_{uv} = \exp\left(-\left\| x_{:,u} - x_{:,v} \right\|_2^2\right), \qquad (2)$$

where $x_{:,u}$ is the u-th column of the input data X. Based on the similarity, we develop the first feature-feature relation-based regularization term as:

$$R_f\left(w^{(t)}\right) = \sum_{u,v=1}^{F} f_{uv} \left\| w_{u,:}^{(t)} - w_{v,:}^{(t)} \right\|_2^2, \qquad (3)$$

where $w_{u,:}^{(t)}$ is the u-th row of $W^{(t)}$ at time point t. Thus, the highly correlated features will get large weights in the above sparsity regularization.

The second regularization is based on the 'subject-subject' relational graph. We know that if the subjects are similar to each other, their corresponding output clinical scores should be also similar to each other. Therefore, similar to the previous term, we use a heat kernel to exploit the 'subject-subject' similarities and define the similarity between the m-th and the n-th subject as below:

$$\phi_{mn} = \exp\left(-\left\|\mathbf{x}_{m,:} - \mathbf{x}_{n,:}\right\|_2^2\right), \tag{4}$$

where $\mathbf{x}_{m,:}$ is the m-th row of input $\mathbf{X}$. Here, 'subject-subject' relational regularization is defined as:

$$R_s\left(\mathbf{W}^{(t)}\right) = \sum_{m,n=1}^{S} \phi_{mn} \left\|\mathbf{x}_{m,:}\mathbf{W}^{(t)} - \mathbf{x}_{n,:}\mathbf{W}^{(t)}\right\|_2^2, \tag{5}$$

The last regularization is based on the 'clinical score-clinical score' relation. For each subject's feature vector $\mathbf{x}_{p,:}$, in our regression framework, different sets of weight coefficients are used to regress the output clinical scores, $\mathbf{y}_{:,p}^{(t)}$. In other words, the elements of each column in $\mathbf{W}^{(t)}$ are related to the elements of each column in $\mathbf{Y}^{(t)}$ through the feature vectors. As a result, in situations that the clinical scores are correlated, we require weight columns in matrix $\mathbf{W}^{(t)}$ to be correlated as well. Similarly, we use a heat kernel to exploit the 'clinical score-clinical score' relation. The similarity between the p-th clinical score and the q-th clinical score is defined using a heat kernel as:

$$\psi_{pqt} = \exp\left(-\left\|\mathbf{y}_{:,p}^{(t)} - \mathbf{y}_{:,q}^{(t)}\right\|_2^2\right), \tag{6}$$

where $\mathbf{y}_{:,p}^{(t)}$ is the p-th column vector of $\mathbf{Y}^{(t)}$. To this end, we define the clinical score relational regularization term as:

$$R_c\left(\mathbf{W}^{(t)}\right) = \sum_{p,q=1}^{C} \psi_{pqt} \left\|\mathbf{w}_{:,p}^{(t)} - \mathbf{w}_{:,q}^{(t)}\right\|_2^2, \tag{7}$$

Therefore, our proposed joint multi-longitudinal learning model using the relational information, as discussed above, would be formulated as follows:

$$\min_{\{\mathbf{W}^{(t)}, t=1,\dots,T\}} \sum_{t=1}^{T} \left\|\mathbf{Y}^{(t)} - \mathbf{X}\mathbf{W}^{(t)}\right\|_F^2 + \lambda_1 \sum_{t=1}^{T} \left(R_f\left(\mathbf{W}^{(t)}\right) + R_s\left(\mathbf{W}^{(t)}\right) + R_c\left(\mathbf{W}^{(t)}\right)\right) + \lambda_2 \|\widehat{\mathbf{W}}\|_{2,1}. \tag{8}$$

This optimization problem could be solved by alternatively solving for one of the optimization variables, while keeping the others fixed, similarly as in [10]. After selecting the most meaningful features, we use a support vector regression model to predict the clinical scores of patients at multiple future time-points. Considering how the patient changes through time, our algorithm benefits from a joint multi-task learning framework, in which multiple relationships are introduced as regularization terms to utilize the local structure similarity in the data. It is the first time to simultaneously incorporate such multi-relational information across multiple time-points into a joint learning model. Due to the sparsity property of the $l_{2,1}$-norm regularization on weight vectors, the optimal weights contain some *zero* or *close to zero* row vectors. In addition, structured sparsity is imposed through penalizing all the regression coefficients corresponding to each single feature, at multiple time points. Thus, the most distinctive and discriminative features will have similar large weights across all time points.

3   Experiments

In our experiments, a set of 445 subjects from the public available ADNI database are used, including 91 normal controls (NC), 202 mild cognitive impairment (MCI) patients, and 152 AD patients. We use T1-weighted MRI data in ADNI with a 1.5 T scanner for each subject. Our goal is to predict the two cognitive measurements (i.e., ADAS-Cog and MMSE) from only baseline MRI data. Specifically, one joint regression model is constructed to predict ADAS-Cog and MMSE changes from the baseline to 2 years follow-up. The widely used Pearson's correlation coefficient (Corr) and root mean square error (RMSE) metrics are used to measure the performance of different methods. The regression model is implemented using LIBSVM toolbox [9] with a sigmoid kernel. We normalize each feature vector into unit norm. A 10-fold cross validation strategy is employed to compute the experimental results, as well as select the best parameters on the training data. For all compared methods, the parameters are determined by cross validation on the training data as well.

We compare our proposed method with three feature selection methods, i.e., Lasso, temporal group Lasso (TGL) [6], and convex fused temporally constrained group Lasso (cFSGL) [5]. Fig. 2 shows performance of different methods on predicting ADAS-Cog/MMSE scores at baseline (T1), 6 months (T2), 12 months (T3), and 24 months (T4). Our experimental results shown in Fig. 2 demonstrate that the proposed method obtains better performance than separate learning method in predicting ADAS-Cog and MMSE scores. We observe that predicting early and 1-year clinical score changes is even more difficult than the later time points since there are less distinct information available for prediction, which was also confirmed by the previous studies [5, 6]. The low correlation values in the early time is mainly because MCI did not progress to early AD, and thus it is more challenging to uncover the essential changes of brain regions in early MCI.

Fig. 3 demonstrates the top 30 most discriminative brain regions with the highest weights for ADAS-Cog and MMSE predictions of our proposed method and cFSGL method, in which darker colors denote large weights, and vice versa. Biomarkers from different time-points are consistently identified, and important MRI patterns are localized. This validates the fact that MRI biomarkers are able to predict the ADAS-Cog and MMSE results effectively. We can observe that the distinctive and important biomarkers selected in our study include hippocampal formation, amygdala, middle temporal lobe, uncus, and corpuscallosum. Actually, hippocampus is the most important region affecting AD by possessing significant structural lesion. Both cFSGL and the proposed method are able to select important biomarkers for AD diagnosis, while our proposed method seems to identify more stable and related features for clinical score measurement. The distinctive information selected by the proposed method is more promising for AD modeling than cFSGL method. This is due to the fact that we adopt the joint learning in a multi-task framework and thus we consider weights for both MMSE and ADAS-Cog jointly, rather than separately. The common and shared high-level information of MMSE and ADAS-Cog scores can be further explored for disease progression modeling. As a result, the most discriminative brain regions such as hippocampus, amygdala, and temporal patterns are commonly selected in our regression model. It can be seen that the identified brain regions are consistent across multiple time points. Weights for ADAD-Cog and MMSE have some similar patterns as well. Moreover, our proposed method further confirms that hippocampus and amygdala are highly correlated with AD.

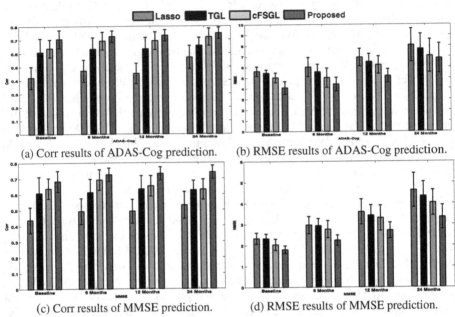

(a) Corr results of ADAS-Cog prediction.   (b) RMSE results of ADAS-Cog prediction.

(c) Corr results of MMSE prediction.   (d) RMSE results of MMSE prediction.

Fig. 2. Comparison of ADAS-Cog and MMSE prediction results by our proposed method and three feature selection methods: Lasso, TGL, and cFSGL, using Corr and RMSE via 10-fold cross validation.

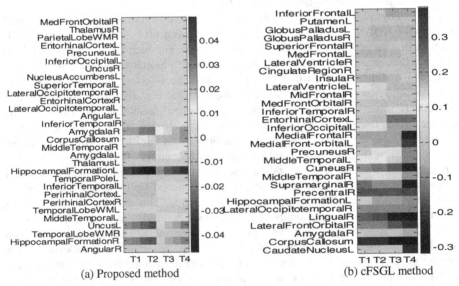

(a) Proposed method   (b) cFSGL method

Fig. 3. The most discriminative regions identified by (a) Proposed and (b) cFSGL method [5]. Note that the propose method learns ADAS-Cog/MMSE jointly, while cFSGL learns them separately.

4   Conclusions

In this paper, we proposed a joint learning of multiple longitudinal prediction models by incorporating the inherent relational information in the training data. We applied our proposed model for AD progression prediction at multiple future time points, using only the baseline data. The feature selection procedure selects the most relevant features for the task of clinical scores prediction at multiple future time-points, followed by SVM regression models for predictions. Experimental results on the ADNI database have demonstrated promising results in estimating clinical cognitive scores.

Acknowledgment. This work was supported partly by National Natural Science Foundation of China (No. 61402296), and National Natural Science Foundation of Guangdong Province (No. S2013040014448).

References

1. Cuingnet, R., Gerardin, E., Tessieras, J., Auzias, G., Lehéricy, S., Habert, M.-O., Chupin, M., Benali, H., Colliot, O.: Automatic classification of patients with Alzheimer's disease from structural MRI: A comparison of ten methods using the ADNI database. NeuroImage **56**(2), 766–781 (2011)
2. Jack Jr., C.R., Knopman, D.S., Jagust, W.J., Shaw, L.M., Aisen, P.S., Weiner, M.W., Petersen, R.C., Trojanowski, J.Q.: Hypothetical model of dynamic biomarkers of the Alzheimer's pathological cascade. The Lancet Neurology **9**(1), 119–128 (2010)
3. Teipel, S.J., Born, C., Ewers, M., Bokde, A.L.W., Reiser, M.F., Möller, H.-J., Hampel, H.: Multivariate deformation-based analysis of brain atrophy to predict Alzheimer's disease in mild cognitive impairment. NeuroImage **38**(1), 13–24 (2007)
4. Vemuri, P., Wiste, H.J., Weigand, S.D., Shaw, L.M., Trojanowski, J.Q., Weiner, M.W., Knopman, D.S., Petersen, R.C., Jack Jr., C.R.: MRI and CSF biomarkers in normal, MCI, and AD subjects: Predicting future clinical change. Neurology **73**(4), 294–301 (2009)
5. Zhou, J., Liu, J., Narayan, V.A., Ye, J.: Modeling disease progression via multi-task learning. NeuroImage **78**, 233–248 (2013)
6. Zhang, D., Liu, J., Shen, D.: Temporally-constrained group sparse learning for longitudinal data analysis. In: Ayache, N., Delingette, H., Golland, P., Mori, K. (eds.) MICCAI 2012, Part III. LNCS, vol. 7512, pp. 264–271. Springer, Heidelberg (2012)
7. Yuan, M., Lin, Y.: Model selection and estimation in regression with grouped variables. Journal of the Royal Statistical Society Series B: Statistical Methodology **68**(1), 49–67 (2006)
8. Belkin, M., Niyogi, P.: Laplacian eigenmaps for dimensionality reduction and data representation. Neural Computation **15**(6), 1373–1396 (2003)
9. Chang, C.-C., Lin, C.-J.: LIBSVM: A library for support vector machines. ACM Trans. Intell. Syst. Technol. **2**(3), 1–27 (2011)
10. Zhu, X., Wu, X., Ding, W., Zhang, S.: Feature selection by joint graph sparse coding. In: SDM 2013, pp. 803–811 (2013)

Author Index

Printed in the United States
by Baker & Taylor Publisher Services